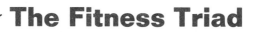

The Fitness Triad

Motivation, Training, and Nutrition

LINDA KELLY DEBRUYNE

FRANCES SIENKIEWICZ SIZER

ELEANOR NOSS WHITNEY

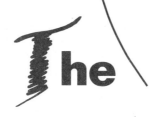The Fitness Triad

Motivation, Training, and Nutrition

West Publishing Company

ST. PAUL • NEW YORK • LOS ANGELES • SAN FRANCISCO

Copyediting • Joan Karnath
Text Design • Melinda Grosser for *silk*
Illustrations • Rolin Graphics
Dummy Artist • David Farr, Imagesmythe, Inc.
Composition • Carlisle Communications
Cover Design • Melinda Grossen for *silk*
Cover Image • John Keely

Printed in the United States of America

98 97 96 95 94 93 92   8 7 6 5 4 3 2 1

Library of Congress Cataloging-in Publication Data

DeBruyne, Linda Kelly.
     The fitness triad: motivation, training, and nutrition / Linda
Kelly DeBruyne,
   Frances Sienkiewicz Sizer, Eleanor Noss Whitney.
       p.   cm.
     Includes index.
     ISBN 0-314-78262-1 (soft)
     1. Physical fitness. 2. Physical fitness—Nutritional aspects. 3. Health.
   I. Sizer, Frances Sienkiewicz.   II. Whitney, Eleanor Noss.   III. Title.
   RA781.D414 1990
   613.7—dc20
                                                    90-42110
                                                       CIP

Text Photo Credits

13 Michael Grecco/Stock Boston;
71 Simon Wilkinson/The Image
   Bank;
87 Courtesy of Universal Gymn
   Equipment, Inc.;
88 ul Courtesy of Universal Gymn
   Equipment, Inc.;

88 ur Courtesy of Nautilus
   Sports/Medical Industries;
88 lr Courtesy of Keiser Sports
   Health Equipment;
88 ll Courtesy of Muscle Dynamics;

90 © David Madison 1988;
122 H. Armstrong Roberts;
124 Ken Levine/Allsport USA;
126 John Gray/TSW-Click, Chicago;
129 Fredrik Bodin/Stock Boston

Chapter Opening Photo Credits

1 © David Madison 1988
2 Alexander Stewart/The Image
   Bank
3 © Allsport USA/Tony Duffy
4 ©Allsport USA/Vandystadt

5 ©Allsport USA/Vandystadt
6 © David Madison 1988
7 Jim Cambon/TSW-Click, Chicago
8 © David Madison 1988
9 © David Madison 1990

10 Karl Weatherly/TSW-Click,
   Chicago
11 Oli Tennet/TSW-Click, Chicago
12 Richard Anderson

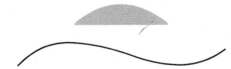

To my brother Dave: whatever you do, don't give up, I'll be right beside you all the way.
Linda

To Roz, Susan, Gary, Mark, Linda, Richard, Jon, and all of you in the film group who delight in good fun and warm my days with friendship.
Fran

To all young people everywhere: I hope you take care of yourselves and your world.
Ellie

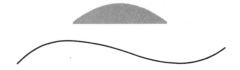

We applaud our reviewers for generously giving their expertise, time, and attention to the book:

Patricia Adlesic
   University of Akron

Sally Almekinders
   North Carolina State University

Thomas Battinelli
   Fitchburg State College

Bob Case
   Sam Houston State University

Ellen Cromwell-Cecrle
   Moorhead State University

Bethann Cinelli
   West Chester University of
   Pennsylvania

Tom Crum
   Triton College

Jean Dudney
   San Antonio College

Harry DuVal
   University of Georgia

Petie Hunt
   University of New Mexico

Jerry Krause
   Eastern Washington University

Thomas Martin
   Wittenberg University

Richard Raklovits
   Western Michigan University

Phyllis Sawyer
   Boise State University

Sarah Short
   Syracuse University

Frank Stanek
   Tulane University of Louisiana

Patricia Taylor
   University of Akron

Raymond Webster
   William Jewell College.

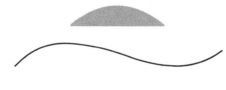

ontents

• **TWO** •

Motivation: The Choice to Be Fit

• **THREE** •

The Elements of Fitness

• **FOUR** •

Conditioning for Flexibility

• FIVE •

Conditioning for Strength and Endurance

• SIX •

Conditioning for Cardiovascular Endurance

• **TWELVE** •

Consumer Choices

• **APPENDIXES** •

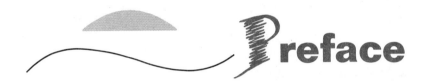

Preface

This text has two missions: First, to present the most current and accurate information available on fitness and nutrition and second, to present this information in a way that both engages and motivates the reader. It can count itself successful only if it motivates its readers to take action in the pursuit of health and physical fitness for themselves.

One can hardly research, write, and instruct others in fitness and nutrition—subjects that so profoundly affect people's lives—without being personally affected. We authors are more motivated than ever to accept the challenges of becoming more fit and making better nutrition choices.

The first two chapters introduce fitness and explore the motivation that makes people seek it. Chapter 1 defines fitness, describes the many rewards that those who pursue fitness experience, and discusses fitness and physical disabilities, pregnancy, and later life. Chapter 2 explores motivation, commitment, and persistence in relation to pursuing and maintaining fitness.

The next four chapters get down to the nitty gritty of fitness. Chapter 3 introduces the elements of fitness, explains conditioning principles, and presents ways to measure fitness. Chapters 4, 5, and 6 expand on three of the elements of fitness: Flexibility, muscle strength and endurance, and cardiovascular endurance.

The next three chapters present the nutrition component of the book. Chapter 7 presents the benefits of sound nutrition, the nutrients in foods, and guidelines for choosing nutritious foods. Chapter 8 describes the fourth element of fitness—body composition—and discusses weight control, thereby bringing fitness and nutrition together. Chapter 9 tells how to eat for sport and how nutrients support physical activity. Chapter 10 shows how physical activity helps the body adapt to stress and offers stress management strategies. Chapter 11 focuses on preventing accidents and healing injuries, and Chapter 12 offers guidelines for evaluating the many health and fitness claims and products available to consumers.

The information in the chapters is based on scientific research, but it is presented to the reader in clear, concise language that invites rather than intimidates. Accordingly, the number of footnotes has been kept to a minimum (however, all references are available from the authors). Each chapter opens with a set of true-false questions designed to dispel common misconceptions concerning the chapter's contents. Within each chapter, the true-false questions are repeated with their answers alongside the paragraphs where they are discussed. The key terms in each chapter are highlighted in bold-faced type and defined in the margins. Key terms that are related to a single topic are boxed together.

The "Quick Tips" in the chapters step away from the text to offer readers practical hints based on certain parts of the chapter's content. The "For Review" questions at the end of each chapter highlight the key points to ease students' studying.

The "Personal Focus" sections at the ends of the chapters and their accompanying "Lab Reports" in Appendix A enable students to assess themselves in the areas of motivation, fitness, nutrition, stress, and consumer awareness, and to apply what they have learned to improve these aspects of their lives if they wish to. Appendix B, The Rockport Fitness Walking Test and Exercise Program, provides an additional means for students to assess and improve their fitness.

Appendix C presents the 1989 Recommended Dietary Allowances, and Appendix D offers an extensive food composition table based on the latest nutrient database prepared by ESHA Research, Inc., of Salem, Oregon.

We hope our informal writing style and dedication to clarity ease students into enjoyment and understanding of the material presented. It is our wish that as readers gain more understanding of how fitness and nutrition can improve the quality of life, they will be motivated to act accordingly.

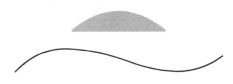# Acknowledgments

Thanks to those who urged us to write this book in the first place—the students and professors who read our other texts. Thanks to our editors: Pete Marshall for his guidance and support, Tom Hilt for his dedication to detail throughout production, and Jane Bacon for her handling of reviews and ancillaries and her enthusiastic attitude. Thanks to Joan Karnath for her expert copyediting, Melinda Grosser for her beautiful text design, and Rolin Graphics for their fine artwork.

We thank our friend and co-worker, Lori Turner, for preparing the last two chapters of the book and the Instructor's Manual; Bonnie Moffatt for her expert advice on exercise form; Elisa Malo for her fast and efficient word processing; Ledean Joyner for helping with so many production tasks; Linda Patton for her skilled library research; and our associate, Sharon Rady Rolfes, for her interest in, and concern for, the book. Her guidance and suggestions along the way were most appreciated. Special thanks to our friends and family members who continue to support our endeavors with their love and enthusiasm.

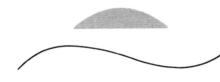

The Fitness Triad

Motivation, Training, and Nutrition

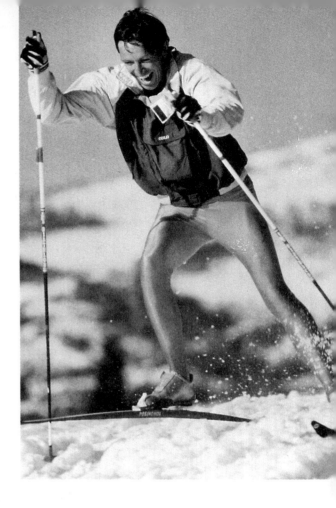

ONE

Contents

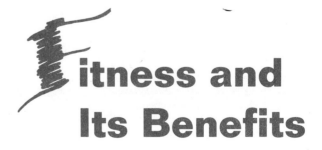

Fitness and Its Benefits

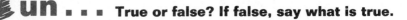
1. The body responds to inactivity by losing muscle and skill (p. 3).

2. The best way to become fit is to become an athlete (p. 3).

3. There is no such thing as too much physical activity (p. 6).

4. Active people build muscles while they sleep (p. 8).

5. Lifelong exercise helps to protect against cancer (p. 9).

6. You can get high from exercising (p. 11).

7. Women should discontinue being physically active when they become pregnant (p. 14).

8. Regular physical activity helps your body to look and function like a much younger body (p. 15).

You are housed in a remarkable body, and it can become remarkably fit, if you choose to make it so. Whatever its outward appearance, your body is magnificently able to adapt to the challenges you present it with. It can learn through practice and become equipped to perform extraordinarily varied tasks, from exquisitely precise movements to great feats of strength. You can choose to develop your body's capacity to perform these wonders to whatever extent you like. To do so is to develop fitness.

Perhaps you are already physically fit. If so, the following description applies to you. You are graceful and move with ease. You are strong and meet physical challenges without strain. You have endurance and your energy lasts for hours. You can meet normal physical challenges with ease and have plenty of energy in reserve to handle emergencies. What is more, you are likely to be well able to meet mental and emotional challenges, too—for physical fitness undergirds mental and emotional, as well as physical, energy and resilience.

If these statements do not describe you as you are today, then you can gain fitness through practice. Pursuing fitness is enjoyable in itself and quickly leads to the rewards of enjoying your body's abilities and activities. Knowing you are fit can enhance your confidence in other areas of your life, too: Social, academic, professional—you name it.

Three Definitions of Fitness

Narrowly defined, the term **fitness** describes *the characteristics of the body that enable it to perform physical activity*. These characteristics include the

fitness: the characteristics of a body that enable it to perform physical activity; more broadly, the ability to meet routine physical demands with enough reserve energy to rise to a sudden challenge; or the body's ability to withstand stresses of all kinds.

flexibility of your joints; the strength and endurance of your muscles, including your heart muscle; and a healthy body composition. These characteristics are defined in Chapter 3. Chapters 4, 5, and 6 tell you how to develop each of them. A broader definition of fitness is *the ability to meet routine physical demands, with enough reserve energy to rise to a sudden challenge.* This definition shows how fitness relates to everyday life: Ordinary tasks such as carrying heavy suitcases, opening a stuck window, or climbing four flights of stairs, which might strain an unfit person, can be well within your capacity if you are fit. Still another definition is *the body's ability to withstand stress,* meaning stresses of all kinds, including psychological stresses. Chapter 10 examines that definition in detail. There is no contradiction between these three definitions; they are three different expressions of the same wonderful condition of the body.

Fitness is the reward of a person who leads a physically active life. The opposite of such a life is a **sedentary** life, which means, literally, "sitting down a lot." Today's world permits many people to lead sedentary lives, and even rewards them for it: It provides elevators, escalators, cars, and golf carts so that people can exert a minimum of physical effort. Unfortunately, people are attracted to labor-saving devices, but the more they use them the more weak and unfit they become, and the less well they feel. The body responds to inactivity by losing muscle and skill, just as it responds to activity by gaining them.

You do not have to become an athlete to become fit. Everyone's capacity for athletic prowess differs. Some people inherit tremendous athletic potential. Others inherit average or less than average potential. Still others, through accidents of heredity or later mischances, become handicapped or disabled. However, everyone can develop fitness; it is not confined to gymnasiums and playing fields. It is part of life, everyone's life, no matter where a person lives or under what circumstances. People with physical handicaps can cultivate fitness. So can pregnant women. People who have inherited particular disease risks have compelling reasons to engage in physical activities, as do all who want to increase their chances of living long, healthy lives.

To evaluate how fit you are, your standard for comparison should not be someone else's capacity, but your own. To develop and maintain the level of fitness that will support your health is certainly a choice worth making, but you can go further if you wish. You can go on to set higher goals and even to become "all that you can be."

A common misconception is that a person who is fit is physically beautiful or perfect. This is not true, although fitness seems to enhance physical beauty in many cases. Different societies define beauty differently, and many associate it with the inactive life of a person whose social class makes physical effort unnecessary. (Such a person might be so unfit as to be short-lived, but might still be seen as beautiful.) As for perfection, of course, it is only an ideal to strive for; you can never achieve perfection. (You can achieve *progress* towards it, though, and that effort brings rewards.) People who *look* beautiful or perfect may not be fit at all. Others who might never think of themselves as beautiful, and who know they are

sedentary: physically inactive (literally, "sitting down a lot").

1. The body responds to inactivity by losing muscle and skill.

   True.

2. The best way to become fit is to become an athlete.

   False.

   You don't have to become an athlete to become fit; many kinds of physical activity lead to fitness.

not perfect, may be very fit indeed. Internally, those who are fit have all the advantages because they feel good.

You can acquire and maintain fitness in any of several different ways. If your life is otherwise sedentary (you are a student or office worker), you can adopt a routine of regular physical activity—either team or solo sports or some other form of activity such as workouts, mountain climbing, or many others. If your job or home life demands heavy physical activity, you may maintain fitness that way. (Fitness has several components, though, so you'll want to inspect your routine to see if it provides *balanced* fitness. Later chapters will help you look at fitness from all sides.) In any case, some form of physical activity is the road to fitness. Even at random moments during the day, you can seize opportunities to be active (see the Quick Tips).

The body that practices a physical activity *adapts* by becoming more able to perform it after each session—more flexible, stronger, more enduring. Moreover, the body that becomes more fit for physical activity also becomes more fit for taking exams in school and taking major responsibilities in society or on the job. Activity promotes fitness; fitness promotes stress resistance in general; and stress resistance benefits health and life in many, many ways.[1]

Fitness is part of a broader state of being: Physical **health,** as shown in Figure 1–1. As the figure shows, physical health also includes rest and sleep, nutritional health, defenses against disease, and accident resistance. Physical health in turn is part of health in general, a large realm that also includes mental, emotional, interpersonal, social, and even spiritual components. This chapter shows how fitness contributes to health, especially physical health, and how physical health contributes to the overall quality of life.

health: a range of states with physical, mental, emotional, interpersonal, social, and spiritual components. At a minimum, health means freedom from negative states in these realms. At a maximum, it means the highest attainable states in these realms.

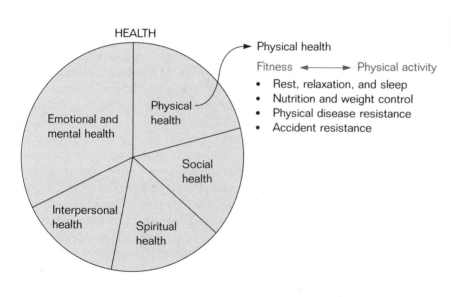

HEALTH

Physical health

Fitness ⟷ Physical activity
- Rest, relaxation, and sleep
- Nutrition and weight control
- Physical disease resistance
- Accident resistance

FIGURE 1–1 Fitness Is Part of Health

Fitness contributes to all aspects of health, as shown in Figure 1–2. That is why books are written about it, courses are taught about it, and programs are devoted to it. The person who fully realizes all the benefits of fitness will naturally want to pursue it. It not only helps you look good, feel good, and have fun, but it gives you many other rewards and can even lengthen your life.

Physical Benefits of Fitness

This section presents some examples of how fitness contributes to all aspects of physical health. The next section provides a few examples of other aspects of health. First under "Physical health" in Figure 1–2 is physical activity.

Physical Activity

Fitness makes it possible to be physically active. Fitness makes activity easy; activity in turn produces fitness, a beneficial cycle (see Figure 1–3). Fitness makes you *feel* like being active, too—a pleasing aspect of the cycle. Activity and fitness are so closely connected that the rest of this chapter makes no distinction between them. The benefits of fitness are the benefits of physical activity, and vice versa.

The proven benefits of regular physical activity are numerous. Because they know this, many more adults in the United States are exercising regularly than in the past. Still, fewer than one-fourth of all adults have made this commitment to themselves. Based on this statistic, you have less than a one-in-four chance of being one of the active ones.

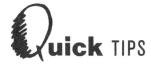

Quick TIPS

Practicing Fitness

To cultivate fitness moment to moment:

- When you sit, stretch.
- When you reach, reach far.
- When you stand, stand straight.
- When you must wait, flex your muscles.
- Do it by hand, not by machine.
- Walk or climb stairs instead of riding.
- Keep your stomach in and buttocks tight.
- Relax often and laugh.
- Breathe deeply.

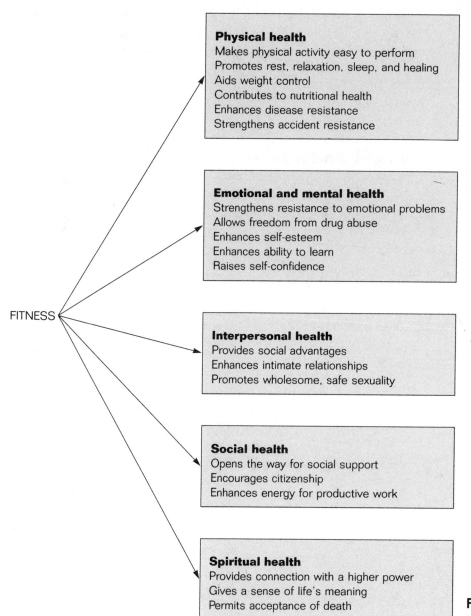

Physical health
Makes physical activity easy to perform
Promotes rest, relaxation, sleep, and healing
Aids weight control
Contributes to nutritional health
Enhances disease resistance
Strengthens accident resistance

Emotional and mental health
Strengthens resistance to emotional problems
Allows freedom from drug abuse
Enhances self-esteem
Enhances ability to learn
Raises self-confidence

Interpersonal health
Provides social advantages
Enhances intimate relationships
Promotes wholesome, safe sexuality

Social health
Opens the way for social support
Encourages citizenship
Enhances energy for productive work

Spiritual health
Provides connection with a higher power
Gives a sense of life's meaning
Permits acceptance of death

FITNESS

FIGURE 1-2 Fitness Contributes to All Aspects of Health

The choice is ultimately yours, but this book will, of course, try to influence it.

Although physical activity is desirable, it can be overdone. It is a form of stress, after all. It requires the body to put forth energy to meet its challenges and then to adapt by growing muscles and other body structures to perform the activity better the next time. (That adaptation, by the way, is exactly what is meant by developing fitness.) The stress of physical activity is a "good stress," though, as long as it is not performed

3. There is no such thing as too much physical activity.

False.

Physical activity can be overdone.

to the point of total exhaustion. (Read about the limits and about avoiding injury in later chapters.) Physical activity in appropriate doses is most beneficial because it increases the body's capacity for a fuller response to the next demand.

Following a good workout, rest is appropriate. Rest permits full recovery from the stress of physical activity.

Rest, Relaxation, and Sleep

Fitness makes it easy to relax and to sleep. Relaxation occurs naturally whenever any stress stops acting on you, and it permits your body to recover from the effort it has made. After you exercise, it is natural to

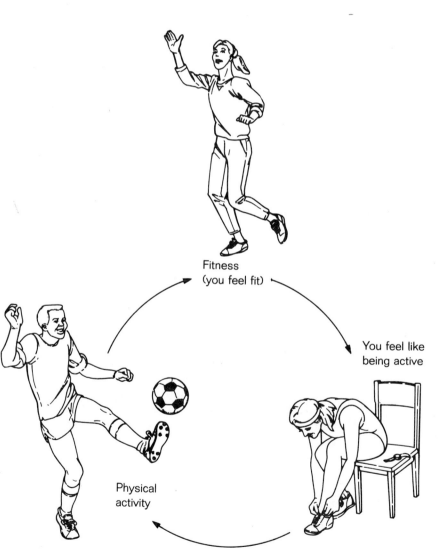

FIGURE 1–3 Physical Activity and Fitness: A Beneficial Cycle

Fitness
(you feel fit)

You feel like
being active

Physical
activity

somatotropin: a hormone secreted by the pituitary gland (a gland in the brain) that directs repair activities during sleep.

rest, relax, and sleep. These activities contribute to fitness and to all aspects of physical health. You'll see later that adequate rest and sleep can even lengthen life, but now consider what sleep does for the body physically.

Sleep (undrugged, natural sleep) is the most profound form of relaxation. Physically, inside the body, several things happen during sleep. The body repairs its damaged parts; it removes and disposes of wastes generated during the day's activity; and it builds new physical structures (for example, muscles and blood vessels). In particular, it builds structures that it "learned" it might need for the next round of physical activity—more flexible joints, stronger muscles, larger lungs, stronger bones, and a more efficient circulatory system. The so-called "growth" hormone, **somatotropin,** is secreted only during sleep, and this hormone directs these repair and building activities. Physical activity stimulates the release of this hormone, thus facilitating healing and development of fitness.

Relaxation and sleep occur naturally after periods of physical activity, but a skillful stress management strategy that includes daily activity can help ensure that you can relax and rest even in the midst of stressful times.[2] Chapter 10 provides the strategies for stress management.

Nutrition and Weight Control

Next under "Physical health" in Figure 1–2 are nutrition and weight control. A fit body differs in composition from an unfit body in many ways. For one thing, it contains more muscle tissue, and muscle tissue burns more calories than other tissues. Fit people, therefore, need to eat more food to meet daily energy needs. If they make wise food choices, they can consume more nutrients, which means that they have less risk of nutrient deficiencies. Fit people also have more nutrients stored up in preparation for times of stress and illness. Thus, fitness contributes to nutritional health.

Nutritional health contributes to fitness, too. The nutrients provide fuel for energy, building blocks for body parts, and other key components to help the exercising body do its work. Chapters 7 and 8 provide details and show how people can adjust their diets to support physical exertion.

Fitness also contributes to weight control. A balanced program of physical activity can reduce fat tissue and augment lean tissue. The fit person can eat and enjoy more food without gaining weight, because lean tissue devours more calories. (An unfit person who eats the same amount of food will gain fat.) Physical activity also helps to control appetite, preventing overeating. Chapter 9 provides details on the relationships between fitness and weight control.

Physical Disease Resistance

You may be surprised to learn that physical fitness enhances disease resistance. For one thing, fitness strengthens the immune system, which provides resistance to infectious diseases of all kinds, from ordinary colds and infections to major diseases. Pneumonia, flu, skin infections (including acne), food poisoning, and many more are less likely, or are overcome more quickly, when the immune system is strong. The immune system helps people resist cancer, too, and researchers now have evidence that lifelong exercise helps to protect against cancer.[3]

Physical activity also helps prevent diseases that occur in later life, such as heart disease, diabetes, and others. Exercise that challenges the heart and the rest of the circulatory system slows the aging of this system and reduces the risk of heart attacks and strokes.[4] It also helps control blood cholesterol and blood pressure, indicators of heart health. These and other benefits of regular physical activity appear in Table 1–1.

Fitness, then, helps you resist *physical* diseases in many ways. Fitness also helps you resist *emotional* problems, as a later section shows.

TABLE 1–1 • Regular Physical Activity Helps to Protect against These Physical Conditions

- Backaches
- Cancer (colon cancer, breast cancer, and others)[a]
- Diabetes[b]
- Digestive disorders (ulcers, constipation, diarrhea, and others)
- Growth failure in children
- Headaches
- Heart and blood vessel disease (heart attacks and strokes)[c]
- High blood cholesterol, high blood pressure
- Infections (colds, flu, and many others)
- Infertility (some forms)
- Kidney disease[d]
- Menstrual irregularities
- Obesity
- Osteoporosis (adult bone loss)[e]

[a]R. E. Frisch and coauthors, Lower lifetime occurrence of breast cancer and cancers of the reproductive system among former college athletes, *American Journal of Clinical Nutrition* 45 (1987): 328–335.

[b]M. J. Franz, Exercise and the management of diabetes mellitus, *Journal of the American Dietetic Association* 87 (1987): 872–880.

[c]L. G. Ekelund and coauthors, Physical fitness as a predictor of cardiovascular mortality in asymptomatic North American men, *New England Journal of Medicine* 319 (1988): 1379–1384.

[d]K. C. Light and coauthors, Psychological stress induces sodium and fluid retention in men at high risk for hypertension, *Science* 220 (1982): 429–431.

[e]B. Krolner and coauthors, Physical exercise as a prophylaxis against involutional vertebral bone loss: A controlled trial, *Clinical Science* 64 (1983): 541–546, as cited in M. E. Nelson and coauthors, Diet and bone status in amenorrheic runners, *American Journal of Clinical Nutrition* 43 (1986): 910–916.

Accident Resistance

The last item under "Physical health" in Figure 1–2 states that the fit person is better defended, even against accidents, than is the unfit person. Of course, many other qualities besides fitness defend you against accidents. Prudence is one; simply knowing how accidents occur and taking precautions to prevent them is another. But certain physical characteristics that come with fitness also help. Skill in movement, coordination, speed of reaction, and acuity of vision and hearing all help you move quickly and appropriately in physical emergencies, reducing the chance of injury. Proper body weight makes it easier to move. And if an accident does occur, the strength and flexibility of your body can make a significant difference in the degree to which you are injured. Accidents and injuries can never be totally prevented, of course, and wisdom dictates that we all learn what to do when they occur. Chapter 11 is devoted to these matters.

Other Benefits of Fitness

The physical benefits of fitness are many, as you have just seen, but there are numerous other benefits. The state of the body also influences the state of the mind and the spirit.

Resistance to Emotional Problems

The more physically fit you are, the better you will feel emotionally. Of course, fitness does not completely prevent mental illness, but it does help to defend against anxiety and depression. Research confirms that this is true; some typical findings are summed up in Table 1–2.

This psychological benefit of fitness applies both when you are under stress and when you are not. If you have to face a breakup, a move, a job change, or any other major life event, physical activity can give you an outlet for your anxiety, and fitness enables you to get through the stressful time with better health and in a better mood than you would if you were unfit. In ordinary times, too, exercise promotes mental health. Regular exercisers, even late in life, report that they feel energetic and have generally good tempers, while sedentary people report that they are more often tired and depressed.[5]

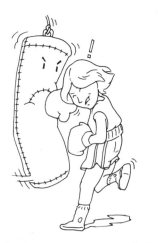

Physical activity can give you an outlet for anxiey, depression, or anger.

Freedom from Drug Abuse

Next in Figure 1–2 is freedom from drug abuse. Needless to say, the person who attempts to mix alcohol or drug abuse with physical activity undermines the effort to acquire fitness. Before a person has attempted to manage this combination for very long, it becomes apparent that the two pull in opposite directions. A choice becomes necessary: Go the drug route or the fitness route; you can't do both. Examples of both choices are well known. Some choose alcohol or drug abuse, of course, and these

TABLE 1-2 • Regular Physical Activity Benefits People Psychologically (Sample Research Findings)

- Physically active people experienced less anxiety and depression than sedentary people.[a]
- Fit people dealt better with emotionally stressful events than sedentary people.[b]
- Depressed people who adopted a routine of regular running became well within three weeks and stayed well for ten weeks of observation—a result as good as that achieved with psychotherapy.[c]

[a]D. L. Roth and D. S. Holmes, Influence of physical fitness in determining the impact of stressful life events on physical and psychologic health, *Psychosomatic Medicine* 47 (1985): 164–173.

[b]R. M. Hayden, Relationship between aerobic exercise, anxiety, and depression: Convergent validation by knowledgeable informants, *Journal of Sports Medicine* 24 (1984): 69–74.

[c]J. H. Griest, Running as treatment for depression, *Journal of Comprehensive Psychiatry*, January/February 1979, pp. 41–54.

sooner or later undermine their health to the point where they cannot stay in top form. Some even die: Famous basketball stars have succumbed to cocaine abuse; famous baseball players to alcoholism; and so forth. Others come to value their own fitness so much that they become willing to give up the use of substances that impair it. A jogger quits smoking in order to improve her daily time and distance; a swimmer quits using alcohol because his performance improves without it.

People use alcohol and other mind-altering drugs because they make them feel good; they produce a "high." Unfortunately, because these drugs have multiple side effects, they harm health. Fit people seek the same good feeling from exercise. Not only can they get it, but they can get it free of side effects and with fringe *benefits* instead. Brainwave patterns and brain chemistry change during certain kinds and intensities of exercise to produce a high similar to that produced by mind-altering drugs.[6] Some exercisers find these effects so pleasing that they literally become "addicted to exercise." Beyond that, the joy of turning in your best performance can produce a "high" like nothing you can get from any drug.

6. You can get high from exercising.

True.

Other Aspects of Health

Fitness and fitness activities contribute to all aspects of health in many more general ways than those just described. For example, one of the chief indicators of mental health is self-esteem—and the person who is fit is likely to have more of it. The sense of achievement that comes with meeting physical challenges promotes self-confidence and a strong self-image. The person who strives to meet the physical challenges of daily exercise is better equipped to meet the emotional challenges of daily life, as well. Table 1–2 has already shown that people who exercise regularly enjoy more freedom from anxiety and depression and generally cope better with life's challenges than do sedentary people.

Other mental health advantages come directly from the good effects fitness has on the circulatory system. The brain is very dependent on its oxygen nutrient supply, brought to it by the blood, pumped by the heart. The brain of a person with a fit body is seldom deprived of these vital materials and can learn better and longer than that of a person who is out of shape.

All of these qualities, from emotional strength to improved learning ability, are aspects of "Emotional and mental health," but the benefits of fitness do not stop there. Take "Interpersonal health," next. An obvious fitness benefit is in the area of sexuality. Mature people know that sexual love is not *just* a matter of physical activity, but certainly activity plays a part in it, and physical fitness contributes to its enjoyment.

Take "Social health" next. Physically active people have more energy and need less sleep than sedentary people. They can thus give energy and time to those around them and can thereby enlarge their social networks. How you spend your energy is a personal choice, of course, but many fit people choose to involve themselves in social activities. By giving more of themselves to others, they ensure that others will give more to them in return. In times of need, mutually supportive relationships among people ensure that needs are met.

Even the last-named aspect of health in Figure 1–2, "Spiritual health," receives a boost from physical fitness. No matter what their personal religious convictions may be, most people can relate to the concept of a higher power, by one name or another—the power of a group, of two people's love for each other, of loyalty to a cause, or of dedication to an ideal. If willing, an individual can gain power from outside the isolated self, and this lesson can be learned in any realm of life first and then transferred to the other realms. In sports, the "team spirit" can enable individuals to do more than they dream they could do otherwise. A person who has climbed a physical mountain gains the self-confidence to become able to climb other kinds of mountains as well, such as finishing challenging intellectual tasks or keeping promises when times are hard. Thus, physical fitness, in its broader aspect, contributes to spiritual health.

Fitness throughout Life

Fitness begins at the very beginning of life, when a healthy man and woman conceive a new individual. The new life is supported by the mother's balanced nutrition, healthy circulation, and a lifestyle free of drugs (including alcohol). At birth, an infant that has been given such a start on life is easy to recognize: Alert, active, hungry, and energetic. Thereafter, the infant becomes ready to learn to crawl, then walk, then run and jump, and wise parents provide daily opportunities for this learning to take place.

Infants normally are spontaneously active. People who care for children can provide opportunities for them to exercise by giving them freedom of movement and the stimulation of play. An active infant is on the way to becoming an active child and a fit adult and can expect to be free of many problems that plague sedentary people's lives.

Children, too, are naturally inclined to exercise, but need their parents and schools to make sure they do so daily. Otherwise, many children today grow up more under the influence of car travel and television entertainment than of sports and outdoor play.

In the teen years, the habit of regular activity, voluntarily undertaken, should become firmly established, and by the time a person has reached college age, a daily or every-other-day fitness routine should be as much a part of life as meals and sleep. Thereafter, maintaining fitness should remain a habit, never abandoned.

Fitness and Physical Disabilities

Sometimes, circumstances make physical activity seem nearly impossible. Factors such as physical disabilities or obesity can place conventional get-up-and-run routines out of reach. But people in these circumstances need fitness *more* than other people, not less: A strong body and an active mind are essential to meet the challenges they face. People who have confronted such limitations have developed excellent, if unconventional, activity programs to keep fit nonetheless.

Swimming is well suited to many people's needs. Joints that on land are stressed by the body's weight work better when weight is supported by water. For example, people who are overweight or poorly coordinated can swim more safely than they can run, and they find it less exhausting, too.

People who are blind, deaf, or use wheelchairs climb mountains, swim, ski, play football, and engage in other activities tailored to their

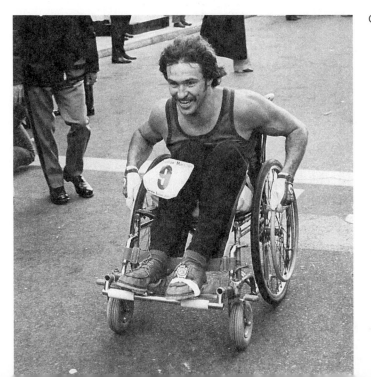

Circumstances need not deprive anyone of fitness.

13

limitations. People who have had heart attacks can do special exercises and work up from one level to the next as they recover. Mentally handicapped people can compete in sports at the community, state, national, and international levels through the Special Olympics. Fitness is important for everybody—don't let circumstances deprive you of it.

Fitness and Pregnancy

Physical activity improves a woman's chances of a healthy pregnancy. For one thing, it helps maintain the bones, which give up calcium to the fetus as it grows. With physical activity, bones store more calcium and become denser, stronger, and able to carry more weight. Physical activity also develops the lean body tissue that serves as a storage site for iron and other nutrients needed in large doses in pregnancy. A healthy circulatory system developed in response to physical activity will be efficient at transporting nutrients to both mother and fetus. Women should, therefore, continue enjoying their customary physical activities during pregnancy to the greatest extent compatible with comfort and safety.

A woman who wants to be physically active while she is pregnant can begin a program gently and work up to more vigorous exercise under supervision, but it is best if she has been physically active *beforehand*. Labor is physically demanding, and a fit woman will find it less exhausting and will heal faster from childbirth than an unfit woman. Women who are physically active prior to and throughout pregnancy find it much easier to resume a demanding routine after recovery from the birth. Thus, all young women who want to enjoy healthy pregnancies later should be physically active now.

Fitness and Health in Later Life

To this point, this chapter has emphasized the present and near-future benefits of fitness. If you undertake a program of regular physical activity, you can expect to see results within only a few weeks—only a few days for some. But if you keep your program up for all of your adult life, rewards await you "way at the other end," as well. The benefits of fitness extend through time to later life.

Researchers have studied how regular exercise, together with other healthy lifestyle choices, affects the quality of later life. Their findings are dramatic.[7] They studied nearly 7,000 adults in California and noticed that some people seemed young for their age; others seemed old for their age. To find out what made the difference, the researchers focused on health habits and identified seven factors that had maximum impact on **physiological age:** Regular, adequate sleep; breakfast eating; regularity of meals; regular physical activity; abstinence from smoking; abstinence from, or moderation in, alcohol use; and weight control (control of body fat content). The effects of these factors were cumulative. That is, those who followed all seven positive practices were in better health, even if older in calendar years, than people who failed to do so. In fact, the

7. Women should discontinue being physically active when they become pregnant.

False.

Women should continue being physically active during pregnancy.

physiological age: your age as estimated from your body's health and probable life expectancy. (Normally, when people refer to *age,* they mean *chronological age*—that is, age as measured from date of birth.)

physical health of those who reported all positive health practices was consistently about the same as that of people *30 years younger* who followed few or none.[8]

These findings demonstrate that although you cannot alter the year of your birth, you can certainly alter the quality of your life, and probably even its length. In effect, you can make yourself younger or older by the way you choose to live. You cannot completely halt the aging process, of course, but you can slow it down and even prevent many of its effects. Table 1–3 gives more details.

One benefit of regular physical activity has sparked the interest of even the most inactive individuals: Exercise may add years to life. A typical study lending support to this assertion followed 16,000 people for 12 to 16 years.[9] Those who expended 2,000 or more calories per week

TABLE 1–3 • Regular Physical Activity Can Help to Prevent These Effects of Aging

Aging Has These Effects:[a]	Regular Physical Activity Has These Effects:
Cardiovascular System:	
Blood pressure rises.	Blood pressure rises less.
Resting heart rate rises.	Resting heart rate is unchanged.
Oxygen use falls.	Oxygen use is maintained.
Blood cholesterol rises.	Blood cholesterol remains lower.
Circulation slows.	Circulation remains normal.
Body Composition and Metabolism:	
Lean body mass declines.	Lean body mass is maintained.
Excess body fat accumulates.	Body fatness remains optimal.
Energy metabolism slows.	Metabolism remains normal.
Other Physical Characteristics	
Body becomes stiff, inflexible.	Body remains flexible.
Teeth are lost.	Teeth remain healthy.
Gum disease occurs.	Gums remain healthy.
Bone loss (osteoporosis) occurs.	Bone loss slows.
Body becomes bent, stooped.	Posture remains good.
Other:	
Thinking becomes confused.	Thinking remains clear.
Sex drive diminishes.	Sex drive remains healthy.
Self-esteem diminishes.	Self-esteem remains high.
Interest in work declines.	Interest in work remains high.
Depression, loneliness set in.	Spirits remain good.

[a]F. S. Sizer and E. N. Whitney, *Life Choices* (St. Paul, Minn.: West Publishing, 1988), Table 14–2, p. 398

TABLE 1-4 • Benefits of Exercise and Fitness (Summary)

- Sound, beneficial rest and sleep
- Improved nutritional health
- Reduced fatness and increased lean body tissue
- Improved resistance to colds, other infectious diseases, and cancer
- Reduced risk of heart and blood vessel disease, diabetes, and other diseases
- Reduced probability of accidents; fewer and less severe injuries
- Reduced incidence and severity of anxiety and depression
- Freedom from drug (including alcohol) abuse
- Improved self-image and self-confidence
- Better learning ability
- Greater interpersonal, social, and spiritual strengths
- Improved quality of life in the later years
- Longer life

exercising had higher survival rates than their peers; they had one-fourth to one-third fewer deaths during the period of observation. (To expend 2,000 calories in a week, you could run or walk about 20 miles that week.) Even if the physically active subjects were smokers, had high blood pressure, or were overweight or underweight, they had a survival advantage over sedentary people matched for those characteristics.

In conclusion, fitness and physical health enhance all of life in many ways, as summed up in Table 1–4. You may engage in a regular activity program because it makes you feel good, or because it makes you look good, or because it's fun—but those are not its only rewards. Late in life, you'll be glad you did for many other reasons, too.

Although fitness is well worth adopting as a personal goal, some people choose it and some do not. Why? Chapter 2 goes on to examine the questions of what motivates people to pursue fitness, and of how they can manage their lives to keep fitness a high priority even in difficult times.

PERSONAL FOCUS   How Physically Active Are You?

Forms for recording your answers to this and other end-of-chapter Personal Focus sections are in Appendix A, Lab Reports.

"The road to fitness is physical activity." How physically active are you? For each question answered yes, give yourself the number of points indicated. Then total your points to determine your score. Don't take this quiz too seriously; it is intended only to help make you aware of opportunities that your life offers you to develop your capacity for fitness. Later Personal Focus sections examine ways to achieve different aspects of fitness such as flexibility, strength, endurance, and a healthy body composition.

A. Formal, Vigorous Exercise Routines

1. I participate in active recreational sports such as tennis or handball for an hour or more:
   a. About once a week (*2 points*)
   b. About twice a week (*4 points*)
   c. Three times a week (*6 points*)
   d. Four times a week (*8 points*)

(Adjust your point score if your answer is less or more than these. For example, if you play sports *six* days a week, give yourself more points— say, 12 points. If you play once a week for only 30 minutes, give yourself 1 point. Note: Any session of less than 20 minutes counts as zero.)

2. At least once a week, I participate in vigorous fitness activities like aerobic dancing, jogging, or swimming (at least 20 continuous minutes each session):
   a. About once a week (*3 points*)
   b. About twice a week (*6 points*)
   c. Three times a week (*9 points*)
   d. Four times a week (*12 points*)

(Adjust your point score upward or downward if your answer is slightly different from these. For example, if you work out *six* days a week, give yourself more points—say, 18 points.)

B. Other Formal Exercise Routines

3. At least two times a week, I perform floor workouts (sit-ups, push-ups) for at least ten minutes:
   a. Two sessions a week (*2 points*)
   b. Three sessions a week (*3 points*)
   c. Four or more sessions a week (*4 points*)

(No points for a session of less than ten minutes; no points for only one session a week; maximum is 4 points.)

4. At least two times a week, I participate in yoga or perform stretching exercises for at least ten minutes:
   a. Two sessions a week (*2 points*)
   b. Three sessions a week (*3 points*)
   c. Four or more sessions a week (*4 points*)

(No points for a session of less than ten minutes; no points for only one session a week; maximum is 4 points.)

5. At least two times a week, I work out with weights for at least ten minutes:
   a. Two sessions a week (*2 points*)
   b. Three sessions a week (*3 points*)
   c. Four or more sessions a week (*4 points*)

   (No points for a session of less than ten minutes; no points for only one session a week; maximum is 4 points.)

C. Occupation and Daily Activities

6. I walk to and from school, work, and shopping (one-half mile or more each way), two or three times a week or more. (*1 point*)
7. I climb stairs rather than using elevators or escalators, every other day or more. (*1 point*)
8. My school, job, or household routine involves physical activity that fits the following description:
   a. It is mostly desk work or light physical activity. (*0 points*)
   b. It is mostly farm activities, moderate physical activity, brisk walking, or the like. (*4 points*)
   c. Many of my typical days include several hours of heavy physical activity (shoveling, lifting, or the like). (Don't include sports practice here. See part A.) (*2 points per day*)

   (Section C maximum: 12 points)

D. Leisure Activities

9. I do several hours of gardening, lawn work, or equally active hobby work each week. (*1 point*)
10. I fish or hunt once a week or more on the average. (These must involve active work such as rowing a boat or tracking game. Dock and truck sitting don't count.) (*1 point*)
11. At least once a week I dance vigorously (folk or square dance) for an hour or more. (*1 point per hour*)

    (Section D maximum: 4 points)

12. In season, I play 9 to 18 holes of golf at least once a week, and I do not use a power cart. (*2 points*)
13. I walk for exercise or recreation:
    a. 1 to 2 hours a week (*1 point*)
    b. 3 to 4 hours a week (*2 points*)
    c. 5 hours or more a week (*3 points*)

14. In *addition* to the above, I choose to engage in other forms of physical activity:
    a. 1 to 2 hours a week (*1 point*)
    b. 3 to 4 hours a week (*2 points*)
    c. 5 hours or more a week (*3 points*)

    (For Section D, don't count sports practice. See part A.)

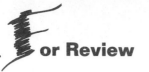

For Review

1. Define *fitness* in three ways. (p. 3)
2. Explain how fitness contributes to each of the following physical aspects of health:
   a. Ability to exercise (p. 5)
   b. Profound, restful sleep (p. 8)
   c. Physical disease resistance (p. 9)
   d. Nutrition (p. 8)
   e. Weight control (p. 8)
   f. Accident resistance (p. 10)
3. Explain how fitness contributes to each of the following other aspects of health:
   a. Resistance to emotional problems (p. 10)
   b. Freedom from drug abuse (p. 10)
   c. Others (p. 11)
4. Can the following people cultivate fitness? Explain how:
   a. A disabled person (p. 13)
   b. A pregnant woman (p. 14)
   c. An older person (p. 14)
5. Name the daily behaviors that, over a lifetime, can alter a person's physiological age by up to 30 years (p. 14).

Chapter Notes

1. H. Steinberg and E. A. Sykes, Introduction to symposium on endorphins and behavioral processes; review of literature on endorphins and exercise, *Pharmacology Biochemistry and Behavior* 23 (1985): 857–862.
2. H. Benson, *The Relaxation Response* (New York: Morrow, 1975).
3. R. E. Frisch and coauthors, Lower lifetime occurrence of breast cancer and cancers of the reproductive system among former college athletes, *American Journal of Clinical Nutrition* 45 (1987): 328–335.
4. L. G. Ekelund and coauthors, Physical fitness as a predictor of cardiovascular mortality in asymptomatic North American men, *New England Journal of Medicine* 319 (1988): 1379–1384.
5. B. Larsson and coauthors, Health and aging characteristics of highly physically active 65-year-old men, *International Journal of Sports Medicine* 5 (1984): 336–340.
6. H. Wagemaker and L. Goldstein, The runner's high, *Journal of Sports Medicine and Physical Fitness* 20 (1980): 227–229.
7. N. B. Belloc and L. Breslow, Relationship of physical health status and health practices, *Preventive Medicine* 1 (1972): 409–421.
8. Belloc and Breslow, 1972.
9. R. S. Paffenbarger and coauthors, Physical activity, all-cause mortality, and longevity of college alumni, *New England Journal of Medicine* 314 (1986): 605–611.

T W O

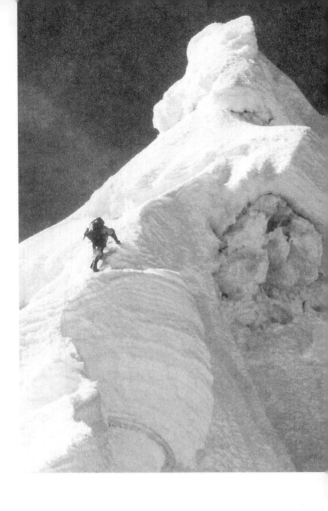

Contents

Motivation:
The
Choice to
Be Fit

1. People will be most motivated to engage in physical activity if they perceive that it will benefit their health (page 24).

2. The ideal time frame for your self-improvement program is one you construct for yourself (page 24).

3. As soon as you know how to change a health habit, it is easy to do so (page 27).

4. Simple enjoyment keeps people from dropping out of fitness programs (page 28).

5. To help a person keep a fitness resolution, a good friend will remind the person to practice daily (page 30).

6. When you get started on a fitness routine, you should make all possible healthful changes in your diet at the same time (page 30).

7. The best fitness goals are lofty goals (page 31).

8. It is best to work out by yourself so that you don't have to depend on other people to make it happen (page 33).

motivation: the desire and impulse to act.

The knowledge of how to become fit is hardly beneficial if it merely enables people to make A's on tests. It is valuable only if people *use* it to become fit—to change their behavior. You may make a commitment to fitness with the long-term future in mind, but to achieve your fitness goal, you must choose to engage in physical activity today. Then you have to make the same choice again tomorrow and the next day, to gain the rewards you are seeking. Fitness doesn't come fast.

Because fitness doesn't happen overnight, people who usually know what they *should* do often do not do it. For the same reason, some people who *do* change their behavior fail to maintain it. Furthermore, the **motivation** to get started is different from the motivation to continue with a fitness behavior.

More and more people each day learn about the benefits of physical activity and make the choice to become fit. However, only about half of those who begin fitness programs stay with them. Chapter 1 emphasized the importance of fitness to physical health, and it also showed how fitness benefits all aspects of health. This chapter goes beyond that point. First, a discussion of motivation and commitment can help you to start becoming physically active. Next, you need motivation to *persist* long enough to reap potential rewards. As you will see, the lessons of this chapter are down-to-earth common sense, but common sense is rare, even in intelligent people's make-up.

Motivation: Benefits versus Costs

In general, **motives** are forces that move people to act. They may be either instinctive or learned. Instinctive motives, or **drives,** are strongest: Hunger, thirst, fear, and fatigue propel you to take the actions necessary to meet your needs for food, water, safety, and sleep. Instinctive drives can also propel you to act in relation to others. The sex drive, protectiveness toward family members, and aggression are examples of instinctive drives. Learned motives may also be powerful—consider the desire for possessions, recognition, or achievement. A powerful motive virtually impels a person to act.

You get your motivation to perform a given act from the balance between the benefits you experience from it and the costs you associate with it. A psychologist explains motivation using the analogy of a black box with a reward inside. Suppose you were told, "If you put a dollar in the slot, you can take $1,000 out." Most people would not hesitate for a moment. They would drop their dollar in. But suppose you were told, "If you put a dollar in the slot today, you can take $1,000 out twenty years from now." Now you might think a minute. Today's dollar may mean more to you than the deferred gratification of many more dollars years from now. Still, you might decide to drop your dollar in. Now suppose you were told, "If you put a dollar in, you may take $1,000 out, but when you touch the box, you'll get an electric shock." Most people want to know, "How much will it hurt?" Or suppose you were told, "If you put a dollar in, there's a one-in-100 *chance* you can take $1,000 out." People are motivated to act in circumstances like these only if they feel that the benefits outweigh the costs.

The situations just described illustrate that motivation is modified by three factors. One is the *value* of the reward: How big is it in relation to its costs? A second modifier is the *immediacy* of the reward: How soon will it come or how soon will the price have to be paid? A third modifier is the *probability* of the reward: How likely is it and how certain is the price? These modifiers produce many variations on the ways in which people make choices. A reward provides positive value, but the costs detract from that value.

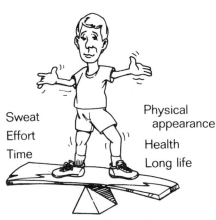

Sweat
Effort
Time

Physical appearance
Health
Long life

Your motivation depends on the balance you perceive between costs and benefits.

Value

The value of a reward depends on your assessment of it. Each person values rewards differently. In the case of physical activity, people tend to value it if it enhances their self-esteem and to devalue it if it detracts from their self-esteem.

Some people have negative feelings toward physical activity, even though they understand the importance of fitness for health. These peo-

competence: the ability to do something well.

ple say that taking up an activity isn't really "them"—it's not in their self-concept, or life-script. People who have these feelings probably base their self-esteem on accomplishments outside of the physical realm. They pride themselves on intelligence, personality, or manual dexterity, not on physical prowess. When people feel this way, it usually means that during the years of development, when the self-concept and self-esteem were in the budding stage, they were not made to feel competent in the physical arena. Perhaps they were even made to feel incompetent by unthinking adults or peers.

The self-concept and self-esteem are so important to mental health that children will devalue areas of life in which they do not receive signals of their own **competence.** Gangly, long-legged Frances at twelve could not quite get all her parts moving in synchrony to succeed in sports, so she avoided playing them and instead honed her library skills to excellence. In healthy self-defense, she devalued the area of life that threatened to rob her self-esteem (sports), and replaced it with another area in which she shined (academics).

It is amazing how sensitive children are to subtle cues and how they mold their lives in response to them. Unfortunately, many people are presented with standards to which they cannot possibly measure up because of the level of difficulty, inborn traits, or like poor Frances, because they are developmentally not ready. In addition, they may criticize themselves when they are unable to perform the impossible. In fact, just a lucky few survive the tender years of building self-concept and self-esteem with mostly positive messages about their abilities. Is it any wonder that some people have written physical activity out of their life-scripts?

Happily, the problem is solvable. Figure 2–1 shows that competence raises the physical self-concept, which in turn bolsters self-esteem. As far as physical activity is concerned, anyone can do better when improvement is measured on a personal scale. The task for the adult is to kick old negative messages into a corner of life with other dusty, useless things that do not matter, and to let a new, healthy concern for physical health shine through. In adult life, Frances managed to devalue old messages that tended to stop her from jogging for fitness by tossing out her old performance standard and adopting a new one—competence. As she gained competence, she also gained in physical condition and her body image improved.

Anyone can do it. Strive to do better today than you did last week or last month (*you* control the time frame and the reward system now), and you will find that not only your body but your self-esteem will benefit.[1]

The person with high self-esteem may care enough to invest energy and effort in fitness from the start. The person with low self-esteem can begin to build it through fitness.

Immediacy

The immediacy of a reward alters the balance a person perceives between the benefits and the costs. If you can enjoy the reward right away, you are

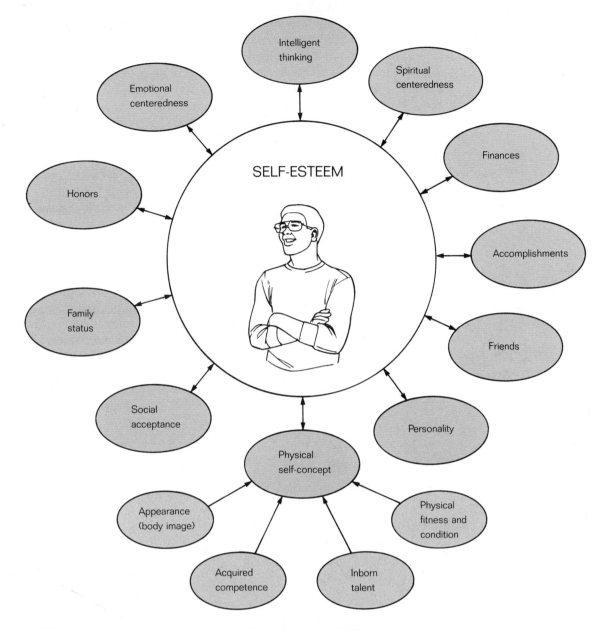

FIGURE 2-1 **Physical Self-Concept Contributes to Self-Esteem**

more motivated to pursue it; if you do not have to pay until later, you are even more motivated. (This is the "buy now, pay later" principle that so often promotes sales successfully.) On the other hand, if you must pay now and don't receive your reward until later (pay now, buy later), you are less motivated. Thus, another pointer for the person developing a fitness program is to make it as enjoyable as you can, not punishing. Also, tune in to the rewards that are available as you go along. Although the ultimate reward of an improved physique may not come after one day's workout, signs do point to your progress. Deep breathing feels good and tells you that your lungs are expanding. A flushed complexion makes you glow and tells you that your blood is nourishing and energizing your skin. Abundant, clean sweat cools you, cleanses your skin, and proves that you are one of the fitness seekers you admire. You have paid with hard work and the rewards have made your effort worth it.

Probability

Probability adds another modifier to motivation. The more certain the outcome, the stronger the motivation to pursue it. If you follow proven guidelines, the results you seek will come automatically. Follow scientifically validated advice, because science gives you rules that work. For example, people seeking to lose weight can do so successfully, not if they follow fraudulent fad diets, but if they follow proven programs. Knowing you can trust a program permits you to put all your effort into following it and none into wondering whether it will work. Following a program, not wishing, is what will get you there.

The fitness guidelines in this book are based on science and ensure that your effort will get you where you want to go. Your motivation will be high, then, because you can be certain of the reward.

This discussion has illustrated the basic elements that affect a person's motivation. These elements are at work in the steps that lead to commitment.

The elements of behavior change.

Commitment

The steps that lead to behavior change seem to be these:

- Awareness: "I could choose to change."
- Cognition: "I know how to change."
- Emotion: "I want to change."
- Decision: "I will change."
- Action: "I am changing."

They don't always appear in the same order, but they do always seem to appear. The following story provides an example.

Being overweight is a problem familiar to many people. (If you can't identify with this problem, substitute some other problem while reading this.) Suppose you know a man who wants to lose weight. He has taken the first two steps: He is *aware* of the need, and he *knows how,* at least to some extent. Still, he is taking no action. Perhaps he doesn't really *want* to. Like many others, he gets stuck at this point. Eating fattening foods brings him great pleasure, for one thing. For another, without being aware of it, he may receive some benefits from being fat. (He doesn't have to cope with many sexual advances, for example.) He may claim he wants to lose weight, and he may be chronically upset with himself for not getting thinner, yet deep inside he may not really want to change.

3. As soon as you know how to change a health habit, it is easy to do so.

False.

Knowing how is not enough to change a health habit; you also have to decide to do it.

Wanting is emotional, and when the emotions become positively involved, a rush of energy enables the person to act. Still, no amount of emotion, by itself, is enough to change behavior. We all can name people who know how to diet and exercise and who desperately want to lose weight, but still do nothing. The person has to make a decision—a step in which the *will* is involved.

Even psychologists don't fully understand how people make decisions. But everyone knows how it feels to arrive at a decision point. One day, you are ready and you know that you will undertake the thing you have wanted to do. At this point—when you say, "I will do it"—the wanting and the knowing how flow together into action and bring about the desired change. One day, your friend who needs to lose weight says, "I'm going to eat wisely from now on and exercise regularly," and from that point on, possibly for months, he will *act*. Now, he will restrict calories, exercise, and lose weight until he seems to have become a completely different person.

In a sense, he is a different person. He has had to let go of his old habits completely. His self-image has had to change. He was an overeater; he is now an ex-overeater, an abstainer. He was an inactive person; he is now an active person. He was a person who avoided facing certain problems by overeating; now he knows himself better, and he asserts himself more effectively. He is *committed*.

Action

Once you are committed, you have to act. The next two sections show you how to undertake and maintain a behavior change. The first one describes ways you can look inside yourself for motivation; the second shows how you can arrange your environment to reinforce your behavior.

Cultivating Intrinsic Motivation

intrinsic motivation: motivation supplied from inside a person, from the way the person feels (as opposed to behavior modification, which provides external motivators).

No one will stay with a program unless it produces *internal* rewards. This is as true of fitness programs as of any others: People drop out. Research indicates that those who persist are the ones who find **intrinsic motivation** in the chosen program. They do not need to be persuaded to participate. The experience itself is rewarding—it is fun, challenging, interesting, exciting, or satisfying enough in any of many other ways to keep them coming back again and again. However, what is intrinsically motivating for one person may not be for another. You may find solitary running to be both interesting and relaxing; your friend finds it boring and prefers to compete in team sports.

Health professionals are concerned about the dropout rate from fitness programs and have researched the factors that induce people to stay in. Intrinsic motivators are most effective; external pressures are less so. Many people start fitness programs to lose weight or to meet compatible people, rather than to become fit. If they don't achieve their chosen goals within a short time, they usually won't persist. One study showed that 92 percent of the people who had not achieved these goals in a fitness program by the end of six months dropped out.[2] What keeps people from dropping out seems to be simple enjoyment.

In choosing a fitness program, it is important to ask yourself what you, personally, really enjoy or can most easily learn to enjoy. Some clues to what people enjoy are reflected in the following statements:

- "I find it interesting" (not "I should do it").
- "It makes me feel good" (not "I know it's good for my
- heart").
- "I chose it for myself" (not "My parents or teachers have pressured me to do it").
- "I have chosen my own program" (not "I'm trying to abide by their program").
- "I like the style of the leaders in the program" (not "The program has a good reputation").

This doesn't mean, incidentally, that anything is wrong with following a coach's directions—but you do that after choosing, for yourself, a particular program or a particular coach.

Intrinsic motivation is important at all levels of athletic performance and is the driving force even for world-class athletes. Athletes work at their sport because they enjoy the process so much that they remain focused even when faced with opposition. They are just like the rest of us: One of the chief things they enjoy is progressing toward their own self-chosen goals.

Employing Behavior Modification Principles

Behavior modification techniques provide external motivation, in contrast to the intrinsic motivators just described. You can choose to use them for yourself to reinforce your own chosen activity pattern.

The strategy of **behavior modification** uses external reinforcers to make changes in many small, individual daily behaviors. Behavior modification experts see each behavior as part two of a three-part sequence. Its **antecedents** precede it, and its **consequences** follow it:

behavior modification: the changing of behavior by the manipulation of *antecedents* (cues, or environmental factors that trigger behavior), the behavior itself, and *consequences* (the penalties or rewards attached to behavior).

A (antecedents) ⟶ B (behavior) ⟷ C (consequences)

A behavior occurs in response to antecedents (cues or stimuli); the more intense the antecedents are, the more likely the behavior will occur. The behavior leads to consequences, and the more positively or negatively intense these are, the more or less likely the behavior is to occur again. To make behavior modification principles work for you, you manipulate the antecedents and consequences to favor the repeated occurrence of a desired behavior and to extinguish the occurrence of unwanted behaviors.

Figure 2–2 illustrates strategies to modify antecedents, behaviors, and consequences to cement a desired behavior in place. In this example,

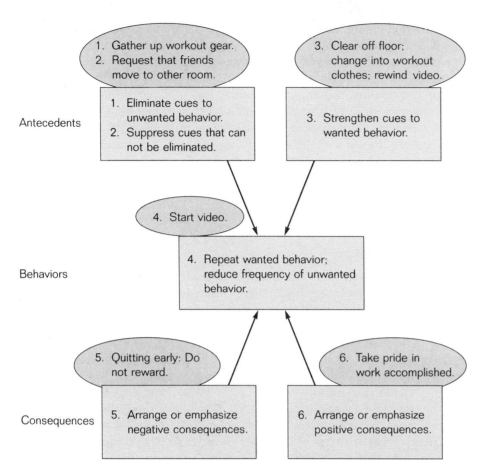

Antecedents

1. Gather up workout gear.
2. Request that friends move to other room.

1. Eliminate cues to unwanted behavior.
2. Suppress cues that can not be eliminated.

3. Clear off floor; change into workout clothes; rewind video.

3. Strengthen cues to wanted behavior.

Behaviors

4. Start video.

4. Repeat wanted behavior; reduce frequency of unwanted behavior.

Consequences

5. Quitting early: Do not reward.

5. Arrange or emphasize negative consequences.

6. Take pride in work accomplished.

6. Arrange or emphasize positive consequences.

FIGURE 2-2 Behavior Modification Example: How to Exercise Effectively

the person is using behavior modification to achieve a fitness goal. Kristin needs to prepare to audition for an aerobic dance instructor position, but she lacks enough motivation to practice her aerobic dance routine. Conditions are unfavorable: Her workout gear is scattered throughout the house, two friends have dropped in and are conversing in the room she dances in, the floor is too cluttered to walk across, much less dance on, and her workout video needs rewinding. It is tempting to procrastinate (unwanted behavior). Knowing the principles of behavior modification, though, Kristin modifies the antecedents. Gathering up her workout gear eliminates one cue to procrastination (strategy 1 in the figure). Requesting that the friends talk in another room suppresses another (strategy 2). Clearing off the floor, changing into her dance clothes, and rewinding the video provide cues to the desired behavior (strategy 3). Once Kristin starts her video, the tendency to procrastinate fades and the aerobic dancing gets under way (strategy 4). Self-congratulation is now in order (strategy 6).

A note about emphasizing negative consequences (strategy 5): Kristin could have asked her friends to bug her if she procrastinated. But oddly enough, bugging is a positive consequence, because it is a form of

5. To help a person keep a fitness resolution, a good friend will remind the person to practice daily.

False.

It is more effective to ignore procrastination and reward only positive behaviors, such as practicing, with attention.

attention-giving, and it reinforces procrastination. The most effective negative consequence you can arrange to eliminate an unwelcome behavior is to have your friends ignore it. Being ignored is a negative consequence, and after you have learned that you cannot get attention by procrastinating, you are more likely to seek it by exhibiting the preferred behavior—in Kristin's case, practicing her dance routine.

Behavior modification techniques equip people with a means to effectively change their behavior if they want to. A particularly attractive feature of these strategies is that they don't involve blaming oneself or putting oneself down—a point of importance in the fostering of self-esteem.

Persistence

Sometimes, even after what seems to be a *firm commitment* to changed behavior, a person slips back. Why? Once you have instituted a change in your life, you will persist in maintaining that change only if the reward-versus-cost balance continues to favor it.

The progress to fitness is not without setbacks. Let's look at a hard-working, over-achieving, highly social college student to examine the broader application of behavior-change principles. She has decided to take up a fitness routine for 30 minutes a day. During the first session, all she can think about are the 101 other things she "should be doing." After two days, she is frustrated, her muscles are sore, and she is driving her friends crazy with her anxiety over trying to fit her new routine into her crowded schedule. At this time, the long-distant rewards of becoming fit and reducing stress have receded far into the background in her thinking, and all that she is aware of is her need to be doing something else.

To succeed, this person needs to have *realistic expectations*. She needs to know from the outset how hard it will be at first to relax during her daily routine and especially how long it will take before her frustration subsides and the rewards begin to come in. It helps, too, to have *awareness of the immediate rewards*—immediate in terms of days, not years. After a week, she is free of thoughts about other things she might be doing during her activity sessions. She is beginning to feel more energetic and stronger and finds she gets more work accomplished in less time. If she notices these changes, she may make it through the hard part.

6. When you get started on a fitness routine, you should make all possible healthful changes in your diet at the same time.

False.

It is best to work on one or a few new behaviors at a time.

People need to know, too, that they can't undertake too large a change and expect to succeed. Suppose a person, in a rush of enthusiasm, decides to do everything at once. "I'm going to start jogging a mile every morning and doing sit-ups every night. I'm going to give up cookies and cakes and candies and colas and all sugar sources," the person tells you. "I'm going to avoid all fatty foods. I'm giving up smoking and all alcoholic beverages, switching from whole milk to nonfat milk—and never using cream—and giving up salt. I plan to go to church every Sunday and spend at least two added hours each day on homework. . . ." The person may be in for a rude surprise. All these changes can be made, but not all at once. After only a few days, such a person will be exhausted and will give it all up. It is important not to bite off more than you can chew. New behaviors require energy. A person undertaking them needs to *work on one or a few new behaviors at a time.*

For example, consider the effort needed just to switch from whole milk to nonfat milk. A "rule of three" can help people learn to like something new. Try nonfat milk once and you will not like it; try it a second time and you will say to yourself, "This isn't as good as whole milk, but I can drink it"; try it a third time and you will say, "This is about the same as whole milk; I guess I don't really care which I have." At that point, the habit can finally maintain itself because the preference for whole milk is gone.

Goal-setting can be an effective motivating technique to help people develop fitness. The way the goal is stated has much to do with its effectiveness. Researchers find that *specific small daily goals* (I will run for 15 minutes) are more effective than imprecise long-term goals (I will exercise more).[3]

Another important aspect of goal-setting is that the goals must be flexible. You must expect to encounter and deal with barriers because they are bound to interfere. What will you do if an unavoidable conflict keeps you from going to your preferred activity programs? What if the gym is closed for repairs? What if it rains when you were planning to play ball? What if you get sick or just feel too tired for physical exercise?

No plan is perfect, no person is perfect. To expect perfection is to set yourself up for failure. Allow yourself some slack. It is fine to aim for a

7. The best fitness goals are lofty goals.

False.

The best fitness goals are specific, small, daily goals.

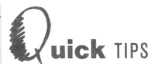

Quick TIPS

Goal-Setting for Best Results

- Not "I will get better at dancing," but "I will attend all my dance classes and practice as instructed."
- Not "I will lose weight this week," but "I will write down everything I eat every day."
- Not "I will prepare better for exercising," but "Each Saturday morning, I will wash, dry, and fold my exercise clothes for the week."
- Not "I will do well on the test next Thursday," but "I will study (practice) for the test in the library (gym) every evening from seven to eight o'clock."
- Not "I will exercise with friends so that I'll enjoy it more," but "Each Sunday evening I'll call and make dates for at least three workouts the next week."
- Not "I will make progress at my chosen activity," but "I will keep a daily log of my improvement."

sterling Plan A (I will run for an hour every day this week), but if Plan A fails, don't give up altogether. Pull Plan B out of your sleeve (I will run for at least 15 minutes, at least four days this week. If it rains, I'll do calisthenics). Research findings show that *flexible goals* promote adherence to and improved performance of fitness programs better than rigid goals.[4] Table 2–1 displays an array of barriers with strategies for overcoming them.

The maintenance of a new behavior sometimes depends on *not forgetting* that a return to the old behavior would be worse. Research on older people supports this point. Heart patients in a medically supervised program who actually have chest pains while exercising are more likely to stay with the program than those who have no symptoms.[5] The symptoms remind them of their condition and motivate them to continue exercising.

TABLE 2–1 • Overcoming Fitness Barriers

Barriers	Solution
I lack energy.	Physical activity will give you a second wind and more energy in the long run.
I fear my surroundings.	Take a friend with you, or change the location of your workout.
I'm too embarrassed.	Begin by working out in your home, alone, or by walking or jogging when few people are around.
I don't know how.	Begin by walking.
I don't think I can.	Try. You'll be surprised — don't sell yourself short.
I don't like the way my body feels when I'm working out.	Your sensations will become familiar and pleasing.
People will laugh.	They aren't laughing at you; they're identifying with you. Laugh back.
I don't like to sweat.	Learn to view sweat as positive proof of your healthful behavior and as a means of cleansing the skin. Learn to like to sweat.
Exercise is boring.	Find a different way to work out. With hundreds of ways to be physically active, maybe it is you that is boring, not the exercise. Use your imagination.
I don't have time.	Find time. Reassess your priorities and remember that physical activity brings many rewards, among them more time to live.
The weather is bad.	Work out indoors.
None of my friends are physically active.	Take up some physical activity; you'll make some new friends.
I don't have a partner to work out with today.	Learn to enjoy working out by yourself.

Many factors influence people's persistence in a fitness program. The ones we have discussed so far are personal factors and include:

- A firm commitment.
- Realistic expectations.
- Awareness of immediate rewards.
- Realistic expectation of rewards to come.
- Working on one or two changes at a time.
- Specific, small, daily goals.
- Flexible goals.
- Remembering penalties of slipping back.

Researchers find that external factors also affect people's adherence to physical activity plans.[6] A major predictor of persistence is *injury prevention*. One study found that about 20 percent of participants who dropped out of a 20-week running program did so because of injury.[7] Most injuries are avoidable; Chapter 11 discusses their prevention.

Other important external influences on persistence are *convenience* and the *size of the group*. Researchers find that a convenient location promotes persistence.[8] People exercising in small groups are more likely to persist at it than are those exercising alone or in large groups. This is probably because small groups facilitate social relationships that reinforce adherence.

The effects of your daily choices are compounded by time. Today's choices, repeated for a week, will have seven times the impact. Repeated every day for a year, they will have 365 times the impact on your health. Over years, the effects accumulate still further. It seems worthwhile, then, to cultivate the motivation to make the beneficial choices today and every day. Make physical activity as much a part of your day as eating or sleeping.

8. It is best to work out by yourself so that you don't have to depend on other people to make it happen.

False.

People exercising in small groups are more likely to persist than are those exercising alone.

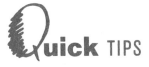
Quick TIPS

Exercise Persistence

To help you stick to it:

- Plan not to get hurt.
- Pick a place that's easy to get to.
- Go with a manageable number of friends.

How's Your Fitness Motivation?

In order to begin a fitness program, you must know *why* you want to do it in the first place and have realistic expectations of what is ahead. Once you are doing it, you need to be aware of the rewards that come with exercising so you can keep going and remind yourself of what the consequences are if you do not keep going. The questions below are designed to help you tune in to your own motivation for exercising. The second part of this section helps you set attainable goals. The third part encourages you to plan some rewards to keep you going, and the fourth part warns you to anticipate possible barriers and plan to overcome them.

A. Discover Your Own Motivation

Learn why you want to exercise by studying the list below. Then, rate each item with a 1 if it is something that is VERY IMPORTANT to you, a 2 if it is SOMEWHAT IMPORTANT to you, and a 3 if it is NOT IMPORTANT at all. The better you know yourself and what motivates you, the more easily you will stay motivated and overcome obstacles.[9]

By exercising and developing fitness, I hope to . . .

_____ make myself more attractive.

_____ lose weight and improve my body composition.

_____ meet new people.

_____ enjoy better health.

_____ feel more self-confident.

_____ enjoy more energy and stamina.

_____ feel more in control of myself and of my life.

_____ improve my stress resistance.

_____ sleep better.

_____ have more fun.

_____ other (you describe) _____

_____ .

Now that you have pinpointed what motivates you to exercise, write your two most important motivators on this chapter's Lab Report form, Section A (see Appendix A).

B. Practice Setting Specific, Realistic Goals

You will learn more about how to design your own individualized fitness program in the chapters to come. For now, start with what you already know, just for practice.

Make your goals specific. "I will exercise three times a week," rather than "I will try to exercise more often." Make them realistic, too. "I will jog (walk, work out) at least 15 minutes every other day," rather than "I will climb a mountain every morning."

Write down two or more goals on the Lab Report, Section B. You are not contracting to achieve these goals (although you may choose to go ahead and do so). You will set more formal goals later and have the opportunity to carry them out. If you need help in goal-setting, consult the Quick Tips in the chapter.

C. Reward Yourself

Some of the changes that motivate you in the checklist of Part A may take a while to come about. In the meantime, plan some immediate rewards for yourself. Make them repeatable, realistic, and really attractive to *you*.

Examples:

1. Each time I complete my routine, I'll treat myself to an orange sherbert.
2. Each week, if I have kept to my fitness plan, I will treat myself to a good movie (or an hour of fun reading).
3. Each month, if I have kept to my plan,* I will buy myself a new piece of equipment (running shorts, sweatband, swim goggles).

Write down on the Lab Report, Section C, exactly what behaviors you will reward, how often, and how.

D. Anticipate Possible Barriers and Plan to Overcome Them

What might keep you from sticking to your plan? How can you overcome each barrier?

Examples:

If it rains, I can't jog.	I'll dress for the rain and jog anyway.
If there's a hurricane, I can't swim.	I'll do a half-hour workout with my exercise tape that day.
If I'm sick, I can't play tennis.	I'll rest.
If I get exhausted, I can't finish my session.	I'll revise my plan (it wasn't realistic).

Record your possible barriers and strategies for overcoming them on the Lab Report, Section D.

*I will allow myself to skip one exercise session in the month without penalty.

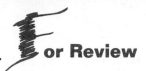# or Review

1. Name two kinds of motives and give examples of each (page 23).
2. Describe three modifiers of motivation (page 23).
3. Describe and give an example of intrinsic motivation (page 27).
4. Briefly describe the strategy of behavior modification (page 28).
5. List some of the personal and environmental factors that enhance persistence in fitness programs (page 30–33).

hapter Notes

1. The ideas here were presented by Kenneth Fox, AAHPERD annual meeting, Boston, Mass., April 1989.
2. R. R. Danielson and R. S. Wanzel, Exercise objectives of fitness program dropouts, in *Psychology of Motor Behavior and Sports— 1977,* eds. D. M. Landers and R. W. Christina (Champaign, Ill.: Human Kinetics, 1978), pp. 310–320, as cited in R. J. Vallerand, E. L. Deci, and R. M. Ryan, Intrinsic motivation in sport, *Exercise and Sport Sciences Review* 15 (1987): 389–425.
3. E. A. Locke and G. P. Latham, The application of goal-setting to sports, *Journal of Sport Psychology* 7 (1985): 205–222, as cited in Vallerand, Deci, and Ryan, 1987.
4. C. E. Thompson and L. M. Wankel, The effect of perceived activity choice upon frequency of exercise behavior, *Journal of Applied Social Psychology* 10 (1980): 436–443; C. J. Alexander, W. J. Schuldt, Effects of achievement standards and choice on a basketball skill, *Journal of Sport Psychology* 4 (1982): 189–193, as cited in Vallerand, Deci, and Ryan, 1987.
5. R. K. Dishman, Motivation and exercise adherence, in *Psychological Foundations of Sport,* eds. J. M. Silva and R. S. Weinberg (Champaign, Ill.: Human Kinetics, 1984), pp. 420–434.
6. Dishman, 1984.
7. M. L. Pollock and coauthors, Effects of frequency and duration of training on attrition and incidence of injury, *Medicine and Science in Sports* 9 (1977): 31–36, as cited in Dishman, 1984.
8. G. M. Andrew and coauthors, Reasons for dropout from exercise programs in post-coronary patients, *Medicine and Science in Sports and Exercise* 13 (1981): 165–168, as cited in Dishman, 1984.
9. This exercise was inspired by, and parts were adapted from, *The Quick Success Program,* Weight Watchers International, Inc., 1987, 1988.

THREE

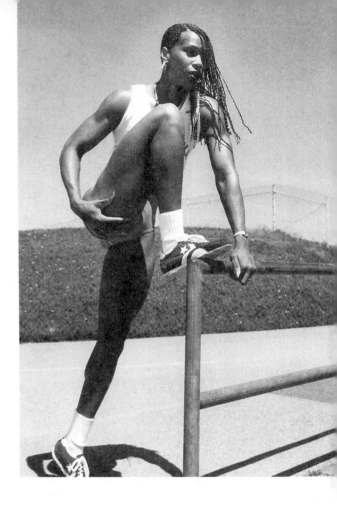

Contents

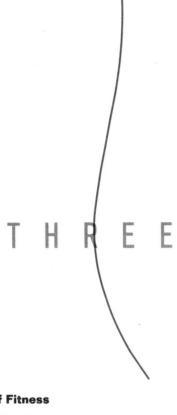

The Elements of Fitness

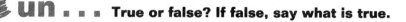
People decide to pursue fitness for many reasons: To lose weight, to gain strength, to minimize risks of heart disease, to compete in sports, and simply to have fun. Whatever the reason, the decision to become physically fit is a sound one in terms of health.

This chapter introduces the basic elements of fitness and presents ways of assessing your own body's fitness. Some of the information presented is intended for people who are just learning that fitness is important; other information is intended to help the seasoned athlete. As fitness expert Dr. George Sheehan says, "We are all athletes, it's just that some of us are in training and others are not."[1]

Chapter 1 discussed the many benefits that come with regular physical activity and a fit body. Science cannot promise that you will receive all of the benefits if you pursue fitness, but almost every active person reaps at least some of them. If even half of the rewards were yours for the asking, wouldn't you step up to claim them? The only cost to you is the effort to plan fitness activity into your days.

The Foundations of Fitness

To be physically fit, you do not have to be spectacular-looking. You do not have to develop an Olympic athlete's body. Rather, what you need is a reasonable weight and body composition and enough flexibility, muscular strength, and endurance to meet the everyday demands life places on you, plus some to spare.

Physical fitness expresses itself in body characteristics. Some are health-related, some are skill-related. One of the health-related characteristics is **body composition**—the proportions of muscle, fat, bone, and other tissue that make up a person's total body weight. Physical activity augments desirable lean body tissue and eliminates excess body fat. A second characteristic is **flexibility,** which is important to the joints. **Muscle endurance** and **strength** are important to the muscles. Endurance is also important to the heart and lungs: This type of endurance is called **cardiovascular endurance.** As you become physically fit, improving your body composition, flexibility, muscle strength and endurance, and cardiovascular endurance, you improve the health of your entire body.

The person who wants to go beyond general health and enhance athletic *performance* in specific sports will also value *skill-related* components of fitness such as **agility, balance, coordination, power, speed,** and **reaction time.** The importance of each characteristic varies widely with individual sports, and athletes practice endless hours to develop them. In a way, you might say the skill-related components arise from the application of health-related fitness components to a task—strength confers grace and agility on a figure skater; flexibility facilitates balance in a gymnast; muscle endurance gives a pitcher the coordination to aim and throw again and again on the mark. The skills a person gains from practicing a sport have little impact on a person's health; they are essential, however, in achieving excellence in sports performance. The focus of this book is fitness and its importance to personal health, and the emphasis here is on the health-related components—flexibility, strength,

1. The skills a person gains from practicing a sport have little impact on the person's health.

True.

ıₙₙₙₙₙₙₙₙₙₙₙ Health-Related Components of Fitness

body composition: the proportions of muscle, bone, fat, and other tissue that make up a person's total body weight.

flexibility: the ability to bend and recover without injury; it depends on the elasticity of muscles and tendons and on the condition of the joints. One kind, *dynamic flexibility,* is the ability to bend the body while in motion, such as the motions required to dunk a basketball; another, *static flexibility,* is the ability to bend while standing, sitting, or lying still.

muscle endurance: the ability of a muscle to contract repeatedly within a given time without becoming exhausted.

muscle strength: the ability of muscles to work against resistance.

cardiovascular endurance: the ability of the cardiovascular system to sustain its oxygen-delivery work over a long time.

and endurance. (Body composition results from food intake and activity taken together and will be a major subject in Chapter 8.)

Principles of Conditioning

Whatever component of fitness you seek to develop—flexibility, strength, or endurance—certain principles apply. The principles of **conditioning** have to do with the way your body adapts to perform the work you ask of it. Conditioning is the microscopic nuts and bolts of fitness. The way you achieve conditioning is by training, primarily by applying overload.

Overload

Your body does physical work every day. The stronger and more fit you are, the less strain it takes to do that work. If your body is weak, you cannot trade it in as you might trade in a car too small to do its job—and fortunately, you do not need to. Unlike a small car, which will break down when consistently overloaded, your body responds to **overload** in a positive way—it gets itself into better shape to meet the demand next time.

If you work a muscle or group of muscles beyond the normal level of demand, hormones that regulate building of muscle tissue are stimulated. In 24 to 48 hours, nature repairs any slight injuries the muscles may have incurred during exercise. It also remodels and builds extra tissue to a point that makes the muscles better conditioned than they were before the workout. This ensures that next time the muscles will meet the more vigorous challenge more easily. To gain fitness, you should work within your capacity but close to it—at around 80 percent of maximum.

conditioning: the physical effect of *training*; improved flexibility, strength, and endurance.

training: practicing an activity, which leads to conditioning. Training is what you do; conditioning is what you get.

overload: an extra physical demand placed on the body; an increase in the frequency, duration, or intensity of exercise.

2. To gain fitness you should never work any muscle or group of muscles beyond the normal level of demand.

   False.

   To gain fitness, you *should* work your muscles close to capacity—but not to the point of injury, of course.

~~~~~~~~ Skill-Related Components of Fitness

> **agility:** the ability to move the entire body quickly.
>
> **balance:** the ability to maintain equilibrium in a fixed position or in motion.
>
> **coordination:** the harmonious functioning of the senses and the muscles to accurately perform complex movements, such as hitting a baseball or juggling two or more objects.
>
> **power:** the combination of strength and speed that allows a person to move quickly and forcefully, such as in jumping, shot-putting, or spiking a ball.
>
> **speed:** the ability to move fast, as in running or swimming.
>
> **reaction time:** the amount of time between a stimulus and a response to the stimulus, such as when starting a race.

progressive overload principle: the training principle that a body system, in order to improve, must be worked at frequencies, durations, or intensities that increase by increments over time.

frequency: the number of occurrences per unit of time (for example, the number of exercise sessions per week).

intensity: the degree of exertion while exercising (for example, the amount of weight lifted or the speed of running).

duration: length of time (for example, the length of time spent in each exercise session).

3. If you hate hard work, you can't gain fitness.

   False.

   If you hate hard work, you can gain fitness by exercising longer.

specificity: the principle that only those body systems that are stressed by exercise will achieve higher levels of physical fitness.

The overload effect applies equally to flexibility, muscle strength and endurance, and cardiovascular endurance. It acts not only on the muscles and joints, but also on other body systems. For example, to develop strong, dense bones, you must start by demanding that the bones bear slightly more stress than they are used to. The bones respond by accumulating more minerals, becoming stronger until, eventually, a maximum is reached. People can develop their body systems to an amazing extent by applying overload progressively, more each time they train. The elite athletes of today have done this to their full genetic potential.

You can achieve overload by using the **progressive overload principle** in several different ways. You can perform the activity more often—that is, increase its **frequency;** you can perform the activity more strenuously—that is, increase its **intensity;** or you can do it for longer times—that is, increase its **duration.** All three strategies work well, and you can pick one or a combination, depending on your preferences. For example, if you really love your workout, do it more often. If you do not have much time, increase intensity. If you hate hard work, take it easy and go longer. If you desire continuous improvements, remember to overload progressively as you gain higher levels of fitness.

When you are increasing the frequency, intensity, or duration of your workout, exercise to a point that only *slightly* exceeds your comfortable capacity to work. It is better to progress too slowly than to risk serious injury by overexertion. Allow enough, but not too much, time for recovery between periods of similar exercise (at least, but not more than, 24 to 48 hours). It does not make sense to start with activities so demanding that pain stops you within two days. Learn to enjoy your small steps toward improvement. Fitness builds slowly.

Here are other pointers about applying overload:

- Exercise regularly.
- Train hard only once or twice a week, not every time you work out. Between times, do light workouts.
- Listen to your body and cooperate. If you feel energetic, work hard; but if you are tired or in pain, go lightly or stop, even if that was not in your original plan.

The metabolic and performance changes that occur with overload are specific to the component of fitness being challenged. In other words, stretching develops flexibility and has no effect on cardiovascular endurance. Taking this principle of **specificity** one step further, a person who wants to condition the body for swimming will achieve the best results by doing just that—swimming. A swimmer could improve cardiovascular endurance by running, and it would carry over into swimming, of course, but by swimming, the swimmer will train the individual muscles needed for the activity and gain the skills as well. This advice does not imply that you should concentrate solely on one type of exercise at the expense of the others, but only that you can tailor your program to achieve the results you want. In brief, practice by doing what you want to become proficient at.

Muscle Fibers and Work

use-disuse principle: the principle that fitness develops in response to demand and diminishes in response to the lack of demand.

Fitness develops in response to demand and wanes when demand ceases—the **use-disuse principle.** Muscles enlarge after being called upon repeatedly to do a certain type of work.* Certain cells in the muscles gain bulk and improve their capacity to work. When the activity is stopped for a few days, the muscles diminish in size and lose strength.** Just as the muscles adapt to greater work demands, so do they adapt to lesser ones.

Muscles respond according to the kinds of demands placed upon them. They are made up, largely, of two different types of contractible cells called **muscle fibers—slow-twitch muscle fibers** and **fast-twitch muscle fibers.** Each of these fiber types is best suited to a specific kind of work—slow-twitch fibers to **aerobic** work and fast-twitch fibers to **anaerobic** work. The different fibers can adapt in size and work capacity to the kind of work you ask your muscles to do.

muscle fibers: muscle cells.

slow-twitch muscle fibers: muscle fibers best suited to producing energy by aerobic processes for prolonged endurance exercise.

fast-twitch muscle fibers: muscle fibers best suited to producing energy by anaerobic processes, to perform high-intensity, short-duration work.

aerobic (air-ROE-bic): refers to energy-producing processes involving the immediate use of oxygen (aero = air).

anaerobic (AN-air-ROE-bic): refers to energy-producing processes that do not involve the immediate use of oxygen (an = without).

The way your muscles adapt also depends partly on your heredity. A person's athletic potential or talent is inborn, partly because every person is born with a set number of each type of fiber. In a sense, you are born to be either a sprinter or a long-distance runner. A person born with tremendous capacity who chooses to develop it to the full can become a great athlete. But even if you were not born with the "right stuff" to be an elite athlete, you can still choose to develop within your own limitations by choosing the right exercises.

High-intensity, short-duration activity depends mostly on fast-twitch muscle fibers and on glucose, the body's sugar, for its anaerobic energy fuel. Activity of lower intensity and longer duration depends more on slow-twitch muscle fibers and on fat, the body's other fuel, to provide energy aerobically.

Imagine a track meet. A sprinter bursts across the starting line in an explosion of energy. The burst lasts only a few seconds, followed by exhaustion at the finish line. Now envision a distance runner on an endless stretch of beach. The runner's steady stride paces off miles of sand with only slight changes in speed, maximizing the distance covered.

4. When your muscle fibers start to twitch, it is time to stop exercising.

   False.

   Twitching is what muscle fibers do.

The sprinter is engaging in mostly anaerobic activity, which is associated with strength, agility, and split-second surges of power. The jump of the basketball player, the slam of the tennis serve, the weight lifter's heave at the barbells, and the fullback's blast through the opposing line are all anaerobic work.

5. Some people are born to be great athletes.

   True.

The distance runner is engaging largely in aerobic work, which is associated with endurance. The ability to continue swimming until you reach the far bank, to continue hiking until you are at camp, or to continue pedaling until you are home reflects aerobic capacity. This capacity is also crucial to improving the health of the heart and circulatory system. The relationships outlined in the margin recur again and again throughout this book, and they bear heavily on how the exercise you

*This is called muscle **hypertrophy** (high-PER-tro-fee).
This is called **atrophy (AT-ro-fee).

These go together:

- Muscle fibers—fast-twitch.
- Major fuel—glycogen made available as glucose.
- Energy production—anaerobic.
- Exercise—high intensity, short duration.

These go together:

- Muscle fibers—slow-twitch.*
- Major fuel—fat.
- Energy production—aerobic.
- Exercise—lower intensity, longer duration.**

warm-up: five to ten minutes of light exercise, such as easy jogging or cycling, to warm up the body in preparation for vigorous exercise.

cool-down: five to ten minutes of light exercise following a vigorous workout to gradually cool the body's core to near-normal temperature.

epinephrine (ep-ih-NEFF-rin): one of the stress hormones. It is secreted whenever emergency action is called for; it readies body systems for fast action and mobilizes fuel to support that action. Epinephrine used to be called *adrenalin*.

6. Stretching is a good way to end a cool-down after a workout.

   True.

choose affects your appearance and your health and on how well the foods you eat support your chosen activities.

Warm-Up and Cool-Down Activities

Training, if done properly, overloads the system as already described. Sudden intense activity could cause injury, and abrupt discontinuance could hamper recovery, so it is best to ease into and out of activity sessions. The body needs fair warning of physical activity ahead, and after activity, it needs an easy transition into inaction. All strenuous workouts should therefore be fitted inside a frame composed of **warm-up** and **cool-down** activities.

A warm-up facilitates gradual warming of the body and also begins the hormonal changes that liberate the needed fuels from storage. Most importantly, the onset of exercise stimulates the release of the hormone **epinephrine,** which mobilizes fuels needed for the exercise to come.[2] Chapter 4 gives further details about the importance of the warm-up.

Cool-down activity eases the transition from exercising to normal functioning. A few minutes of light activity facilitates the relaxation of tight muscles and enhances the circulation of blood through them. The circulation in turn brings accumulated heat from the body's core to the surface where it can radiate away. As you approach the end of your workout, gradually ease up on the intensity of the activity (for example, if you are running, begin to slow to a light jog) reaching a minimum intensity over 5 to 10 minutes. Stretching exercises to promote flexibility are particularly well suited to the end of the cool-down.

Cool-down activities can also help to prevent symptoms—dizziness, for example—that you may experience if you abruptly stop exercising.[3] A cool-down facilitates a gradual drop in blood pressure; an abrupt drop would stress the heart. It can also help to prevent muscle cramps that might otherwise occur.

Up to now, this chapter has introduced the elements of fitness and described the principles of training that will enable you to develop those elements of fitness. The next few sections provide ways to measure your fitness so that you can plan a fitness program to take you from where you are now to where you want to be.

Measuring Fitness

The tests for measuring fitness are described here. If you wish to use them, follow the instructions in the Personal Focus section at the end of the chapter, and use the Lab Report form to record your results. These tests can help you determine how fit you are, at least in a general way.

---

*Fast- and slow-twitch are the two best known muscle fiber types. There are others.

**Higher intensity aerobic exercise, although using fat as a partial source of energy, depends primarily on glucose.

You can use the results to guide you in designing a personal fitness program. If you score high in strength but low in cardiovascular fitness, for example, you can plan more aerobic work into your activity routine; if you can run, but lack flexibility, this is a signal to stretch more, and so on.

Before you take these tests, take a moment to answer the health questions listed in Table 3–1. Ordinary exercises are not hazardous to any healthy person, but if you have health problems, you should proceed with caution. You do not want a medical condition to impair your fitness program. If, during testing, you notice *any* change in your functioning, or any pain, stop exercising and consult your health care provider before continuing. The rest of this chapter assumes your exercise program will go well. Chapter 11 discusses preventing sports injuries and heat stroke.

The tests included in this section are intended for the person who has no access to standard equipment of the type used for assessment in clinics. You do need a few items (ask your fitness instructor for them if necessary): A tape measure or yardstick, a fatfold caliper, a hand dynamometer (dine-a-MOM-me-ter), and a stopwatch. If you also have access to such facilities as a treadmill, a bicycle ergometer, or a machine to measure your oxygen consumption, use them too. They will increase the probability of accurate measurements.

Body Composition

Techniques for estimating body fat percentage include underwater weighing, electrical impedance, body girth measurements, and fatfold thickness. These techniques vary in their complexity. For example, underwater weighing, recognized as one of the most accurate ways to measure body composition, requires considerable time, expensive equipment, and skilled technicians. Underwater weighing determines body density, from which you can calculate body fat percentage (lean tissue is denser than fat tissue). Electrical impedance requires expensive equipment. Electrodes are placed on a person's hand and foot on the same side

---

TABLE 3–1 • **Cautions on Getting Started**

If you answer yes to any of the questions that follow, consult with a health care provider trained in fitness before beginning an exercise program.

- Are you over 35?
- If you are over 35, have you been sedentary for a long time?
- Are you more than 20 pounds heavier than you should be?
- Do you now smoke more than a pack and a half of cigarettes per day?
- Do you have any chronic illness?
- Has a health care provider ever said you had heart trouble?
- Did you ever have, or do you now have, a heart murmur?
- Have you ever had a diagnosed or suspected heart attack?
- Do you have chest pains at any time?

---

7. To estimate whether you are too fat, you can pinch the back of your arm.

True.

pinch test: an informal means of measuring body fatness by lifting a fold on the back of one arm with the fingers and estimating its thickness.

fatfold test: a clinical test of body fatness in which the thickness of a fold of skin and underlying fat on the back of the arm (triceps), below the shoulder blade (subscapular), or in other places is measured with an instrument called a caliper. The older, less preferred term for this is **skinfold test.**

of the body, and a small current is transmitted. This method is based on the principle that lean tissues are full of electrolyte-containing fluids that readily conduct an electrical current. Fat, on the other hand, is a poor conductor. Body girth measurements to estimate body fat require only a measuring tape, to measure body circumference at various points. The limitation of this technique is that it may be invalid for people who are thin or obese.[4] Other, simple techniques permit a ballpark estimate of whether a person is too fat or not. The accompanying Quick Tips provide rules of thumb such as the **pinch test** to assess body fatness.

A direct and practical method for estimating body fatness is to use a fatfold caliper—a device that measures the thickness of a fold of fat on the back of the arm, below the shoulder blade, on the side of the waist, or elsewhere. About 50 percent of the body's fat lies beneath the skin, and its thickness reflects total body fat. The **fatfold test** is a practical diagnostic procedure in the hands of trained people and is in wide use. Table 3–2 presents standards for fatfold measures at one location, the back of the arm (over the triceps muscle). Generally speaking, people whose fatfold measurements exceed the 95th percentile are considered obese.*

*A percentile is one of 100 equal divisions of data. For example, if a value, such as a person's test score, is higher than that of 75 percent of the rest of the population, then it is at the 75th percentile in the range of test scores. A person whose weight is at the 75th percentile weighs more than 75 percent of the population being used for comparison.

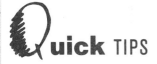

Rules Of Thumb to Assess Body Fatness

These methods for estimating how much body fat you have are just for fun:

- A crude measure of body fatness is the pinch test (this is a fatfold measure without the equipment to make it accurate). Pick up the skin and fat at the back of either arm with the thumb and forefinger of the other hand. Keep your fingers still, so as not to lose the "measurement" when you pull them away from your arm. Measure the thickness on a ruler. A fatfold over an inch thick reflects obesity.
- Another shortcut method is to compare your waist and chest (not bust) measurements. Every inch by which your waist measurement exceeds your chest measurement is said to take two years off your life.
- Another crude measure is to lie down, relax, and place a ruler across your abdomen from one hipbone to the other. If the ruler does not easily touch both bones while you're relaxing, you're too fat.

TABLE 3-2 • Triceps Fatfold Standards (Millimeters) for Males and Females (Percentiles)

Age	Male					Female				
	5th	25th	50th	75th	95th	5th	25th	50th	75th	95th
1– 1.9	6	8	10	12	16	6	8	10	12	16
2– 2.9	6	8	10	12	15	6	9	10	12	16
3– 3.9	6	8	10	11	15	7	9	11	12	15
4– 4.9	6	8	9	11	14	7	8	10	12	16
5– 5.9	6	8	9	11	15	6	8	10	12	18
6– 6.9	5	7	8	10	16	6	8	10	12	16
7– 7.9	5	7	9	12	17	6	9	11	13	18
8– 8.9	5	7	8	10	16	6	9	12	15	24
9– 9.9	6	7	10	13	18	8	10	13	16	22
10–10.9	6	8	10	14	21	7	10	12	17	27
11–11.9	6	8	11	16	24	7	10	13	18	28
12–12.9	6	8	11	14	28	8	11	14	18	27
13–13.9	5	7	10	14	26	8	12	15	21	30
14–14.9	4	7	9	14	24	9	13	16	21	28
15–15.9	4	6	8	11	24	8	12	17	21	32
16–16.9	4	6	8	12	22	10	15	18	22	31
17–17.9	5	6	8	12	19	10	13	19	24	37
18–18.9	4	6	9	13	24	10	15	18	22	30
19–24.9	4	7	10	15	22	10	14	18	24	34
25–34.9	5	8	12	16	24	10	16	21	27	37
35–44.9	5	8	12	16	23	12	18	23	29	38
45–54.9	6	8	12	15	25	12	20	25	30	40
55–64.9	5	8	11	14	22	12	20	25	31	38
65–74.9	4	8	11	15	22	12	18	24	29	36

Source: Adapted from A. R. Frisancho, New norms of upper limb fat and muscle areas for assessment of nutritional status, *American Journal of Clinical Nutrition* 34 (1981): 2540–2545.
© American Society of Clinical Nutrition.

The major limitation of the triceps fatfold test, by itself, is that fat may be thicker under the skin in one area than another. A pinch at the side of the waistline may not yield the same measurement as a pinch on the back of the arm. This limitation can be overcome by taking fatfold measures at several (often three) different places on the body, as described in Figures 3–1A and 3–1B.

The average body fat percentage for men 18 to 22 years of age is 15 percent; for women of the same age, it is 25 percent.[5] Male athletes have an average of 12 percent body fat, and female athletes have an average of 18 percent body fat. The minimum amount of body fat recommended for

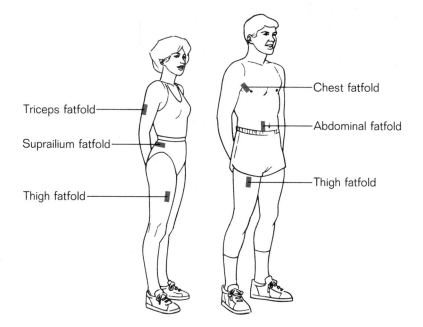

Triceps fatfold

Suprailium fatfold

Thigh fatfold

Chest fatfold

Abdominal fatfold

Thigh fatfold

The fatfold sites for men are:

- **The chest** (a diagonal fold midway between the shoulder crease and nipple).
- **The abdomen** (a vertical fold just to the side of the umbilicus).
- **The thigh** (a vertical fold on the front of the thigh midway between the hip and the knee).

For women, the sites are:

- **The triceps** (a vertical fold on the back of the upper arm, midway between the shoulder and the elbow).
- **The suprailium** (just above the hipbone, in line with the middle of the armpit).
- **The thigh** (a vertical fold on the front of the thigh midway between the hip and the knee).

FIGURE 3-1A Fatfold Sites for Women and Men

men is between 3 and 7 percent; the minimum for women is between 10 and 20 percent.[6] Below a certain threshold, some individuals develop symptoms such as infertility, depression, or abnormal hunger regulation. The threshold differs according to an individual's characteristics and may vary for each symptom even within an individual. Much remains to be learned about the hazards of extremely low levels of body fat.

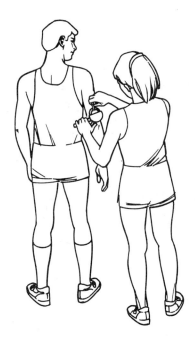

All fatfold measurements should be taken on the right side of the body while the person is standing, using the fatfold sites for men and women shown in Figure 3-1A. The procedure is as follows:

1. Grasp, between the thumb and the forefinger, a fold of skin and fat that lies just under the skin. To confirm that muscle is not included, have the person contract and relax the involved muscle.
2. Place the fatfold calipers perpendicular to the fold. Measure each fatfold site three times and take the average of the two closest measures as the final value.
3. Derive percent of body fat by adding the three fatfold values and looking them up on Table 3-3 for women, and Table 3-4 for men. Compare with the standards for body fat percentages in Table 3-5.

FIGURE 3-1B How to Take a Fatfold Measure
Fatfold calipers are available for as little as a few dollars to over $150. Accurate measures can be obtained with either cheap or expensive instruments, as long as they are used correctly.

MEASURING FITNESS

TABLE 3-3 • Women: Sum of Three Fatfolds (Triceps, Suprailium, and Thigh) Used to Estimate Percent of Body Fat

Find the sum in the left-hand column and the age at the top of the table. Read off the percent fat where the column and the row meet. Example: For a sum of 50–52 mm, a woman aged 22 has 20.6 percent body fat.

| Sum of Fatfolds (mm) | Age to the Last Year | | | | | | | | |
	Under 22	23 to 27	28 to 32	33 to 37	38 to 42	43 to 47	48 to 52	53 to 57	Over 58
23–25	9.7	9.9	10.2	10.4	10.7	10.9	11.2	11.4	11.7
26–28	11.0	11.2	11.5	11.7	12.0	12.3	12.5	12.7	13.0
29–31	12.3	12.5	12.8	13.0	13.3	13.5	13.8	14.0	14.3
32–34	13.6	13.8	14.0	14.3	14.5	14.8	15.0	15.3	15.5
35–37	14.8	15.0	15.3	15.5	15.8	16.0	16.3	16.5	16.8
38–40	16.0	16.3	16.5	16.7	17.0	17.2	17.5	17.7	18.0
41–43	17.2	17.4	17.7	17.9	18.2	18.4	18.7	18.9	19.2
44–46	18.3	18.6	18.8	19.1	19.3	19.6	19.8	20.1	20.3
47–49	19.5	19.7	20.0	20.2	20.5	20.7	21.0	21.2	21.5
50–52	20.6	20.8	21.1	21.3	21.6	21.8	22.1	22.3	22.6
53–55	21.7	21.9	22.1	22.4	22.6	22.9	23.1	23.4	23.6
56–58	22.7	23.0	23.2	23.4	23.7	23.9	24.2	24.4	24.7
59–61	23.7	24.0	24.2	24.5	24.7	25.0	25.2	25.5	25.7
62–64	24.7	25.0	25.2	25.5	35.7	26.0	26.7	26.4	26.7
65–67	25.7	25.9	26.2	26.4	26.7	26.9	27.2	27.4	27.7
68–70	26.6	26.9	27.1	27.4	27.6	27.9	28.1	28.4	28.6
71–73	27.5	27.8	28.0	28.3	28.5	28.8	28.0	29.3	29.5
74–76	28.4	28.7	28.9	29.2	29.4	29.7	29.9	30.2	30.4
77–79	29.3	29.5	29.8	30.0	30.3	30.5	30.8	31.0	31.3
80–82	30.1	30.4	30.6	30.9	31.1	31.4	31.6	31.9	32.1
83–85	30.9	31.2	31.4	31.7	31.9	32.2	32.4	32.7	32.9
86–88	31.7	32.0	32.2	32.5	32.7	32.9	33.2	33.4	33.7
89–91	32.5	32.7	33.0	33.2	33.5	33.7	33.9	34.2	34.4
92–94	33.2	33.4	33.7	33.9	34.2	34.4	34.7	34.9	35.2
95–97	33.9	34.1	34.4	34.6	34.9	35.1	35.4	35.6	35.9
98–100	34.6	34.8	35.1	35.3	35.5	35.8	36.0	36.3	36.5
101–103	35.3	35.4	35.7	35.9	36.2	36.4	36.7	36.9	37.2
104–106	35.8	36.1	36.3	36.6	36.8	37.1	37.3	37.5	37.8
107–109	36.4	36.7	36.9	37.1	37.4	37.6	37.9	38.1	38.4
110–112	37.0	37.2	37.5	37.7	38.0	38.2	38.5	38.7	38.9
113–115	37.5	37.8	38.0	38.2	38.5	38.7	39.0	39.2	39.5
116–118	38.0	38.3	38.5	38.8	39.0	39.3	39.5	39.7	40.0
119–121	38.5	38.7	39.0	39.2	39.5	39.7	40.0	40.2	40.5
122–124	39.0	39.2	39.4	39.7	39.9	40.2	40.4	40.7	40.9
125–127	39.4	39.6	39.9	40.1	40.4	40.6	40.9	41.1	41.4
128–130	39.8	40.0	40.3	40.5	40.8	41.0	41.3	41.5	41.8

Source: **Tables 3–3 and 3–4** from M. L. Pollock, D. H. Schmidt, and A. S. Jackson, Measurement of cardiorespiratory fitness and body composition in the clinical setting, *Comprehensive Therapy* 6 (1980): 12–27. Courtesy of the Laux Company, Inc., Maynard, Mass. **For Tables 3–3 and 3–4,** percent fat = $[(4.95/BD) - 4.5] \times 100$, where BD = body density from W. E. Siri, Body composition from fluid spaces and density, in *Techniques for Measuring Body Composition*, eds. J. Brozek and A. Hanschel (Washington, D. C.: National Academy of Sciences, 1961), pp. 223–224.

TABLE 3-4 • Men: Sum of Three Fatfolds (Chest, Abdomen, and Thigh) Used to Estimate Percent of Body Fat

Find the sum in the left-hand column and the age at the top of the table. Read off the percent fat where the column and the row meet. Example: For a sum of 53–55 mm, a man aged 23 has 15.7 percent body fat.

Sum of Fatfolds (mm)	Age to the Last Year								
	Under 22	23 to 27	28 to 32	33 to 37	38 to 42	43 to 47	48 to 52	53 to 57	Over 58
8–10	1.3	1.8	2.3	2.9	3.4	3.9	4.5	5.0	5.5
11–13	2.2	2.8	3.3	3.9	4.4	4.9	5.5	6.0	6.5
14–16	3.2	3.8	4.3	4.8	5.4	5.9	6.4	7.0	7.5
17–19	4.2	4.7	5.3	5.8	6.3	6.9	7.4	8.0	8.5
20–22	5.1	5.7	6.2	6.8	7.3	7.9	8.4	8.9	9.5
23–25	6.1	6.6	7.2	7.7	8.3	8.8	9.4	9.9	10.5
26–28	7.0	7.6	8.1	8.7	9.2	9.8	10.3	10.9	11.4
29–31	8.0	8.5	9.1	9.6	10.2	10.7	11.3	11.8	12.4
32–34	8.9	9.4	10.0	10.5	11.1	11.6	12.2	12.8	13.3
35–37	9.8	10.4	10.9	11.5	12.0	12.6	13.1	13.7	14.3
38–40	10.7	11.3	11.8	12.4	12.9	13.5	14.1	14.6	15.2
41–43	11.6	12.2	12.7	13.3	13.8	14.4	15.0	15.5	16.1
44–46	12.5	13.1	13.6	14.2	14.7	15.3	15.9	16.4	17.0
47–49	13.4	13.9	14.5	15.1	15.6	16.2	16.8	17.3	17.9
50–52	14.3	14.8	15.4	15.9	16.5	17.1	17.6	18.2	18.8
53–55	15.1	15.7	16.2	16.8	17.4	17.9	18.5	18.1	19.7
56–58	16.0	16.5	17.1	17.7	18.2	18.8	19.4	20.0	20.5
59–61	16.9	17.4	17.9	18.5	19.1	19.7	20.2	20.8	21.4
62–64	17.6	18.2	18.8	19.4	19.9	20.5	21.1	21.7	22.2
65–67	18.5	19.0	19.6	20.2	20.8	21.3	21.9	22.5	23.1
68–70	19.3	19.9	20.4	21.0	21.6	22.2	22.7	23.3	23.9
71–73	20.1	20.7	21.2	21.8	22.4	23.0	23.6	24.1	24.7
74–76	20.9	21.5	22.0	22.6	23.2	23.8	24.4	25.0	25.5
77–79	21.7	22.2	22.8	23.4	24.0	24.6	25.2	25.8	26.3
80–82	22.4	23.0	23.6	24.2	24.8	25.4	25.9	26.5	27.1
83–85	23.2	23.8	24.4	25.0	25.5	26.1	26.7	27.3	27.9
86–88	24.0	24.5	25.1	25.7	26.3	26.9	27.5	28.1	28.7
89–91	24.7	25.3	25.9	25.5	27.1	27.6	28.2	28.8	29.4
92–94	25.4	26.0	26.6	27.2	27.8	28.4	29.0	29.6	30.2
95–97	26.1	16.7	27.3	27.9	28.5	29.1	29.7	30.3	30.9
98–100	26.9	27.4	28.0	28.6	29.2	29.8	30.4	31.0	31.6
101–103	27.5	28.1	28.7	29.3	29.9	30.5	31.1	31.7	32.3
104–106	28.2	28.8	29.4	30.0	30.6	31.2	31.8	32.4	33.0
107–109	28.9	29.5	30.1	30.7	31.3	31.9	32.5	33.1	33.7
110–112	29.6	30.2	30.8	31.4	32.0	32.6	33.2	33.8	34.4
113–115	30.2	30.8	31.4	32.0	32.6	33.2	33.8	34.5	35.1
116–118	30.9	31.5	32.1	32.7	33.3	33.9	34.5	35.1	35.7
119–121	31.5	32.1	32.7	33.3	33.9	34.5	35.1	35.7	36.4
122–124	32.1	32.7	33.3	33.9	34.5	35.1	35.8	36.4	37.0
125–127	32.7	33.3	33.9	34.5	35.1	35.8	36.4	37.0	37.6

TABLE 3-5 • Body Fat Percentage Ratings for Men and Women 18 to 30 Years of Age[a]

Classification	Men	Women
Excessively lean	< 5%	< 10%
Lean	5–12%	10–18%
Normal	13–19%	19–25%
Overfat	20–24%	26–34%
Obese	25% or higher	35% or higher

[a]If you are over 30, you can use these standards, but you can relax them a little. It is probably normal to grow a little fatter as you grow older.

Source: Adapted from E. A. Fox, L. M. Boylan, and L. Johnson, Clinically applicable methods for body fat determination, *Topics in Clinical Nutrition*, October 1987, pp. 1–9; M. L. Pollack, D. H. Schmidt, and A. S. Jackson, Measurement of cardiorespiratory fitness and body composition in the clinical setting, *Comprehensive Therapy*, 6 (1980): 12–27; T. G. Lohman, Body composition methodology in sports medicine, *Physician and Sportsmedicine* 10 (1982): 47–58; M. H. Williams, *Nutritional Aspects of Human Physical and Athletic Performance*, 2d ed. (Springfield, Ill.: Charles C. Thomas, 1985), p. 361.

Flexibility

The flexibility tests in Figure 3–2 are divided into three parts: Upper trunk, lower back and hamstrings, and shoulders. It is impractical to test the flexibility of all movable joints; these tests assess those used most frequently in physical activity. After you complete the tests, compare your results to the standards in Table 3–6.

TABLE 3-6 • Flexibility Ratings

	Men			Test C[a]		Women			Test C[a]	
	R Test A	L	Test B	R up	L up	R Test A	L	Test B	R up	L up
Excellent	33		17	7	7	28		17	8	8
Very good	28		13	6	5	25		14	7	6
Marginal	20		8	5	2	18		9	5	2
Poor	13		4	0	−2	13		4	0	−2
Very poor	11		0	−2	−5	11		0	−2	−1

[a]If you are left-handed, switch L and R in these columns.

Source: Adapted from E. A. Fleischman, *The Structure and Measurement of Physical Fitness* (Englewood Cliffs, N. J.: Prentice-Hall, 1964), pp. 78–79.

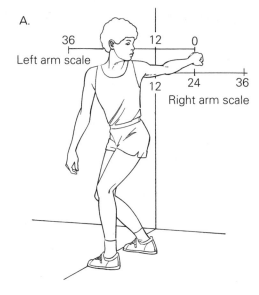

A.

36 12 0
Left arm scale

12 24 36
Right arm scale

A. UPPER TRUNK FLEXIBILITY

Attach two measuring tapes or yardsticks horizontally to the wall at shoulder height as shown. Draw a vertical line that intersects the yardsticks at the 12-inch line, extending this line down the wall and out onto the floor for about 4 feet.

1. Stand with your toes touching the line on the floor. Your right side should face the flexibility scale on the wall.
2. Stand far enough from the wall so that your closed fist can just touch the wall when your right arm is extended horizontally.
3. Extend your left arm to the side at shoulder height with fist closed. Keeping your feet stationary (knees can bend), twist the trunk of your body counter-clockwise and reach as far as possible along the scale.
4. The score is the point touched on the wall scale. Hold for at least two seconds. Table 3-6 (Test A), on p. 50, interprets this score.
5. Repeat in the other direction, left side to the wall, using the right arm and twisting in clockwise direction.

B. FLEXIBILITY OF LOWER BACK AND HAMSTRINGS

Turn a bench or a box on its side so that it forms a platform approximately 12 inches high. Put your feet flat against it, and lay a yardstick on top with the first 6 inches extending toward you.

1. Sit on the floor with your knees together and your feet flat against the bench.
2. Keeping your knees straight, reach forward with your arms fully extended.
3. Measure the distance your fingertips reach (refer to the yardstick fixed on the bench).

C. SHOULDER FLEXIBILITY

1. Stand with your nose, chest, and abdomen against a projecting corner or a vertical pole.
2. Raise your right arm, bend your elbow, and reach down across your back as far as possible.
3. At the same time, extend your left arm down and behind your back and try to reach up and cross your fingers over those of your right hand.
4. Have a partner measure the overlap to the nearest half-inch. If fingers overlap, score as a plus; if they fail to meet, score as a minus; use a zero if your fingertips just touch.
5. Repeat with your arms crossed in the opposite direction.

FIGURE 3-2 How to Measure Flexibility

B.

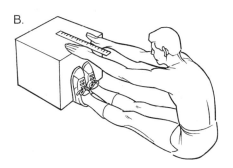

C.

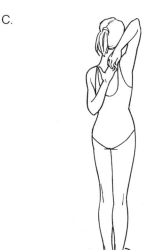

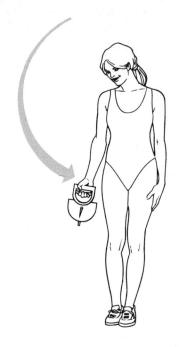

Hold the hand dynamometer in one hand (your dominant hand). The hand dynamometer can be adjusted to fit any hand size. Once you have fitted it to your hand, grip it and raise your arm overhead. As you steadily lower your arm to your side, tighten your grip. The indicator needle will stop at your maximum grip squeeze. Read your score in kilograms and record the best of two trials. Table 3–7 interprets your grip score.

FIGURE 3–3 How to Measure Muscle (Grip) Strength

Muscle Strength and Endurance

An exact strength assessment of the major muscle groups of the body entails considerable time and equipment. For each muscle group tested, the maximum weight that can be lifted one time is determined by trying different weights. A more practical way to measure strength is to test grip strength by way of a hand dynamometer, as shown in Figure 3–3. The hand dynamometer measures the muscular strength of the hand and forearm. This test correlates with tests of general body strength. The best of two measures of grip strength of a person's dominant hand are recorded. Table 3–7 interprets your grip score.

Traditional push-ups and sit-ups can be used to evaluate muscle endurance. Do as many push-ups in a row (untimed) as you can to test upper body muscle endurance and as many sit-ups as you can (in 60 seconds) to test abdominal muscle endurance. Figure 3–4 shows how to

TABLE 3–7 • Grip Strength Ratings (Kilograms)

Males	Strength Rating	Females
62 or above	Excellent	38 or above
56–61	Good	34–37
45–55	Average	25–33
Below 45	Poor	Below 25

Standard push-ups

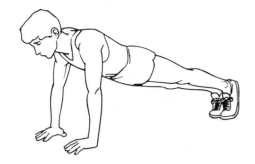

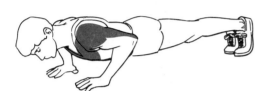

A. Push-ups

Traditionally, push-ups have been done differently by men and women because of the differences in weight distribution between the sexes. People of either sex who have trouble with standard push-ups may do well performing modified push-ups—that is, supporting their weight on their knees and hands instead of on their toes and hands. This exercise will help them build up to doing standard push-ups. Perform either type of push-up as many times in a row as you can; do not time yourself. Place your hands about shoulder width apart, fingers pointing straight ahead. Consult Table 3–8 for ratings.

Sit-ups

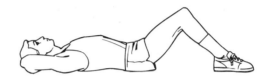

Modified push-ups

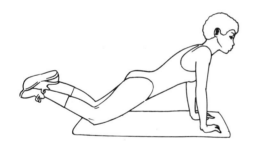

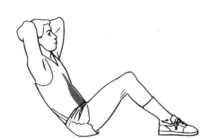

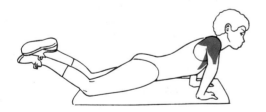

B. Sit-ups

Everyone should do sit-ups the same way—with knees bent, feet flat on the floor (not hooked under a piece of furniture to hold them down), and hands locked behind the head. Do not push your head forward as you come up, however. Keep your neck straight, using your hands only as a support for your head. Raise your upper body only as far as necessary to move your lower back off the floor. Do as many sit-ups as you can in 60 seconds. Consult Table 3–8 for ratings.

FIGURE 3–4 How to Measure Muscle Endurance

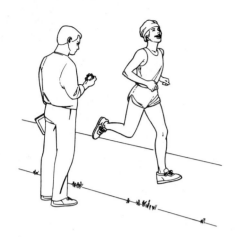

perform these exercises correctly. Your score for sit-ups and push-ups compared with the values provided in Table 3–8 will give you an idea of the general state of your muscle endurance, although laboratory tests are more specific.

Cardiovascular Endurance

Figure 3–5 provides a test of cardiovascular condition. Your score here reflects the ability of your heart and lungs to deliver oxygen to your tissues, as well as your muscles' ability to use fuels aerobically. You can compare your test results with those listed in Table 3–9.

FIGURE 3–5 How to Measure Cardiovascular Endurance *Cooper's Test.* This test requires you to walk, jog, or run as far and as fast as you comfortably can for 12 minutes. You may need to measure out the route using a car's odometer, or you may have access to a measured track. Be sure to use a stopwatch to get an accurate time measurement. Table 3–9 provides ratings for men and women.

TABLE 3-8 • Muscle Endurance Ratings

Standard Push-ups–Number of Repeats[a]

Age	Excellent	Good	Average	Fair	Poor
20s	55 or more	45–54	35–44	20–34	0–19
30s	45 or more	35–44	25–34	15–24	0–14
40s	40 or more	30–39	20–29	12–19	0–11
50s	35 or more	25–34	15–24	8–14	0–7
60+	30 or more	20–29	10–19	5–9	0–4

Modified Push-ups–Number of Repeats[b]

Age	Excellent	Good	Average	Fair	Poor
20s	49 or more	34–48	17–33	6–16	0–5
30s	40 or more	25–39	12–24	4–11	0–3
40s	35 or more	20–34	8–19	3–7	0–2
50s	30 or more	15–29	6–14	2–5	0–1
60+	20 or more	5–19	3–4	1–2	0

Sit-ups–Number of Repeats in 60 seconds[c]

Age	Excellent	Good	Average	Fair	Poor
20s	46 or more	41–45	35–40	31–34	0–30
30s	38 or more	33–37	27–32	23–26	0–22
40s	33 or more	28–32	22–27	18–21	0–17
50s	28 or more	23–27	17–22	13–16	0–12
60+	23 or more	18–22	12–17	8–11	0–7

[a]For men or muscular women.

[b]For women or less muscular men.

[c]Generally, men are assumed to be able to do a few more repetitions than women because they develop stronger muscles. Men and muscular women should add 2 to these numbers; other women and less muscular men should subtract 2.

TABLE 3-9 • **Cardiovascular Endurance Ratings (Distance in Miles Covered in 12 Minutes)**

Fitness Category	13-19	20-29	30-39	40-49	50-59	60+
Very poor						
(men)	1.30 or less	1.22 or less	1.18 or less	1.14 or less	1.03 or less	0.87 or less
(women)	1.0 or less	0.96 or less	0.94 or less	0.88 or less	0.84 or less	0.78 or less
Poor						
(men)	1.30-1.37	1.22-1.31	1.18-1.30	1.14-1.24	1.03-1.16	0.87-1.02
(women)	1.00-1.18	0.96-1.11	0.95-1.05	0.88-0.98	0.84-0.93	0.78-0.86
Fair						
(men)	1.38-1.56	1.32-1.49	1.31-1.45	1.25-1.39	1.17-1.30	1.03-1.20
(women)	1.19-1.29	1.12-1.22	1.06-1.18	0.99-1.11	0.94-1.05	0.87-0.98
Good						
(men)	1.57-1.72	1.50-1.64	1.46-1.56	1.40-1.53	1.31-1.44	1.21-1.32
(women)	1.30-1.43	1.23-1.34	1.19-1.29	1.12-1.24	1.06-1.18	0.99-1.09
Excellent						
(men)	1.73-1.86	1.65-1.76	1.57-1.69	1.54-1.65	1.45-1.58	1.33-1.55
(women)	1.44-1.51	1.35-1.45	1.30-1.39	1.25-1.34	1.19-1.30	1.10-1.18
Superior						
(men)	1.87 or more	1.77 or more	1.70 or more	1.66 or more	1.59 or more	1.56 or more
(women)	1.52 or more	1.46 or more	1.40 or more	1.35 or more	1.31 or more	1.19 or more

Source: Adapted from *The Aerobics Program for Total Well-Being* by Kenneth H. Cooper, M.D., M.P.H. Copyright 1982 by Kenneth H. Cooper. Used by permission of Bantam Books, a division of Bantam, Doubleday, Dell Publishing Group. New York, New York, p. 1502.

A Sample Fitness Program

Now that you know some of the underlying principles of fitness and how to begin and end exercise sessions, you are ready to get down to work with specific exercises. The next few chapters provide details about developing each of the three components of fitness: flexibility, muscle strength and endurance, and cardiovascular endurance.

To develop a lifelong fitness program, tailor it to your own personal abilities and ambitions. As mentioned earlier, your athletic potential or talent is inborn, and if you choose to develop your inborn capacity, you can reach that potential. But health and well-being do not depend on developing to your potential. Remaining active is more important to health than attaining your ultimate potential.

Plan out your program and keep it reasonable. Do not work so hard that you become discouraged within a few days. Some people get so carried away with becoming physically fit that they actually endanger their health instead of improving it.

TABLE 3-10 • **Sample Fitness Program (45 Minutes a Day)**

Monday, Wednesday, Friday:

- 10 minutes of warm-up activity and stretching.
- 25 minutes of aerobic exercise.
- 10 minutes of cool-down activity.

Tuesday, Thursday:

- 10 minutes of warm-up activity and stretching.
- 25 minutes of weight training.
- 10 minutes of cool-down activity.

Saturday or Sunday:

- Softball, walking, hiking, biking, or swimming.

To give you a sense of what your program might look like, Table 3-10 shows a sample fitness program. Whether you spend 2 hours a day or 45 minutes every other day on fitness, you will want to allocate your efforts to the various components according to your goals. One ambitious person, whose goal is overall fitness, allocates 45 minutes a day, as shown in Table 3-10. Someone wanting more cardiovascular fitness might spend more time on aerobic activities; if more muscle strength is the goal, additional or more intense weight work is in order.

How Fit Are You?

To develop better fitness, you need to know how fit you are in the first place. By following the instructions below and recording your answers on this chapter's Lab Report in Appendix A, you will gain an idea of how fit you are, and which of the health-related fitness components you want to work hardest on improving. You need to use the scores and ratings you record on this chapter's Lab Report as the baselines to judge your progress on later Lab Reports. Before you turn this chapter's Lab Report in, copy your scores and ratings into the appropriate places on Lab Reports 4, 5, and 6.

A. Body Composition

Estimate your percent of body fat by following the instructions in Figures 3–1A and 3–1B and record your results on this chapter's Lab Report in Appendix A.

B. Flexibility

1. Follow the instructions in Figure 3–2, Part A, to measure the flexibility of your upper trunk, and record your results on the Lab Report.
2. Follow the instructions in Figure 3–2, Part B, to measure the flexibility of your lower back and hamstrings, and record your results on the Lab Report.
3. Follow the instructions in Figure 3–2, Part C, to measure the flexibility of your shoulders, and record your results on the Lab Report.

C. Muscle Strength

Follow the instructions in Figure 3–3 to measure your grip strength. Record your results on the Lab Report.

D. Muscle Endurance

1. Follow the instructions in Figure 3–4, Part A, to measure the endurance of your upper body muscles, and record your results on the Lab Report.
2. Follow the instructions in Figure 3–4, Part B, to measure the endurance of your abdominal muscles, and record your results on the Lab Report.

E. Cardiovascular Endurance

1. Follow the instructions in Figure 3–5 to measure your cardiovascular endurance, and record your results on the Lab Report.
2. Take your resting pulse rate. (If you don't know how to do this, turn to Figure 6–2 in Chapter 6, p. 117.) Record your result on the Lab Report.

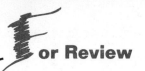

For Review

1. Describe the health-related components of fitness (page 39).
2. Describe the terms *overload* and *use-disuse,* and explain how they relate to physical fitness (page 40, 42).
3. Name and describe two kinds of muscle fibers (page 42).
4. Discuss the importance of warm-up activities before, and cool-down activities after, an exercise session and describe some activities appropriate to each (page 43).
5. Name and describe two ways to measure body composition (page 44).
6. Name and describe three ways to measure flexibility (page 51).
7. Name and describe one way to measure muscle strength (page 52).
8. Name and describe two ways to measure muscle endurance (page 53).
9. Name and describe one way to measure cardiovascular endurance (page 54).

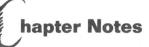

Chapter Notes

1. G. Sheehan, *Tallahassee Democrat,* 1988.
2. M. H. Williams, Human energy, in *Nutritional Aspects of Human Physical and Athletic Performance* (Springfield, Ill.: Charles C. Thomas, 1985), pp. 20–57.
3. C. A. Milesis, M. G. Fougeron, and H. Graham, Effect of active vs. passive recovery on cardiac time components, *Journal of Sports Medicine* 22 (1982): 147–153.
4. E. A. Fox, L. M. Boylan, and L. Johnson, Clinically applicable methods for body fat determination, *Topics in Clinical Nutrition,* October 1987, pp. 1–9.
5. T. G. Lohman, Body composition methodology in sports medicine, *Physician and Sportsmedicine* 10 (1982): 47–48, 51–53, 56–58.
6. Lohman, 1982.

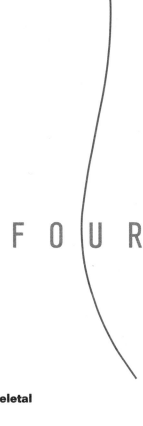

F O U R

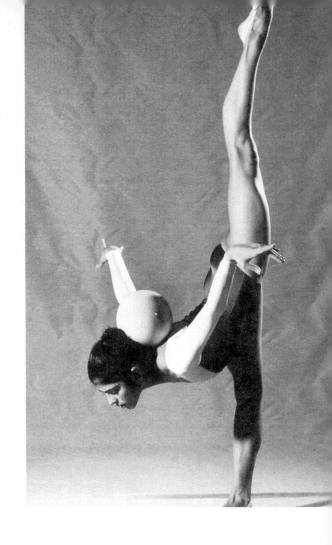

Contents

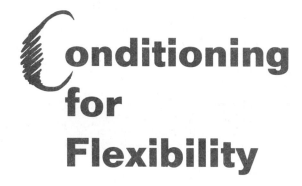

Conditioning for Flexibility

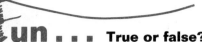
1. Excess body fat reduces flexibility (page 63).

2. If you are flexible in one joint, you are probably flexible all over (page 65).

3. Flexibility can enhance sports performance (page 65).

4. When you sleep, lie flat on your back to give maximum support to the spine (page 66).

5. To get the most out of a stretch, stretch as far as you possibly can, and then bounce to stretch farther (page 68).

6. Using a partner to help you stretch can be dangerous (page 68).

7. People may vary in flexibility at first, but with practice, everyone should be able to bend their joints about the same amount (page 70).

8. Although advances in strength may be somewhat unpredictable, people can make steady progress in gaining flexibility. (page 70).

9. The best way to get ready for a workout is to stretch so that you won't tear your muscles or injure your joints (page 70).

10. If you have limited time for a flexibility workout, stretch each muscle only once, but be sure to stretch them all (page 76).

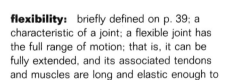

Have you noticed that some people find reaching movements difficult? For some, even tying their shoes can be a challenge. Occasionally, such limited movement results from a disease such as arthritis, but more commonly the cause is failure to maintain **flexibility.** For a person who lacks flexibility, it is uncomfortable even to reach to the ground to retrieve a dropped item. Contrast this person with a dancer of the same age taking a graceful bow after a performance, hands almost brushing the floor. These people represent both ends of the flexibility spectrum. The first person is stiff from years of limited movement. The second person has worked for years to maintain flexibility.

Flexibility and the Skeletal System

Flexibility depends on the condition of the skeletal system: The **joints,** the attached **muscles,** and the **connective tissues**—the **tendons, cartilage,** and **ligaments.** If you try to bend an inflexible joint, the motion is

flexibility: briefly defined on p. 39; a characteristic of a joint; a flexible joint has the full range of motion; that is, it can be fully extended, and its associated tendons and muscles are long and elastic enough to allow mobility.

joints: places where two or more bones meet.

connective tissues: fluid, gelatin-like, fibrous, or strap-like materials that bind, support, or protect other body tissues or organs; the most common tissues of the body.

limited and tissues attached to the joint may tear. In contrast, a flexible joint bends easily without injury. Figure 4–1 shows how body joints are bound together by connective tissue loosely enough to permit movement, yet tightly enough to withstand the stress of even vigorous exercise. Take a look at Figure 4–2, as well; it shows the muscles for later reference. Later figures in this chapter show individual muscles being stretched, and the next two chapters continue to emphasize the use of individual muscles.

cartilage: connective tissue that resembles bone but has no embedded minerals; in joints, cartilage reduces friction and cushions the ends of bones.

ligaments: flexible straps of connective tissue that connect bones to each other and support joints.

muscles: tissues made of many fibers (long, thin cells) that have the ability to contract. The muscles of interest here are the **skeletal muscles**, which move the bones. (Other muscles are the heart muscle and the muscles of internal organs.)

tendons: elastic, flexible straps of connective tissue that anchor the ends of muscles to bones.

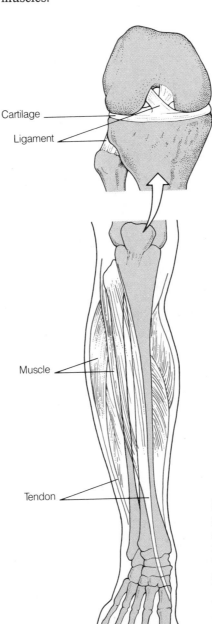

Cartilage
Ligament
Muscle
Tendon

FIGURE 4–1 A Joint and Its Connective Tissue The bones of a joint do not actually touch each other. As a muscle contracts, it pulls the two bones to which it is attached closer together, creating movement. Ligaments strap bones to each other and offer protection and support to joints. Tendons anchor muscles to bones and permit muscles to pull on bones, generating movement. Cartilage cushions the bones of a joint.

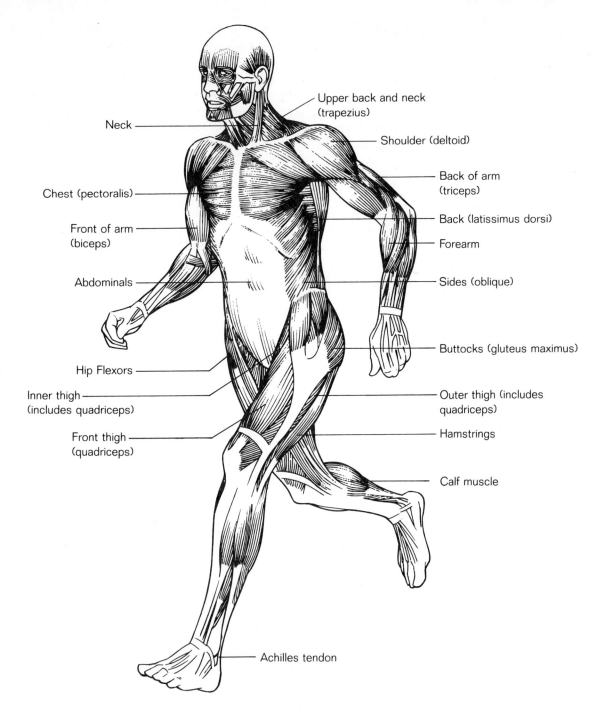

Neck

Chest (pectoralis)

Front of arm
(biceps)

Abdominals

Hip Flexors

Inner thigh
(includes quadriceps)

Front thigh
(quadriceps)

Upper back and neck
(trapezius)

Shoulder (deltoid)

Back of arm
(triceps)

Back (latissimus dorsi)

Forearm

Sides (oblique)

Buttocks (gluteus maximus)

Outer thigh (includes
quadriceps)

Hamstrings

Calf muscle

Achilles tendon

FIGURE 4-2 The Body's Skeletal Muscles

A joint is a place where one bone meets another. Some joints permit no movement (for example, the fused joints between the bony plates of the skull); some permit only a little movement (for example, between the bones of the spine); and others are freely movable (for example, the hip and shoulder joints). Movable joints are of several different types, permitting different ranges of motion (see Figure 4–3). The simplest movable joints are gliding joints in which one bone point glides over another, such as between the ribs and the vertebrae. The elbow is a hinge-like structure; it allows movement in only one direction and allows no movement backward beyond the straight-arm position. The shoulder joint acts like a ball in a socket, allowing movement in almost any direction, even circular movement. The more complicated the movement, the more complicated is the structure of the joint.

The bones of joints do not actually touch each other. They are separated by a cushion of cartilage and strapped together by ligaments, which protect and strengthen the joint and determine its **range of motion.** Cartilage acts as a pad between the bones of a joint, reducing the friction and bearing the brunt of wear and tear. Cartilage is lubricated by a thin, syrup-like fluid that further reduces friction. Ligaments are connective-tissue cords that join two bones and provide strength and support to the joint. For instance, internal ligaments are important stabilizers at the knee joint. Ligaments can be found in the joint cavity, along the outside of the cavity, or in both places. Tendons are bundles of connective tissue that anchor muscles to the bones. They permit the muscles to pull on bones, generating motion; and like ligaments, they also provide support and protection to joints.

Several characteristics determine the range of motion of a joint. The joint structure itself, including the bone structure and the way the connecting tissues are attached to it, determines the direction in which it can bend and limits how far it can bend or straighten. The condition of the muscles and connective tissues—the **elasticity** of the tendons and the length and elasticity of the muscles (cartilage and ligaments are not elastic)—also affect the range of motion. The knee and elbow, for example, cannot bend backward, because the shape of the bones and the connecting tissues do not permit that. A joint that has a maximum range of motion (see Figure 4–4) has unimpaired extensibility of the tissues, maximum elasticity of the tendons and muscles, and unconstricted muscle length. In short, it has flexibility.

Flexibility Factors

Flexibility is influenced by many factors. Certain body types are more flexible; for example, excess body fat limits flexibility by hindering bending. Age is a factor; children are more flexible than adults because tendons lose their elasticity as we age, and muscles shorten because of disuse. Gender is a factor; women tend to be more flexible than men because the hormones that permit women's tissues to stretch during

range of motion: the mobility of a joint; the direction and the extent to which it can bend.

- Cartilage lubricates joints and cushions bones.
- Ligaments connect bones to other bones.
- Tendons connect bones to muscles.

elasticity: the characteristic of being easily stretched or bent and able to return to original size and shape.

1. Excess body fat reduces flexibility.

   True.

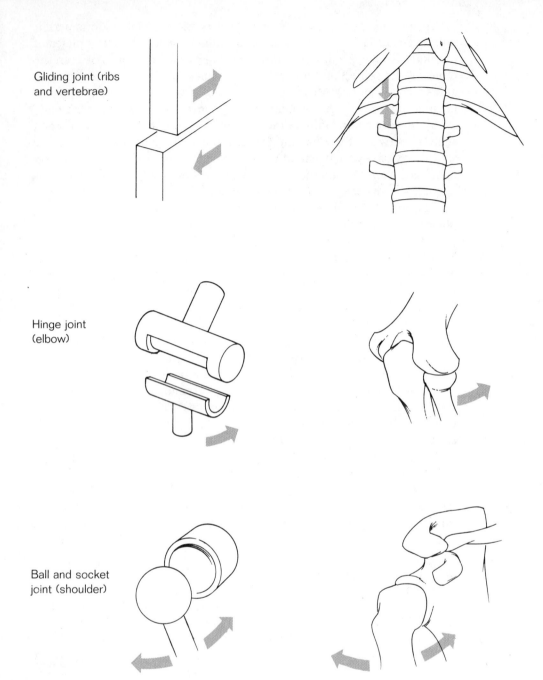

Gliding joint (ribs and vertebrae)

Hinge joint (elbow)

Ball and socket joint (shoulder)

FIGURE 4–3 Movable Joints

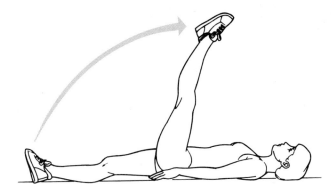

FIGURE 4-4 Range of Motion A joint is flexible when it has its full range of motion.

childbirth facilitate all body stretching. Past injuries can impair flexibility because, once over-stretched, tendons do not regain elasticity. Lifestyle can improve flexibility, and some physical activities enhance it.

Improvement in the flexibility of a joint results from stretching the muscles and tendons associated with that joint. Flexibility in one area of the body, therefore, does not guarantee flexibility in another. Exercises to enhance flexibility of the legs do little for shoulder flexibility.

Most sports demand more flexibility in one area of the body than in others. Swimming, for example, requires flexibility of the arms and shoulders; cycling requires flexibility of the knees and hips. Regardless of how flexible one part of the body may be, other body parts may be stiff. People need flexibility of all body parts to maximize the body's health and resistance to injury. Therefore, a regular whole-body flexibility routine such as the one described later in Figure 4–8 is recommended for everyone. Such a routine enhances the flexibility of muscles and joints that may not be exercised otherwise and that are probably the least flexible.

2. If you are flexible in one joint, you are probably flexible all over.

False.

The flexibility of one joint does not ensure the flexibility of others.

Benefits of Flexibility

Flexibility confers grace and ease of motion on everyone and minimizes the risk of injury when sudden motion is called for. In addition, flexibility enhances sports performance and posture.

Flexibility and Sports Performance

Standards of flexibility have not been established for individual sports, but limited research shows that flexibility enhances the performance of specific activities, such as throwing or sprinting.[1] Conversely, athletic performance enhances flexibility—especially that of the muscles and joints involved in the activity being performed. Each improves the other.

Flexibility stretching can also help relieve muscle soreness after a strenuous workout. During a workout, you tighten your muscles. Nerves send a message to the muscles, telling them to contract. The nerves

3. Flexibility can enhance sports performance.

True.

continue to promote contraction until they get the message that it is time to relax. Nerves should get that message at the end of the workout; otherwise, the nerves will still be directing the muscles to contract the next day, resulting in muscle fatigue and soreness. Failure to stretch at the end of a workout sets the stage for this delayed reaction. The person who prances out of the gym proud of having done 100 squats will feel differently about it the next morning when it is difficult to walk down the porch steps to pick up the morning paper.

Athletes in training who include stretching after strenuous workouts can make progress faster with less discomfort.[2] Short, tight muscles can impair the grace of ice skaters, gymnasts, and dancers and can limit the golfer's stroke, the tennis player's serve, and the batter's swing—the moves that deliver power. Short calf muscles can strain the feet, disabling not only sports performance but all daily activities.

Flexibility and Posture

posture: position and arrangement of the body.

An erect bearing and graceful movement are partly the result of a person's conscious efforts to walk, stand, sit, and lie correctly. Such **posture** is greatly enhanced by two components of fitness: flexibility and strength (the next chapter will show you how strength helps). Stiff joints and weak muscles contribute to improper posture and to the number one medical complaint in the United States: Back pain. Exercises that develop flexibility release tension and lengthen and condition muscles, thereby improving posture and often alleviating back pain. Many cases of lower back pain are due to strained muscles and torn ligaments.[3]

To correct poor posture and alleviate back pain, you first need to learn how to sleep, sit, stand, and walk. Figure 4–5 illustrates correct and incorrect posture positions. Next, you need to practice stretching to avoid straining muscles and spraining ligaments.

Not only in your daily routines, but also in activity sessions, you need to cultivate correct posture. Many references to "proper form" in later chapters will emphasize this point.

4. When sleeping, it is best to lie flat on your back to give maximum support to the spine.

False.

It is best to sleep on your side, to keep from bending the spine unnaturally.

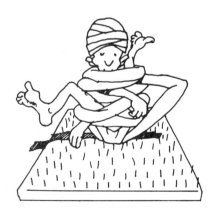

Remember that your goal is to get limber, not to be a contortionist.

Stretching Safely and Effectively

Gains in flexibility can be achieved faster than gains in other components of fitness. When you stretch to gain flexibility, remember that your goal is to get limber, not to be a contortionist. (Observe a cat stretching, and notice the technique—the stretch is long and luxurious, a few moments of pure pleasure.) Choose stretches that are easy to do and stretch only to the point of resistance; that is, until you feel tightness, but not to the point of pain.[4] As you hold a stretch, the feeling of the stretch should become less intense the longer you hold it. If the feeling grows in intensity or becomes painful as you hold the stretch, you are overstretching.

Use smooth motions; do not bounce. Bouncing can overstretch or tear the ligament until it can no longer support its joint, making the joint

FIGURE 4-5 Correct and Incorrect Posture Positions

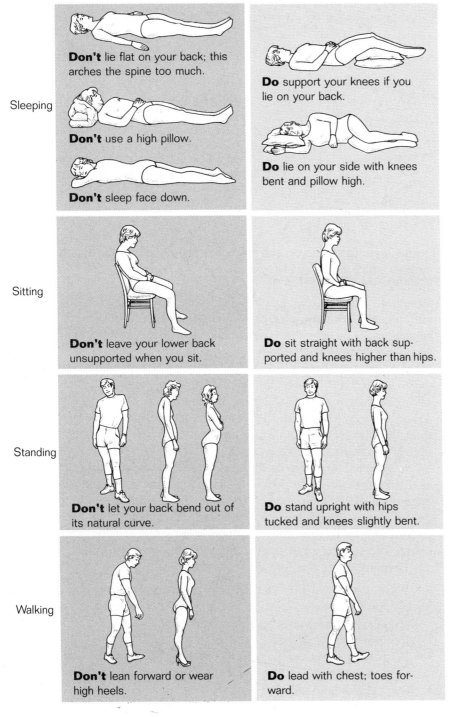

Sleeping

Don't lie flat on your back; this arches the spine too much.

Don't use a high pillow.

Don't sleep face down.

Do support your knees if you lie on your back.

Do lie on your side with knees bent and pillow high.

Sitting

Don't leave your lower back unsupported when you sit.

Do sit straight with back supported and knees higher than hips.

Standing

Don't let your back bend out of its natural curve.

Do stand upright with hips tucked and knees slightly bent.

Walking

Don't lean forward or wear high heels.

Do lead with chest; toes forward.

STRETCHING SAFELY AND EFFECTIVELY   **67**

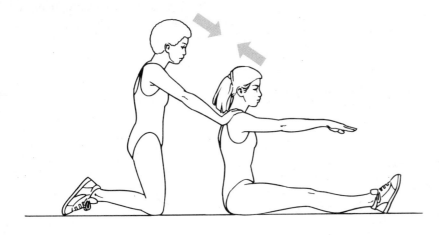

FIGURE 4 – 6 An Example of a PNF Stretch: Dangerous If Not Performed Correctly It is easy to see how an untrained pair could easily incur injury this way. PNF stretches are appropriate only for athletes supervised by professional coaches.

low-force: a recommended stretching technique that lengthens tissues without injury; characterized by long-lasting, painless, pleasurable stretches. Also called **static** stretching.

high-force: a dangerous technique of stretching, characterized by short, choppy, sometimes painful movements, which often pull connective tissues beyond their elastic limits. Also called **ballistic stretching.**

5. To get the most out of a stretch, stretch as far as you possibly can, and then bounce to stretch farther.

   False.

   Stretch only to the point of resistance, not to the point of pain, and do not bounce; bouncing can injure tissues.

6. Using a partner to help you stretch can be dangerous.

   True.

prone to injury. Nerves can overstretch painfully, too, if you are too enthusiastic. Research shows that gentle, long-duration, **low-force** stretches are as effective as, and safer than, short-duration, **high-force** stretches.[5] For the same gains in flexibility, low-force stretching injures and weakens the muscles and joints less than faster, more forceful stretching.[6] The stretches recommended in this text are low-force, not high-force, stretches.

A third stretching technique has a name few people care to learn; we'll call it PNF.* This technique requires a partner and involves alternating contractions and stretching (relaxation), as shown in Figure 4–6. Research suggests that the PNF technique promotes greater flexibility than the stretching techniques just described.[7] However, the inconvenience of needing a partner for PNF stretching, and the potential for harm when partners overdo the stretching, limit the feasibility and safety of this method for most people. Professional athletic trainers frequently employ the PNF technique to improve the flexibility of the joints required for specific athletic activities. Some experts maintain that the PNF technique is dangerous unless both partners know exactly what they are doing. The stretches recommended in this text are not PNF stretches.

Here are other tips for safe workouts:

- Warm up first, gently and lightly stretch muscles you intend to use, do your main workout, and last, do the majority of your stretching. Warm muscles and connective tissues stretch more easily than do cold tissues.
- Progress without comparison to other people; they may be naturally more flexible than you are.
- Start slowly and advance slowly.
- Stretch only to the point of slight discomfort, not pain, even if you stretched farther yesterday; expect to backslide sometimes.
- If you have injured a joint, do not stretch. Seek medical advice.
- Use safe stretches. Avoid those in Figure 4–7.

*The name is proprioceptive neuromuscular facilitation.

FIGURE 4–7 Stretches to Avoid and Recommended Alternatives

NOT RECOMMENDED

RECOMMENDED

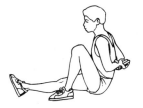

The plough: Dangerous to the back and neck

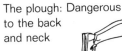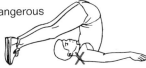

One-leg stretch

Straight-leg toe touch: Stressful to the lower back

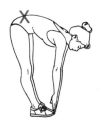

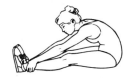

Seated stretch with knees slightly bent

The hurdler's stretch: Dangerous to the knee

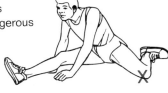

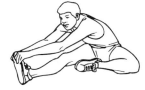

Lateral straddle stretch

Ballistic or high-force kick: Can cause muscle soreness

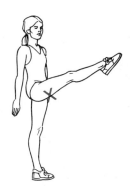

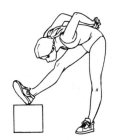

Bent-leg stretch

STRETCHING SAFELY AND EFFECTIVELY

7. People may vary in flexibility at first, but with practice, everyone should be able to stretch their joints about the same amount.

False.

Some people are naturally more flexible than others.

8. Although advances in strength may be somewhat unpredictable, people can make steady progress in gaining flexibility.

False.

Stretching ability varies from day to day and backsliding is not unusual.

9. The best way to get ready for a workout is to stretch so that you won't tear your muscles or injure your joints.

False.

Do not stretch first; warm up first.

You can also take steps to maximize the benefits from your stretching routine by following the recommendations in the Quick Tips.

The Flexibility Routine

This section describes a routine that can improve your overall body flexibility. You can perform it in isolation or as the concluding cool-down routine following a strength workout or a cardiovascular conditioning workout as described in the next chapters. Whatever you do, though, warm up first.

The Warm-up

Muscles and joints stretch more easily when they are warm. The relatively low temperature of the body's tissues before a warm-up period makes the muscles and tendons vulnerable to injury and unable to stretch very far. A warm-up activity increases blood flow to muscles and produces heat that warms the muscles and connective tissues, permitting them to stretch without tearing. Do not stretch first; warm up first.[8] A 5 to 10-minute session of light, gradually progressive exercise, such as brisk walking, light jogging, or cycling, before stretching enables the tissue temperatures to rise, making later stretching safer and more productive.[9] If the environment is cold, it will take longer to warm up enough to start exercising. Another way to warm up is to take a hot shower or bath before stretching. A light sweat indicates that you are ready to work.

Specific warm-ups are appropriate for specific activities. Runners should stretch their calf muscles; swimmers should stretch their shoulders. Each sportsman develops a routine appropriate to the sport. Before

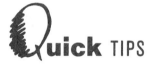
Quick TIPS

Stretching Strategies

For the most effective stretching routine, follow these tips:

- Plan for uninterrupted stretching time.
- Stretch between, not directly after, meals.
- Take the phone off the hook.
- Pretend you're a dancer (unless you are one); enjoy your own grace.
- Play relaxing music or enjoy the silence.
- Wear loose-fitting clothing.
- Breathe deeply and slowly without forcing your breathing; take long, filling breaths that stretch your diaphragm and rib cage.

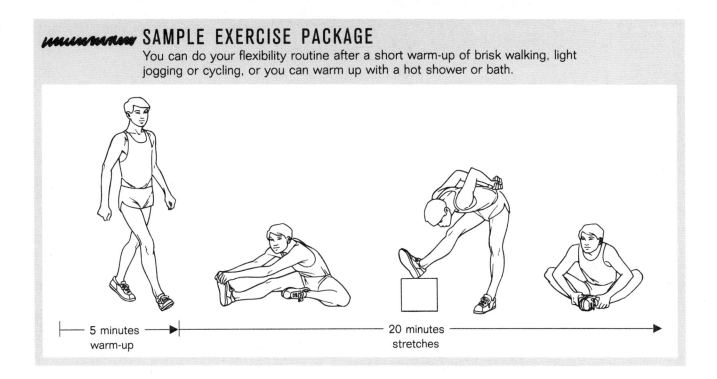

5 minutes
warm-up

20 minutes
stretches

your flexibility routine, warm your whole body for about five minutes in whatever way you choose. Only a few minutes should elapse from the completion of the warm-up to the start of the activity.

Flexibility Exercises (Stretches)

A flexibility training program consists of stretches that work all the major body regions: the neck; the shoulders, elbows, and wrists; all back regions; the pelvic regions; the thighs (inner, front, and back); the calf muscles; and the ankles (see Figure 4-8, A to J). The stretches shown here were chosen for their effectiveness, safety, and ease of instruction, but others serve equally well to stretch the muscles.

Each stretch should be gradual, to fully lengthen the muscles. Relax and allow the body part to move slowly through its full range of motion. Stretch the muscles about 10 percent beyond normal length—to the point of slight discomfort, but not pain. Hold each stretch position for 10 seconds to begin with, and repeat each stretch at least once or twice. Repeat the same stretches on both sides of your body. Remember to breathe normally and, again, resist the urge to bounce. To improve a stretch, add 2 seconds to each time you hold the stretch, until you can hold it for 30 seconds. Gradually, the muscles will lengthen, and the range of motion will increase. Remember that improvements in flexibility will not come overnight, and that rushing the process will only slow you down by damaging muscles and connective tissues.

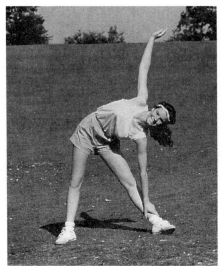

A good stretch is long and luxurious, a few moments of pure pleasure.

FIGURE 4-8 **Flexibility Routine (Long Version)**

A. WHOLE-BODY STRETCH

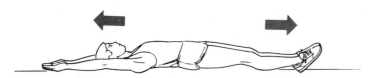

Extend your arms and legs as far as possible, legs together, arms extended past the head, palms facing the ceiling. Hold the stretch for at least 10 seconds, then relax. Repeat three times. When doing this stretch, breathe deeply and slowly. Begin every stretching session with this exercise.

B. NECK STRETCHES*

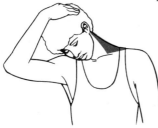

Grasp the back of your head with your right hand, and pull it forward to the right while relaxing your neck muscles. Repeat with the left hand, pulling your head forward to the left.

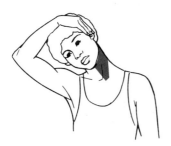

Put your right hand over your left ear, and pull your head to the right while relaxing your neck muscles. Repeat the exercise with your left hand over your right ear and pull your head to the left.

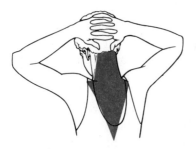

Interlace your fingers behind your head. Push your chin to your chest to stretch the muscles in the back of your neck.

*Note: do not bend your head back; this can compress the spinal bones in your neck and injure the spinal nerves.

FIGURE 4 – 8 – Continued

C. UPPER BODY STRETCHES

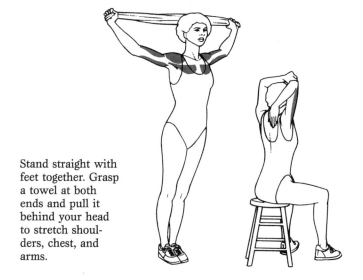

Stand straight with feet together. Grasp a towel at both ends and pull it behind your head to stretch shoulders, chest, and arms.

Sit or stand up straight and place the palm of your right hand behind your neck on the right shoulder blade. Grasp your right elbow with your left hand and pull it toward the back of your head, stretching the tricep muscles of the arm. Relax. Repeat on the same side. Do the same exercise for the left arm.

D. LOWER BACK STRETCHES

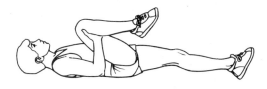
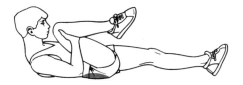

Lie flat on your back and slowly bring one knee up to your chest. Grasp your thigh, not your knee, keeping the other leg, knee slightly bent, on the floor and pull gently. Curl your head up toward your knee. Relax. Repeat with the same leg, then with the other.

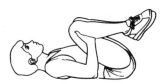
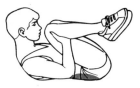

Lie flat on your back and slowly bring both knees up to your chest. Grasp your thighs as shown and curl your head up toward your knees. Relax. Repeat.

FIGURE 4 – 8 — Continued

E. BUTTOCKS STRETCH

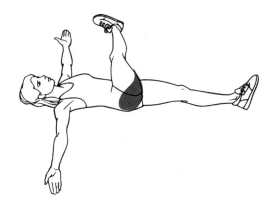

Lie face up on the floor with arms extended out to the sides. Slowly raise your right leg, keeping it straight. Turning only on your hips, and keeping your shoulders and arms on the floor, cross the leg over your body. Your foot need not touch the floor. Do several times for each leg.

F. HAMSTRING STRETCH

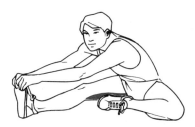

Sit on the floor with one leg extended and the other leg bent at the knee. Keep your back straight and slowly lean forward from the hips (not from the shoulders). Grasp your toes. Be sure to keep the foot of the extended leg upright, not turned to the side, and do not lock your knee.

G. QUADRICEPS AND HIP FLEXORS STRETCH

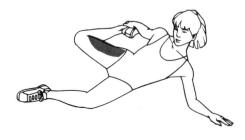

Lie on your left side and grasp your right foot with your right hand as shown, pulling back on your foot until you feel the quadriceps and hip flexors stretch. Relax. Repeat. Then do the other side and repeat.

FIGURE 4 – 8 — Continued

H. INNER THIGH STRETCH

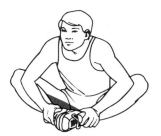

Sit on the floor, bend your knees, and put the soles of your feet together. Grasp your ankles, lean forward from the hips, not from the head and shoulders, looking out in front of you. Gently press down on your shins with your forearms.

I. CALF MUSCLE STRETCH

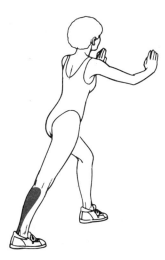

Place the palms of your hands against a wall; bring your left knee forward and extend your right leg behind you. Keep your right leg straight and your heel on the ground. Your feet should be pointed straight ahead, not turned out or in. Feel the stretch in your right calf. Relax. Repeat with the same leg, and then with the other.

FIGURE 4 – 8 — Continued

J. ANKLE AND FOOT STRETCH

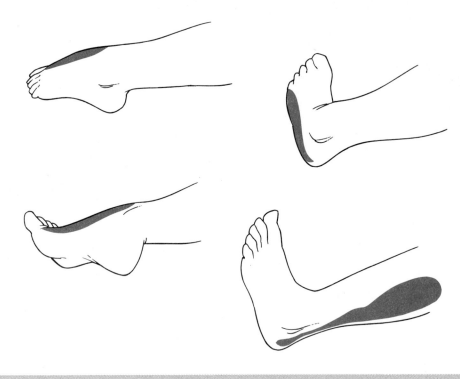

Sit in a chair with one foot off the floor. Begin (*top left*) by extending your toes as far as possible. Feel the stretch along the top of your ankle and foot. Next (*clockwise*) turn your foot in to stretch the muscles along the outside of your foot. Flex your foot, pulling your toes back toward your body and stretching your achilles tendon and calf muscle. Finally, turn your foot out to stretch the muscles along the inside of the foot.

10. If you have limited time for a flexibility workout, stretch each muscle only once but be sure to stretch them all.

False.

If you have limited time for a flexibility workout, concentrate on the muscles that you rely on most.

When you do not have time for a complete flexibility routine, do a few stretches that concentrate on the muscles that you rely on most. This is preferable to hurrying through a complete body routine, or not stretching at all. Moderately active people should concentrate on the hamstrings, quadriceps and hip flexors, calves, and the large trunk and back muscles. This shortened flexibility routine (see Figure 4–9, A to E) stretches the most frequently used muscles; but, for maximum benefit, the whole-body routine is recommended and preferred.

The "Personal Focus" section that follows builds on the baseline flexibility measures that you were instructed to take at the end of Chapter 3. You can go forward from these measures to improve your flexibility as much as you like. At first, in order to make substantial flexibility *progress,* you should stretch four or more days a week. Once you have improved to a personally satisfying point, you can *maintain* flexibility by stretching three days a week. Stretching regularly not only improves flexibility, but is relaxing as well.

FIGURE 4 – 9 **Flexibility Routine (Short Version)**

A. HAMSTRING STRETCH

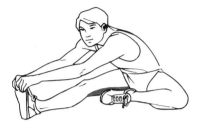

Sit on the floor with one leg extended and the other leg bent at the knee. Keep your back straight and slowly lean forward from the hips (not from the shoulders). Grasp your toes. Be sure to keep the foot of the extended leg upright, not turned to the side, and do not lock your knee.

B. QUADRICEPS AND HIP FLEXORS STRETCH

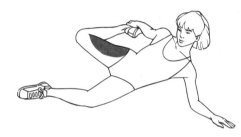

Lie on your left side and grasp your right foot with your right hand as shown, pulling back on your foot until you feel the quadriceps and hip flexors stretch. Relax. Repeat. Then do the other side and repeat.

C. CALF MUSCLE STRETCH

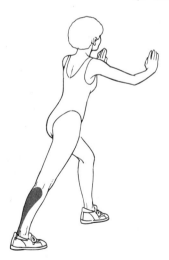

Place the palms of your hands against a wall, bringing your left knee forward and extending your right leg behind you. Keep your right leg straight and your heel on the ground. Your feet should be pointed straight ahead, not turned out or in. Feel the stretch in your right calf. Relax. Repeat with the same leg, and then with the other.

FIGURE 4 – 9 — Continued

D. LOWER BACK STRETCH

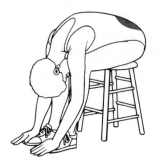

Sit on a chair or stool. Gradually bend your body toward the floor, letting your head drop between your legs and your arms dangle to the floor.

E. UPPER BACK AND SIDE STRETCH

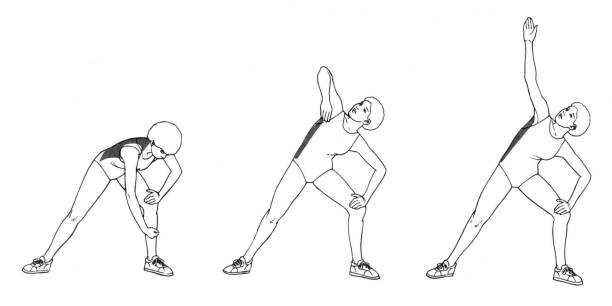

(From left to right) Stand with your legs apart and reach with your right hand toward your left foot. Keep your right leg straight and your left knee bent. Feel the stretch in your back. Then bring your right arm up, starting with your elbow, until your arm is completely extended. Relax. Repeat. Then repeat on the other side.

PERSONAL FOCUS How to Improve Your Flexibility

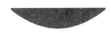

1. You were instructed in Personal Focus 3 to test your flexibility, to record your scores and ratings on Lab Report 3, and to copy those scores and ratings onto Lab Report 4, Part 1. If you haven't already done that, do it now.

2. You will now plan 15 stretching routines for the next month. Plan to stretch about every other day. Decide whether you will do the long routine OR the short one. Perhaps you will want to do the long one when you have time, and the short one when you are pressed for time. In any case, plan the way that you will progress, using part 2 of the lab report. Use pencil so that you can change your mind. Start on day one by doing each stretch once and holding it for 10 seconds. By the 15th time you do your stretches, you will be performing each stretch three times and holding it for 30 seconds. Your instructor may wish to plan your progression or may allow you to plan it for yourself.

3. Now, record the days you actually did these stretches on part 3 of the lab report.

4. At the end of the month, test your flexibility again, following the instructions in Personal Focus 3. Record your scores and ratings on part 4 of the lab report.

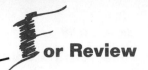

For Review

1. How is flexibility important to health and physical fitness (page 65)?
2. Why is low-force, long-duration stretching preferable to high-force, short-duration stretching (page 68)?
3. What is one disadvantage of the PNF stretching technique (page 68)?
4. Describe some stretches you should avoid (page 69).
5. How far should you stretch your muscles (page 71)?

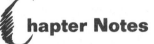

Chapter Notes

1. E. O. Owolabi, Trunk flexibility and vertical jump test scored in different units, and male volleyball ability in Nigerian players, *Scottish Journal of Physical Education* 14 (Spring 1986): 43–48.
2. A. A. Sapega and coauthors, Biophysical factors in range-of-motion exercise, *The Physician and Sportsmedicine* 9 (1981): 57–65.
3. E. Zamula, Back talk: Advice for suffering spines, *FDA Consumer* April 1989, pp. 28–35.
4. B. Anderson, Flexibility, *National Strength and Conditioning Association Journal* August/September 1984, pp. 10–22, 71–73.
5. Anderson, 1984.
6. C. G. Warren, J. F. Lehmann, and J. N. Koblanski, Heat and stretch procedures: An evaluation using rat tail tendon, *Archives of Physical Medicine and Rehabilitation* 57 (1976): 122–126, as cited in Sapega and coauthors, 1981.
7. W. E. Prentice, A comparison of static hip joint flexibility, *Athletic Training* 18 (1983): 56–59.
8. Sapega and coauthors, 1981.
9. Sapega and coauthors, 1981.

FIVE

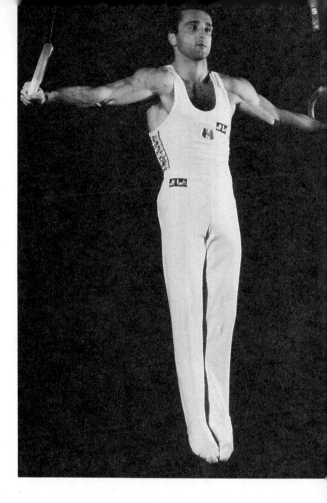

Contents

Conditioning for Strength and Endurance

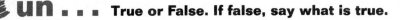
1. A strong person's muscles are large (page 82).

2. White granules seen in a muscle under the microscope indicate a need for medical attention (page 83).

3. If you want strong muscles, you must lift weights (page 84).

4. Strength training is an excellent way to lose body fat (page 84).

5. To gain strength, you must sacrifice some flexibility (page 85).

6. Weak stomach muscles can give you a sore back (page 85).

7. If you want to apply overload when you are strength training, you have to add more weight (page 85).

8. To get strong fast, you should lift weights every day (page 90).

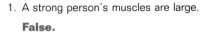

1. A strong person's muscles are large.

   False.

   A person can be strong without having bulging muscles.

tone: the appearance and health of the muscles; not related to contraction but to their condition.

resistance: a force that opposes another; in fitness, the weight or other opposing force against which muscles must work.

When you think of a strong body, do you visualize the huge, bulging muscles of a professional bodybuilder? Certainly, bodybuilders represent an extreme in strength development. For most people, though, a body with enough strength to be fit bears little resemblance to this extreme. It is in the name of competition, not fitness, that a few bodybuilders devote most of their waking hours to intensive training in order to look like they do. Moderate exercise to develop enough muscular strength and endurance to be fit will not make you look overdeveloped. It will, however, **tone** your muscles, giving them a pleasing contour.

Thus, when you embark on a strength-building program, you can expect your appearance to change for the better. Even your fat tissue will appear trimmer as you develop and shape your lean muscle tissue.

Muscle Strength and Endurance Described

Muscle strength is a familiar concept. It is the ability of the muscles to work against **resistance:** To pull weeds from the ground, to push a stalled car, or to open a jar of jam. Many of today's mechanical helpers invented

strength: briefly defined on p. 39; the ability of a muscle to exert force (contract) once against a given resistance.

endurance: briefly defined on p. 39; the ability of a muscle to sustain a contraction for long periods of time or for many repetitions.

Muscle fibers and their fuels were described on p. 42 (Chapter 3).

2. White granules seen in a muscle under the microscope indicate a need for medical attention.

False.

White granules seen in a muscle under the microscope may be fuel stores to support strength work.

to spare our effort rob us of the opportunity to develop strength—for example, the strength that would be gained from chopping firewood instead of turning up a thermostat.

Muscle **strength** is closely related to, but not quite the same as, muscle **endurance.** Muscle strength is the ability of a muscle to exert force (contract) against a given resistance one time. Muscle endurance is the ability of a muscle to sustain a contraction for long periods of time or for many repetitions.

Muscle strength and endurance are a result of structural characteristics inside muscle fibers. Many of these are characteristics of the structures responsible for cellular work.

If you could look through a powerful microscope at a muscle before and after a program designed to build *strength,* you would be able to observe a change in the strength-conferring fast-twitch fibers—you would see an increase in the number of white granules of stored glycogen, which is the fibers' anaerobic fuel. Another change you might observe is the thickening of sheets of contracting proteins responsible for muscle movement.

Suppose you were looking at muscles after a program designed to develop muscle *endurance* instead of strength. You could easily distinguish the microscopic changes from those you had noted with strength. Endurance fibers, the slow-twitch cells, would appear a deeper red because of their increased stocks of oxygen-handling equipment. (Similar equipment also gives blood its red appearance.) Early researchers who first observed that some muscle fibers appeared white and some red did not yet fully grasp the functional implications of the differences, and so they named the fiber types accordingly: red fibers, now known as slow-twitch, and white fibers, now known as fast-twitch.

Most muscles have a mixture of slow- and fast-twitch fibers, but some may contain more of one than another. For example, the muscles that support the weight of the body, those in the back and legs, must maintain their activities for long periods of time—they need endurance conferred by slow-twitch fibers. The muscles of the arm may be called upon to perform short but intense bursts of activity, such as pitching baseballs or lifting heavy weights—they need strength conferred by fast-twitch fibers. Thus, pitchers and weight-lifters rely more on fast-twitch fibers, while long-distance runners call upon slow-twitch fibers to perform.

The percentage of fast- and slow-twitch fibers a person has is genetically determined. Most people have about equal amounts of fast- and slow-twitch fibers, although world-class endurance athletes have larger percentages of slow-twitch fibers.[1] Unfortunately, you cannot change the percentage of fast- and slow-twitch fibers you have; it is set from birth. However, with enough of the right kinds of exercise, you can develop the potential of the fibers you do have. Unless you intend to compete at a high level in a particular athletic event, you do not need to focus your efforts specifically on developing your different kinds of muscle fibers. The necessary changes take place without your conscious effort; you will recognize the process because your work will become easier.

Some of the changes that take place with strength training are visibly apparent, as with the well-developed muscles of people who lift weights. The contractile proteins of the fast-twitch muscle fibers and their associated connective tissues strengthen by thickening their structures and increasing their density. In addition, even the slow-twitch fibers become more like fast-twitch fibers—that is, they develop more of a capacity for anaerobic work, although they never become as good at it as the fast-twitch fibers are.[2]

Up to now, we have been discussing muscle strength and muscle endurance separately, but they tend to develop together and enhance each other. Muscle endurance depends somewhat on muscle strength—a muscle cannot contract repeatedly if it is too weak to contract in the first place. Muscle strength also benefits from muscle endurance, because the more you can repeat a move, the greater the strength you can gain. Many exercises promote both muscle strength and muscle endurance, although, depending on the technique, they can emphasize one more than the other. Two ways to gain muscle strength and endurance are **weight training** and **calisthenics** (weight-free exercising), which are discussed in a later section.

weight training: the use of free weights (dumbbells or barbells) or weight machines to provide resistance for developing muscle strength.

calisthenics: exercises that use a person's body weight to provide resistance for developing muscle strength and endurance.

Benefits of Muscle Strength and Endurance

Muscle strength and endurance confer many advantages on a person. An active daily life, overall good health, satisfactory sports performance, and good posture all attest to their merits.

Daily Challenges

Think of all the times you have had to call upon your body to meet challenges beyond those you expected to encounter in a day. Your car stalled and you had to carry a can of gas for miles along the highway. A friend moved and asked you to help carry boxes. A dresser drawer got stuck and you struggled to pull it open. Everyone can remember times when their strength and endurance were equal to a task, and times when they were not. The rewards of a well-conditioned body are fewer frustrations and more successes in these efforts.

3. If you want strong muscles you must lift weights.

   False.

   Lifting weights is only one way to build strong muscles; calisthenics are another.

Health Benefits

Strength training also promotes the development of lean tissue, which shifts body composition favorably. Strength training does not measurably contribute to loss of body fatness, but it does reduce the likelihood of obesity. It builds lean tissue that requires more energy than fat tissue does. This makes it possible to eat food without gaining weight. If that food is well chosen, the body also receives more nutrients. Overall health improves as a result.

Strong muscles also confer benefits on neighboring body parts. Strong abdominal muscles help hold the digestive organs in place. Strong

4. Strength training is an excellent way to lose body fat.

   False.

   Strength training does not measurably contribute to loss of body fat, but it does build lean tissue.

muscles support and strengthen the bones, creating the stress that bones respond to by building their strength. Strong muscles undergird the joints they support, minimizing the risk of stressing the joints. They surround blood vessels, protecting them from injury, and they perform a special task for the veins, which have no muscles of their own: They squeeze them, helping them return blood to the heart.

Sports Performance Benefits

Strength and endurance training, of course, enhance performance in sports, too. Strong muscles permit sudden bursts of strength needed by such athletes as volleyball players who must jump and spike the ball. Gymnasts rely on strong muscles to facilitate balance and coordination. Muscle endurance also permits muscles to work longer before fatigue sets in. Strength training, properly conducted, even enhances flexibility, for it takes the muscles through their full range of motion, stretching them.

Posture Benefits

Muscle strength and endurance, especially that of the back, abdomen, and legs, facilitate proper posture, a must for a healthy, pain-free back. Weak muscles, especially weak abdominal muscles, cannot support the spine properly. (Yes, that's right: It is weakness of the abdominal muscles, even more than of back muscles, that renders the back vulnerable to pain and injury.) Weak abdominal muscles, together with weak, inflexible back muscles, fail to protect the spine from stress: It can easily be forced to curve abnormally, pinching nerves and causing pain.

Weak abdominal muscles combined with *strong* back muscles can also pose a hazard to the spine. Strong back muscles, especially if they get tight, can pull hard on the spinal bones; if the abdominal muscles that pull the other way are too weak to oppose them, pinching of the nerves is again likely. Thus, when you do your sit-ups, congratulate yourself twice — once for the flat belly you are earning, and once for the comfortable lower back.

Principles of Training for Strength and Endurance

As discussed in Chapter 3, the basis of improving physical fitness is to apply overload. To gain muscle strength and endurance, you can apply overload in four ways: You can work against more and more resistance; you can do more and more repetitions in a **set;** you can increase the number of sets you do; or you can reduce the intervals between sets. The first two types of progression are the basic ones, and your choice of which to do depends on the outcome you seek. The most efficient way to gain *strength* is to increase resistance; for example, a person training with weights progressively increases the weight lifted. The most efficient way to build *endurance* is to increase the number of **repetitions** in a set; for

5. To gain strength, you must sacrifice some flexibility.

   False.

   Strength training, properly conducted, enhances flexibility.

6. Weak stomach muscles can give you a sore back.

   True.

7. If you want to apply overload when you are strength training, you have to add more weight.

   False.

   You can apply overload four different ways when you are strength training.

set: a specific number of repetitions.

repetitions: the number of times an exercise or muscle contraction is consecutively repeated.

example, a person increases the number of times an exercise or muscle contraction is consecutively performed.

Most strength training exercises rely on **isotonic muscle contractions.** Isotonic muscle contractions involve movement; the muscle shortens and lengthens to overcome and control resistance. Lifting weights or doing pull-ups are examples of isotonic muscle contractions. Isotonic contractions strengthen muscles throughout the full range of motion. Other types of contractions are used if a muscle is injured or if special equipment is available.*

Training with Machines and Weights

Training with resistance provided by machines or weights is the most efficient way to develop muscle strength and endurance. Typically, weight training has been portrayed as a man's workout technique, but in reality, it is ideal for both men and women. It need not produce big, bulky muscles; it does so only in people who have the genetic potential to develop such muscles and who follow programs specifically designed to do just that. Nor, as mentioned, will weight training produce muscle-bound inflexibility; that results from improper strength training and omission of flexibility training.

Isotonic training can be conducted in two ways—using machines or free weights to provide the resistance or using the body itself (calisthenics). Machines have a safety advantage over free weights in that the weights are stacked in a frame so that they cannot fall. Among the machines available for weight training are those depicted in Figures 5–1 and 5–2. Among the most commonly used free weights are **dumbbells** and **barbells.**

Rules for Weight Training

Before you begin training, be aware that improper use of weights can be dangerous. Anyone who wishes to include weight training in a fitness program should seek guidance from a trainer with an established reputation for safety and effectiveness. New employees of spas and gyms may be long on enthusiasm but short on knowledge of proper form.

Here are some rules to keep in mind whenever you are doing any kind of weight training:

---

*An alternative kind of strength training involves *isometric muscle contractions.* Isometric contractions occur without movement or muscle shortening. In other words, the resistance is fixed, as when you try to lift or push an immovable object. Isometric strength training is valuable in rehabilitating injured muscles that have been restricted from movement. Another kind of strength training involves *isokinetic muscle contractions.* Isokinetic training, like isotonics, involves movement, but requires special equipment. Unlike isotonic contractions, during which the resistance usually remains fixed, the resistance adjusts to the varying degrees of strength present during isokinetic contractions so that maximum resistance occurs throughout the range of motion.

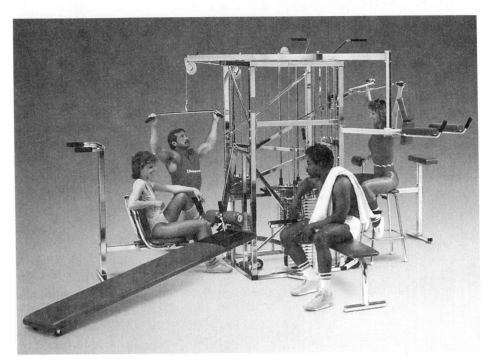

FIGURE 5-1 A Complete Set of Weight Machines This equipment uses adjustable stacked weights to mimic free weight exercises. The user can select the amount of weight that will provide the desired resistance. The equipment in the example shown is Universal Gym Equipment. An advantage of this type of weight training is that the risk of dropping weights is eliminated.

- Never hold your breath when you work with weights or weight machines; it puts pressure on the heart and lungs and can damage them. For most weight training exercises, exhale as you raise or push the weight away (a way to remember is to "blow the weight away from you"), and inhale as you lower it.
- Raise and lower the weight smoothly. Jerking it up or letting gravity pull it down fails to improve strength and threatens to injure your joints.
- Lower the weight extra slowly to develop maximum strength from the smallest number of repetitions.[3] When you have the feeling right, a complete set of ten repetitions of a particular exercise will take about one minute.
- Pay attention to the order in which you do your exercises. Small muscles fatigue quickly and can hinder your continuing the workout, so strengthen the larger muscle groups first, then the smaller ones.

Make sure, too, to distribute the weight work equally over the arms and legs and on both sides of the body—all the muscles. Muscles that work opposite sides of a joint must be of equal strength. Weak muscles on

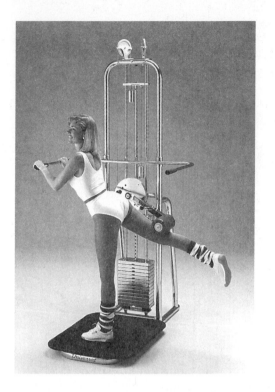
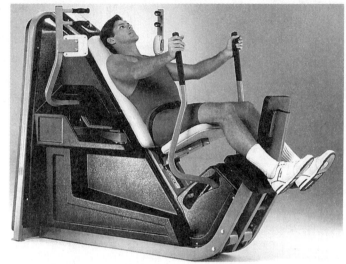
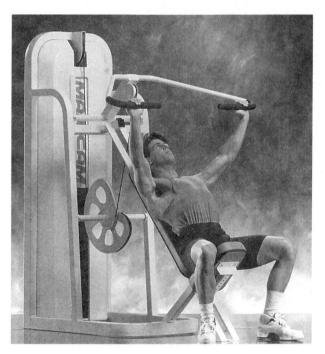
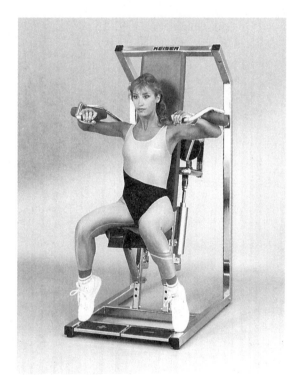

FIGURE 5–2 Examples of Weight Machines Each machine works a specific set of muscles. *Clockwise:* Universal® machine; Nautilus machine; Keiser® compressed air machine (CAM); Muscle Dynamics compressed air machine (CAM) (CAMs have no pulleys, cables, or chains, so they are light, quiet and safe, although expensive).

one side of a joint make the joint prone to injury. If you work your biceps, for example, work the triceps as well; if you work the hamstrings, work the quadriceps too. As is true for flexibility, strength develops only in those muscles actively involved in the work. Overdeveloped muscles in one part of the body can stress other, weaker parts and cause damage.

Getting Started

Each time you learn a new movement, try it first without weights. Just go through the motions for a few repetitions until you feel comfortable with them. Then determine the maximum amount of weight you can move one time. Now decide whether your goal is to increase muscle strength or endurance or a combination of both. Either of the progressions we are about to tell you about will do both, but one emphasizes strength, and the other, muscle endurance.

If your primary goal is to gain muscle *strength,* begin your training by working with 80 percent of the maximum weight you can lift, for four to six repetitions (one set). Perform two to three sets with a rest period of 30 to 90 seconds between sets. Rests longer than two minutes between sets are counterproductive. At the next workout, try to add one repetition per set; at the workout after that, add another, and so on up to 10 repetitions. Once you can do ten repetitions, increase the weight by increments. Then increase the number of sets, up to a maximum of five sets. This may take weeks to achieve.

SAMPLE EXERCISE PACKAGE
Frame your strength routine with a warm-up and stretches.

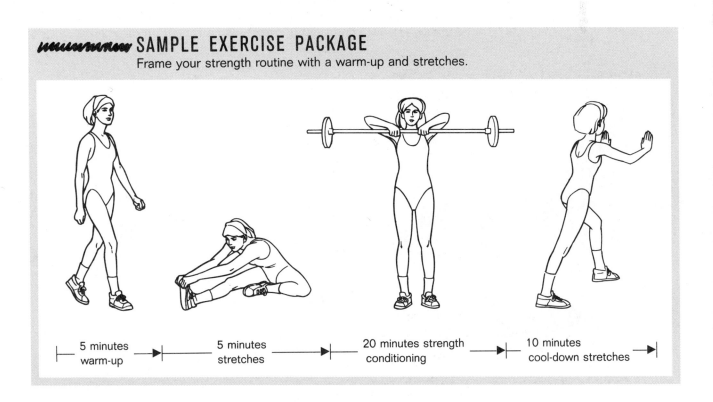

| 5 minutes warm-up | → | 5 minutes stretches | → | 20 minutes strength conditioning | → | 10 minutes cool-down stretches | → |

If your primary goal is to increase muscle *endurance,* work with about 60 to 70 percent of the maximum weight you can lift, completing two to three sets of about 12 repetitions each. In general, if you can do more than 10 repetitions with a weight, you are building more muscle endurance than strength. If you can complete only between 6 and 10 repetitions, you know the weight is sufficient to build both strength and endurance.

Whether your goal is strength, endurance, or both, weight training every other day, or about three to four times a week, seems to produce the best results. Rest is as important as work; muscles use the time between exercise sessions to replenish their fuel supplies and to build themselves up to meet the next challenge, so do not work them every day. Every other day is sufficient for both work and rest. Once you have reached your strength and endurance goal, you can maintain it with just one to two workouts per week.

Training without Weights: Calisthenics

Calisthenics are a series of exercises that develop muscle strength and endurance using gravity to provide the resistance. Familiar examples are sit-ups and pull-ups (try them and you will see that you are lifting weights). Calisthenics were a popular form of exercise long before aerobic dance classes, running, and other fitness activities gained popularity; they are as effective today as ever.[4]

Calisthenics usually include some aerobic activities, such as jumping rope or running in place, but these are done intermittently, so that little, if any, aerobic conditioning occurs. Each repetition of a calisthenic ex-

8. To get strong fast, you should lift weights everyday.

False.

Weight training every other day produces the best results.

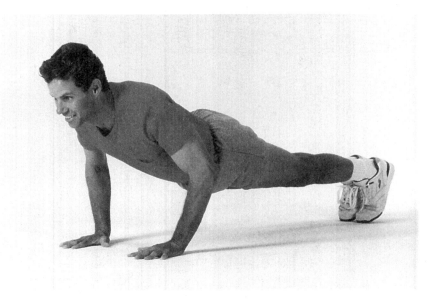

Calisthenics build muscle strength and endurance without the use of weight equipment.

ercise is easy, so improvement results from increasing the number of repetitions and the duration of the workout. Calisthenics are an effective means of increasing muscle endurance and can produce gains in strength, too, although they are less effective than weight training for this purpose. The calisthenic exercises presented here do not include aerobic-type exercises; they are the focus of the next chapter.

Muscle Strength and Endurance Routines

Two routines of training exercises are offered here for developing muscle strength and endurance. The first routine uses free weights or machines (Figure 5–3, A through E). The second routine is a program of calisthenics (Figures 5–4, A through I). You may want to select from both when you design your own conditioning routine. As you proceed, remember that improvements in strength will not happen overnight; go slowly and carefully to prevent injury and minimize muscle soreness. The Quick Tips offer further suggestions.

The exercises recommended here are not the only ones that work the muscles indicated; they were chosen on the basis of their effectiveness, ease of instruction, and safety. If you perform them properly and gradually apply overload as you go along, your muscles will gain in strength and endurance.

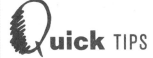

Reminders to Minimize Muscle Soreness

1. Warm up first.
2. Stretch.
3. Work within your capacity.
4. Apply overload within reason.
5. Rest a minute between sets.
6. Stretch each muscle after you have worked it.
7. Rest a day between workouts.

FIGURE 5 – 3 **Training with Weights and Machines**

A. BENCH PRESS

Bench presses work the shoulders, back, upper arms, and chest. Specific muscles that gain strength and endurance include the triceps, deltoids and pectoral muscles. This exercise is done on a bench rather than on the floor to enable your arms to flex below the shoulders. Recommended starting set for strength: 6 repetitions with 80% of the weight you can lift once. Recommended for endurance: 12 repetitions of a lighter weight.

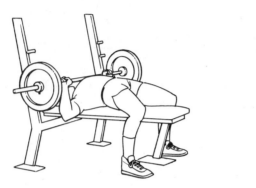 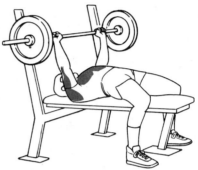

Barbell. Lie flat on the bench with knees bent and feet flat on the floor. Do not arch your back during this exercise. Use a palms-down grip, hands about shoulder width apart. Place the bar at the midline of your chest. Push the bar straight up until your arms are fully extended. Lower the bar to chest position to complete the lift.

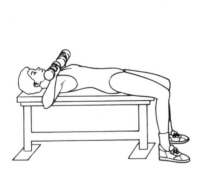 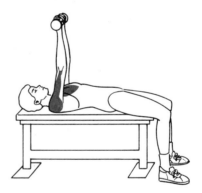

Dumbbells. Lie flat on the bench with knees bent and feet flat on the floor. Use a palms-down grip, hands about shoulder width apart. Place the weights at the midline of your chest. Push the weights until your arms are fully extended. Lower the weights to chest position to complete the lift.

FIGURE 5 – 3 — Continued

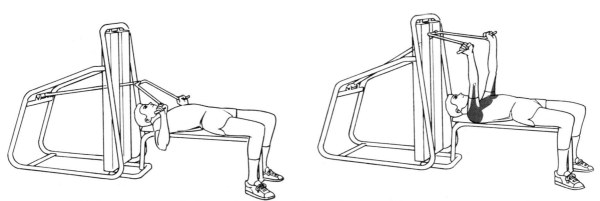

Weight Machine. Lie flat on the bench with your head toward the weights, feet flat on the floor, and the bar above the midline of your chest. Press the bar upward until your arms are completely extended, then return to the starting position.

B. UPRIGHT ROWING

Upright rowing works the shoulders, back, and front of upper arms. Specific muscles that gain strength and endurance include the biceps, deltoids and trapezius. Recommended starting set for strength: 6 repetitions with 80% of the weight you can lift once. Recommended for endurance: 12 repetitions of a lighter weight.

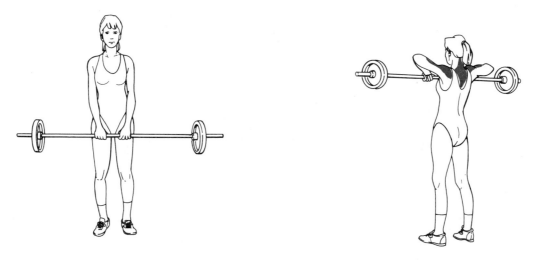

Barbell. From a standing position with feet about shoulder width apart, grasp the bar with your hands about four inches apart, palms down, and allow the bar to touch your thighs. Raise the bar as high as your collarbone, always keeping your elbows higher than the bar. Lower the bar to the starting position to complete one lift.

FIGURE 5 – 3 — Continued

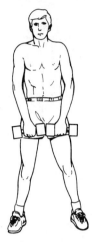 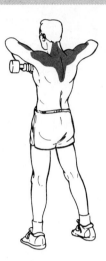

Dumbbells. Stand with your feet shoulder width apart, and hold the weights at thigh level using a palms-down grip. Slowly lift the weights straight up to your collarbone and then lower them to the starting position.

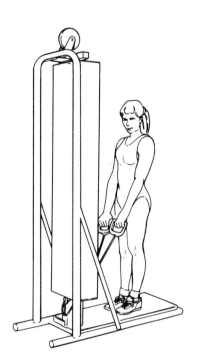 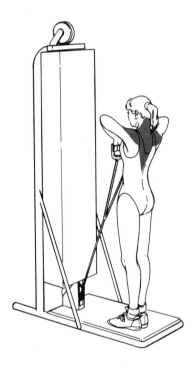

Weight Machine. Stand with your arms extended and grip the handles with your palms down. Pull the handles up to your chin, then return to the starting position.

FIGURE 5 – 3 — Continued

C. BICEPS CURL

The biceps curl works the biceps. Recommended starting set for strength: 6 repetitions with 80% of the weight you can lift once. Recommended for endurance: 12 repetitions of a lighter weight.

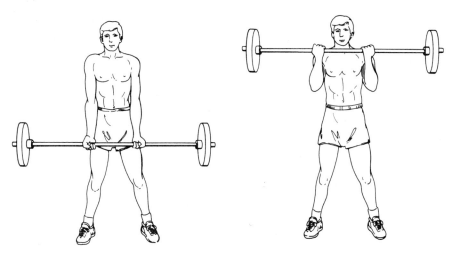

Barbell.   Stand with your shoulders down, back straight, and feet spread shoulder width apart. Extend your arms down, with your elbows close to your sides, holding the barbell with your palms up. Flex your arms and bring the barbell up to your chest without bending forward or arching your back. Keep your upper arms and elbows against your body—the only movement is your elbows bending.

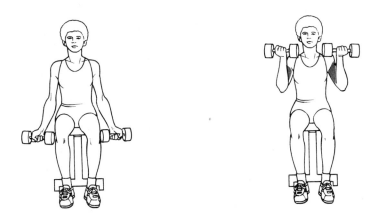

Dumbbell (method 1).   Double biceps curls work both bicep muscles simultaneously. Sit or stand with your shoulders down, back straight, weights held with your palms up, and your arms extended at your sides. Flex your arms and bring the weights all the way up without bending forward or arching your back. Keep your upper arms and elbows against your body—the only movement is your elbows bending.

FIGURE 5-3—Continued

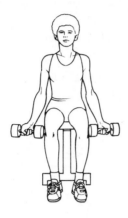 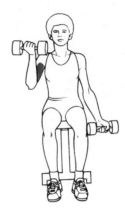

Dumbbell (method 2). Alternating biceps curls work the right and left alternately. Use the same position as in *method 1*. Flex one arm and bring the weight all the way up without bending forward or arching your back; then lower the weight while flexing the other arm. Keep your upper arms and elbows against your body—the only movement is your elbow bending.

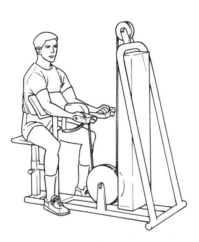 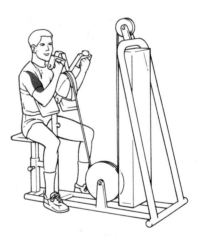

Weight machine. Sit with your back straight and your arms extended in front of you as shown. Use a palms-up grip and curl your arms up as far as you can, then return to the starting position.

FIGURE 5 – 3 — Continued

D. TRICEPS EXTENSION

The triceps extension works the triceps. Recommended starting set for strength: 6 repetitions with 80% of the weight you can lift once. Recommended for endurance: 12 repetitions of a lighter weight. **Note:** Triceps extensions with barbells are not recommended because the best way to do this exercise with free weights is to use one arm at a time.)

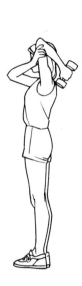 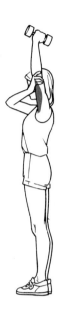

Dumbbell. From a sitting or standing position, grasp the dumbbell in one hand and lower the weight behind your head; extend your arm overhead for one lift. Steady the arm holding the weight by placing your other hand just below the elbow.

FIGURE 5 – 3 — Continued

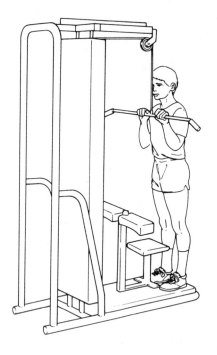 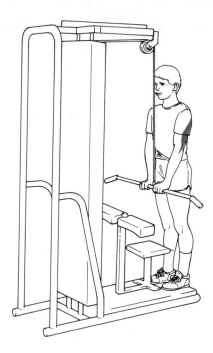

Weight machine.   Grip the bar with your palms down, hands closer together than shoulder width, elbows bent. Completely extend your arms and return to the starting position. Make sure that you keep your elbows and upper arms firmly against your body to ensure maximum use of the triceps during the exercise.

FIGURE 5-3 — Continued

E SQUAT

The squat works the muscles in the legs and back. Specific muscles that gain strength and endurance include the quadriceps, buttocks, hamstrings, and lower back muscles. Recommended starting set for strength: 6 repetitions with 80% of the weight you can lift once. Recommended for endurance: 12 repetitions of a lighter weight. **Note:** Doing the squat using dumbbells is not recommended because you need the stabilizing effect of the bar to maintain control of the weight.

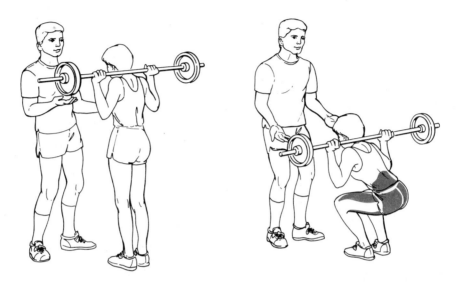

Barbell. Stand erect, head up, and back straight. Place the barbell across your shoulders using the palms-down grip. Your feet should be about shoulder width apart. Squat until your thighs are parallel with the floor. Keep your back flat and your head up. Rise to the starting position to complete the lift. **Note:** A spotter is recommended when doing this exercise.

FIGURE 5-3 — Continued

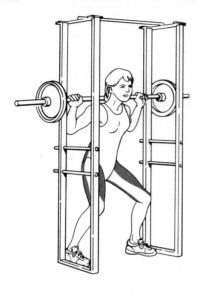

The safest way to do barbell squats is with a squat rack. The pins in the rack are set to prevent you from going too far down, as shown in the drawing.

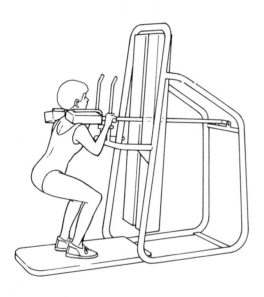 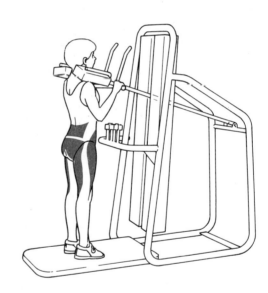

Weight machine. Start with your knees bent and shoulders under the bars. Completely extend your legs (don't lock your knees); then return to the starting position.

FIGURE 5 – 4 Calisthenics

A. STOMACH CRUNCHES

Stomach crunches work the abdominal muscles. They are extremely effective for strengthening abdominal muscles and increasing their endurance if done properly. They are less stressful for the back than sit-ups are. Recommended starting routine: 2 sets of 10 to 20 repetitions.

Method 1

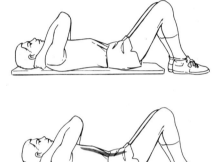

Start from a lying down position, back flat on the floor, knees bent, feet flat on the floor about 18 inches in front of your buttocks (not hooked under anything or held down). Lock your hands behind your head at the base of your skull with the elbows either pointed forward for less exertion (*Method 1*) or spread out (*Method 2*) for more exertion. While you raise your body, do not pull your head forward. Find a spot on the ceiling and focus on it while doing your crunches. Raise your body up, but not too high (about 30 degrees). The bottom of your shoulder blades can still be touching the floor. Then lower yourself back down to starting position.

Method 2

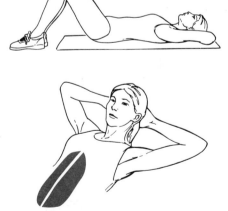

FIGURE 5 – 4 — Continued

B. PUSH-UPS AND MODIFIED PUSH-UPS

Push-ups work the triceps, deltoids, and pectorals. Recommended starting routine: 2 sets of 10 to 20 repetitions.

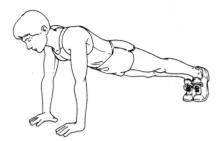 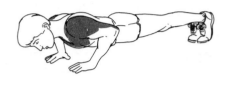

Push-ups.   Start by supporting your weight on your arms (do not lock your elbows). Extend your feet behind you. Keep your body as straight as possible. Flex your elbows and lower yourself to the floor. Then raise yourself back up to the starting position. Do not

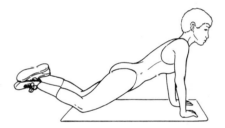 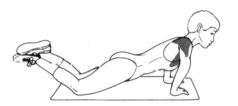

Modified push-ups.   You can work against slightly less resistance if you support your lower body with your knees rather than your feet. Start by supporting your weight on your arms (do not lock your elbows). Keep the trunk of your body as straight as possible. Flex your elbows and lower yourself to the floor. Then raise yourself back up to the starting position. Do not arch your back; keep it flat.

FIGURE 5 – 4 — Continued

C. PULL-UPS AND MODIFIED PULL-UPS

Pull-ups work the biceps, forearm, deltoids, and latissimus dorsi. Recommended starting routine: 3 to 10 repetitions.

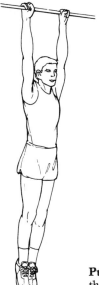 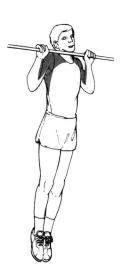

Pull-ups. Suspend yourself from a horizontal bar, using a thumbs-in, palms-down grip. Pull your body up until your chin is above the bar; then lower your body slowly to the starting position.

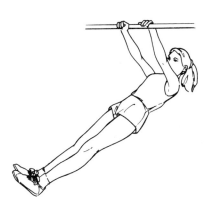 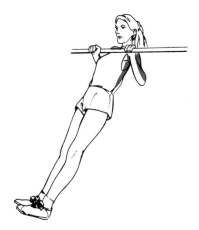

Modified pull-up. You can reduce the resistance by using a lower bar and supporting your lower body with your heels on the floor. Suspend yourself under the bar, resting your heels on the floor. Pull your body up until your chin is above the bar (do not use your legs to help raise yourself). Lower your body slowly to the starting position.

FIGURE 5 – 4 — Continued

D. BACK PUSH-UPS AND MODIFIED BACK PUSH-UPS

Back push-ups work the deltoids and triceps. Recommended starting routine: 3 to 10 repetitions.

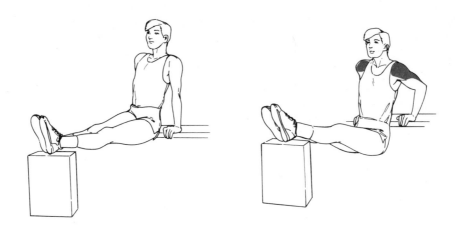

Back push-ups.   Suspend your body in a sitting position with legs straight between two raised supports, feet on one, hands on the other, fingers forward. Lean back on your hands, balancing with your heels. Keep your back straight and shoulders square. Bend your arms and lower yourself without letting your shoulders hunch up. Straighten your arms to push yourself back up.

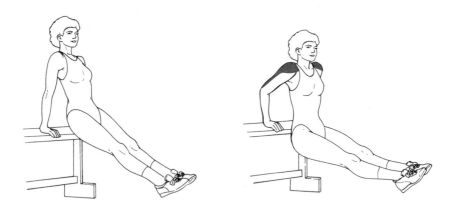

Modified back push-ups.   You can reduce the resistance by resting your heels on the floor. Put a chair, bench, or stool behind you and lean back on your hands, balancing with your heels. Keep your back straight and shoulders down. Bend your arms and lower yourself without letting your shoulders hunch up. Straighten your arms to push yourself back up.

FIGURE 5-4—Continued

E. PELVIC TILT

The pelvic tilt works the buttocks (gluteal muscles). Recommended starting routine: 2 sets of 10 to 20 repetitions.

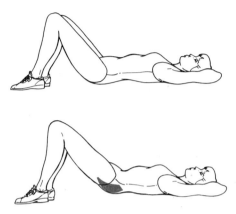

Lie flat on the floor, with your hands under your head, your abdomen in, knees bent, and feet slightly apart and pointed straight ahead. Keep your back on the floor, and gently tilt your hips forward and up, folding at the waistline (try to touch your belly button to your back bone). Contract your buttocks and squeeze them together. Relax. The movement in this exercise is ever so slight, and the back remains firmly on the floor.

F. BENT-LEG LIFT

The bent-leg lift works the outer thigh muscles. Recommended starting routine: 2 sets of 10 to 20 repetitions.

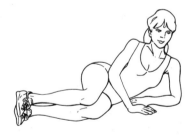 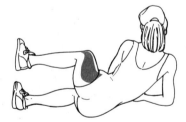

Position yourself on one side of your body, propped up on one elbow as shown, with your other arm in front of your body for support. Lean slightly forward so that you work your leg muscles, not your hip flexors. One leg should be directly on top of the other (stacked), back straight, legs flexed at the knees. Lift the leg on top, still bent, and bring it back down until knees and ankles touch.

FIGURE 5 – 4 — Continued

G. INNER THIGH LIFT

The inner thigh lift works the inner thigh muscles. Recommended starting routine: 2 sets of 10 to 20 repetitions.

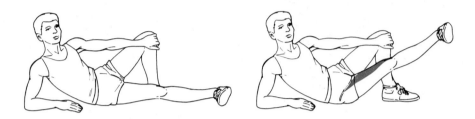

Prop yourself on one hip, leg straight, using your forearm and opposite bent leg to balance you, as shown. Turn your extended leg out and flex the foot, so that the heel faces up and the toe faces down. Raise your extended leg as high as you can without moving your back. Pause, then lower the leg, but do not let it rest on the floor.

FIGURE 5 – 4 — Continued

H. HAMSTRING CURL

The hamstring curl works the hamstring muscles. Caution: Do this exercise in front of a mirror, if possible, so that you can check to make sure you maintain the correct position throughout the exercise. An improper position can strain your lower back. If you feel any discomfort at all, discontinue the exercise. Recommended starting routine is 10 repetitions: 1 set of *Variation 1;* 1 set of *Variation 2.*

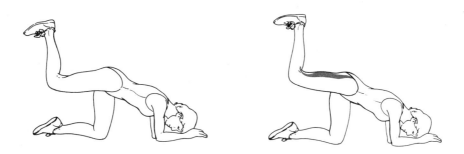

Variation 1. Position yourself on your knees and forearms as shown. Take care to keep your back flat, not arched, head down, and abdomen in. Lift one leg off the floor, knee bent to make a 90 degree angle. Now raise the leg slightly. Repeat with the other leg.

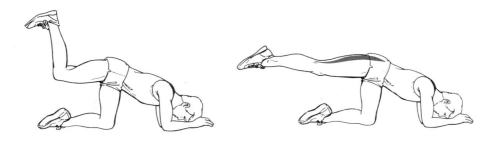

Variation 2. Raise the leg, knee bent as before, and then extend and flex the leg to return to the starting position.

FIGURE 5 – 4 — Continued

I. QUADRICEPS LIFT

The quadriceps lift works the front thigh (quadriceps and hip flexors). This exercise can be done either sitting (*Method 1,* which is more difficult) or lying down (*Method 2,* which is easier). If sitting, make sure you keep your back straight, not hunched forward. If lying down, keep your back flat against the floor. Recommended starting routine: 10 repetitions (1 set of either *Method 1* or *Method 2*).

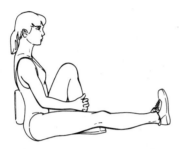 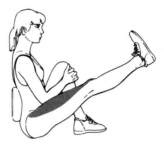

Method 1. Sit up straight against a wall; for extra support, place a pillow behind your lower back. Bend one leg, bring it to your chest, and wrap your arms around it. Extend the other leg out on the floor with the knee just slightly bent. Flex the foot of the extended leg and slowly raise the leg up as high as you can, without going higher than the knee of your other leg. After pausing, lower the extended leg, but do not let your heel touch the floor.

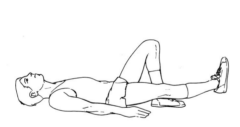 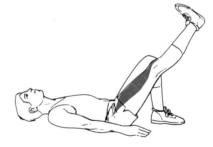

Method 2. Lie down, and make sure your back is flat against the floor. Bend one leg and extend the other on the floor. Flex the foot. Raise the extended leg, but not higher than your other knee. Lower the leg, but do not let your heel touch the floor.

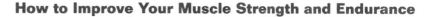

PERSONAL FOCUS

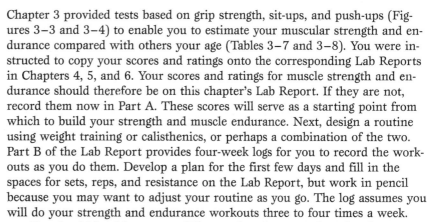

How to Improve Your Muscle Strength and Endurance

Chapter 3 provided tests based on grip strength, sit-ups, and push-ups (Figures 3–3 and 3–4) to enable you to estimate your muscular strength and endurance compared with others your age (Tables 3–7 and 3–8). You were instructed to copy your scores and ratings onto the corresponding Lab Reports in Chapters 4, 5, and 6. Your scores and ratings for muscle strength and endurance should therefore be on this chapter's Lab Report. If they are not, record them now in Part A. These scores will serve as a starting point from which to build your strength and muscle endurance. Next, design a routine using weight training or calisthenics, or perhaps a combination of the two. Part B of the Lab Report provides four-week logs for you to record the workouts as you do them. Develop a plan for the first few days and fill in the spaces for sets, reps, and resistance on the Lab Report, but work in pencil because you may want to adjust your routine as you go. The log assumes you will do your strength and endurance workouts three to four times a week.

You should be able to see a difference in your strength and endurance after about a month. At that time, do the tests in Chapter 3 again, and record your scores and ratings on Part C of this chapter's Lab Report.

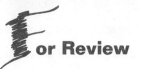

For Review

1. How does muscle strength differ from muscle endurance (page 83)?
2. Describe some of the differences between muscle fibers that develop with strength training and those that develop with muscle endurance training (page 83).
3. Describe some benefits of muscle strength and endurance (page 84).
4. Name and describe two ways to develop muscle strength and endurance (page 84).
5. List four ways to increase overload in muscle strength and endurance training (page 85).
6. Why is it dangerous to hold your breath when lifting weights (page 87)?

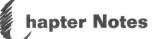

Chapter Notes

1. B. Saltin and P. Gollnick, Skeletal muscle adaptability: Significance for metabolism and performance, in *Handbook of Physiology: Skeletal Muscle,* eds. L. D. Peachey, R. H. Adrian, and S. R. Geiger (Bethesda, Md.: American Physiological Society, 1983), pp. 555–631.
2. Saltin and Gollnick, 1983.
3. K. Hakkinen, M. Alen, and P. V. Komi, Neuromuscular, anaerobic, and aerobic performance characteristics of elite power athletes, *European Journal of Applied Physiology* 53 (1984): 97–105.
4. B. Stamford, What happened to old-fashioned calisthenics?, *Physician and Sports Medicine,* November 1985, p. 149.

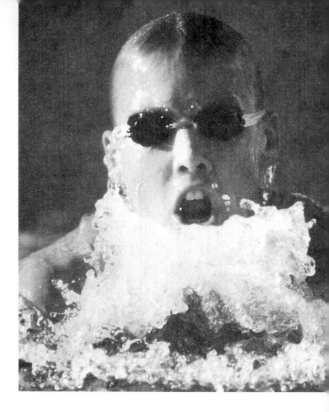

S I X

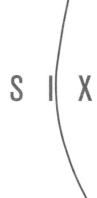

Contents

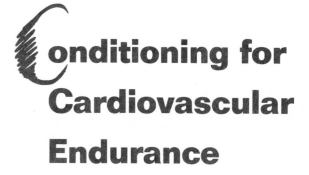

Conditioning for Cardiovascular Endurance

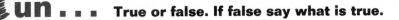

1. A conditioned heart beats faster (page 113).

2. The overload principle does not apply to your heart muscle; you should never overload your heart (page 115).

3. For most people, 30 minutes of vigorous exercise every day is the minimum necessary to gain cardiovascular endurance (page 118).

4. Interval training can improve aerobic condition in professional athletes, but it is not recommended for beginners (page 119).

5. Aerobic training is hard on the knees (page 121).

6. Only a few activities build cardiovascular endurance (page 121).

7. Overexercising can lead to exhaustion, but it is otherwise harmless (page 122).

8. Walking is the most popular form of exercise in the United States (page 123).

9. Using ankle weights when you walk is a safe and effective technique of overloading (page 124).

Chapter 3 introduced the components of fitness and described some basic principles for developing these components. Chapters 4 and 5 offered details about two of them: Flexibility, and muscle strength and endurance. This Chapter's mission is to tell you about a third health-related fitness component, cardiovascular endurance.

Cardiovascular Endurance Described

As you know, the heart beats faster during exercise. How long you can keep exercising with an elevated heart rate—that is, the ability of the heart, lungs, and blood to sustain a given demand—is your **cardiovascular endurance.** With training, you can improve your ability to sustain a vigorous activity such as running, brisk walking, or swimming. Cardiovascular endurance training enhances the ability of the heart, lungs, and blood to deliver oxygen to, and remove waste from, the body's cells.

Working muscles need oxygen to produce energy. Cardiovascular endurance training requires the heart and lungs to work extra hard to deliver oxygen to the muscle cells for a sustained period. Cardiovascular

cardiovascular endurance: a component of fitness; the ability of the cardiovascular system to sustain effort over a long period of time.

endurance training, therefore, is *aerobic* (oxygen-requiring). As the cardiovascular system gradually adapts to the demands of aerobic exercise, the body delivers oxygen more efficiently.

Muscle cells are not alone in their need for oxygen. All of the cells in the body require oxygen to function. When the cells of the body receive more oxygen more readily, both your body and mind benefit.

The changes you gain from aerobic workouts that enhance cardiovascular endurance are called **cardiovascular conditioning.** For example, the total blood volume increases, so the blood can carry more oxygen. The heart becomes larger and stronger, and each beat pumps more blood. As the heart pumps more blood with each beat, fewer beats are necessary, and the pulse rate slows down. The average resting pulse rate for adults is around 70 beats per minute. Thanks to cardiovascular conditioning, active people can have resting pulse rates of 50 or even lower. The muscles that work the lungs become stronger too, so breathing becomes more efficient. Circulation through the body's arteries and veins improves. Blood moves easily, and blood pressure falls. Cardiovascular endurance is the physical achievement that many people appropriately prize the most highly because it reflects the health of the heart and circulatory system, on which all other body systems depend. Figure 6–1 shows the major relationships between the heart, circulatory system, and lungs.

A fringe benefit of aerobic training is its effect on muscles. The more fit a muscle is, the more oxygen it draws from the blood. That oxygen is drawn from the lungs, so the person with more fit muscles extracts from the inhaled air more oxygen than a person with less fit muscles. This improves the efficiency of the cardiovascular system still further, reducing the heart's workload. An added bonus is that muscles that can use more oxygen can burn fat longer—a plus for body composition and weight control. (Chapters 8 and 9 describe these benefits further.)

The Benefits of Cardiovascular Endurance

The previous two chapters included sections that described the benefits conferred by flexibility and muscle strength and endurance. The benefits that accompany cardiovascular endurance greatly enhance the quality of life. Look back to Table 1–3 in Chapter 1. All of the fitness benefits listed there derive directly from cardiovascular endurance training. Some of the benefits, such as sound sleep, increased lean body mass, and improved self-image, can be promoted by way of flexibility or strength training, but cardiovascular endurance training promotes each and every one.

Cardiovascular endurance is, therefore, the single component of fitness most important to health and life. A poorly conditioned cardiovascular system limits a person's performance of daily activities more than a lack of flexibility or muscle strength does. Climbing a flight of stairs should be easy, but for an unfit person, it can be inconveniently difficult. The fit person can leap exuberantly up a flight of stairs, skipping every other step.

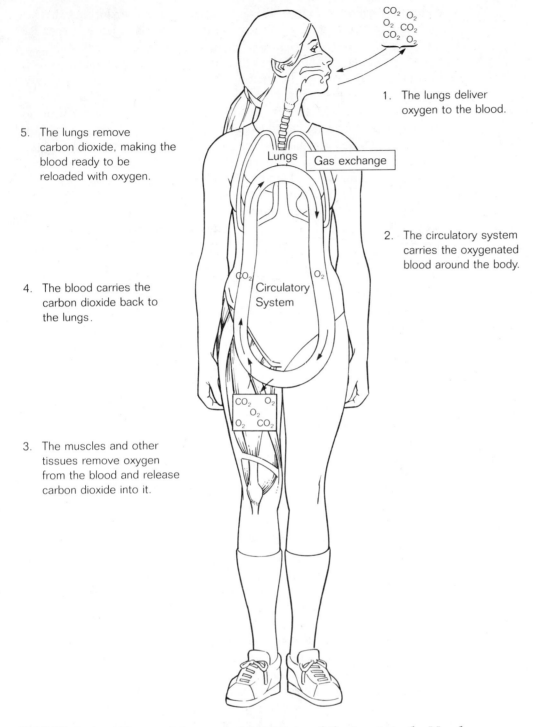

5. The lungs remove carbon dioxide, making the blood ready to be reloaded with oxygen.

1. The lungs deliver oxygen to the blood.

2. The circulatory system carries the oxygenated blood around the body.

4. The blood carries the carbon dioxide back to the lungs.

3. The muscles and other tissues remove oxygen from the blood and release carbon dioxide into it.

FIGURE 6-1 Delivery of Oxygen by the Heart and the Lungs to the Muscles

Principles of Cardiovascular Conditioning

The overload principle applies to the heart muscle in the same way that it does to the other muscles of the body: The heart becomes stronger when the workload increases progressively. You can gradually place more demand upon your cardiovascular system by increasing the intensity, duration, or frequency of your workout. You can adjust any or all of these factors as you choose, depending on your goals and preferences.

Remember as you read the following sections that pacing is important. The caution offered earlier is especially important when the heart is involved. Don't try to progress too fast, for safety's sake; but don't be too lazy or you won't progress at all. Remember, too, to frame your workout with a warm-up and cool-down as depicted in the Sample Exercise Package.

Intensity of Training

The first and most important question you must answer when starting a cardiovascular endurance program is: How hard should I work out? Your age provides part of the answer. Another part of the answer comes from your resting heart rate. To improve your cardiovascular endurance, you must train at an intensity that elevates your heart rate a certain amount beyond its resting level. Your **target heart rate zone** describes the

---

2. The overload principle does not apply to your heart muscle; you should never overload your heart.

False.

The overload principle applies to the heart muscle in the same way that it does to the other muscles of your body.

target heart rate zone: the range of the heartbeat rate that will achieve cardiovascular conditioning for a person—fast enough to push the heart, but not so fast as to strain it.

SAMPLE EXERCISE PACKAGE
Frame your aerobic routine with a warm-up and stretches.

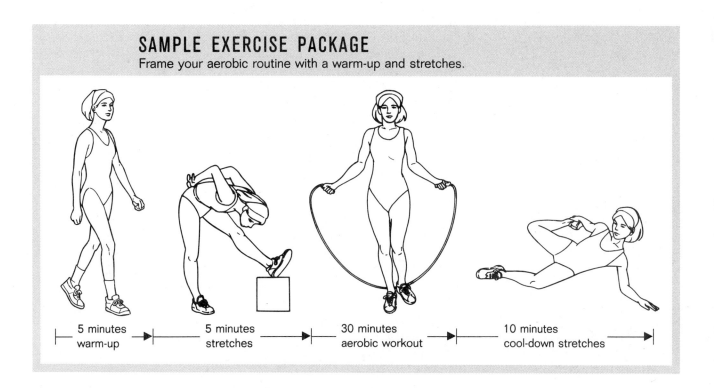

| 5 minutes warm-up | 5 minutes stretches | 30 minutes aerobic workout | 10 minutes cool-down stretches |

boundaries within which you should exercise to achieve and maintain cardiovascular fitness. Exercising below your target zone will not condition the cardiovascular system; exercising above it is dangerous and unnecessary.

You can calculate your target heart rate zone from your age and resting heart rate. The older you are, the lower it will be. Figure 6–2 shows how to take your pulse, and the accompanying box shows how to calculate your target heart rate zone. Figure 6–3 depicts the zone for an example person, aged 25. Another 25-year-old might have a different heart rate zone.

Once you calculate your target heart rate zone, you know how intensely to exercise in order to build cardiovascular fitness. As your cardiovascular fitness improves, you will have to exercise more intensely to reach the same target rate. Be proud; this means you are making progress.

At the same time, keep remembering to be careful. To increase the workload of the heart too fast is counterproductive and potentially dangerous. One group of researchers studied changes in aerobic capacity and skeletal muscle in people during endurance training.[1] When the researchers increased the intensity of the activity arbitrarily, the participants were unable to perform the activity for the expected length of time. When the researchers increased the workload systematically, according to each individual's heart rate, cardiovascular endurance improved.

Admittedly, it is inconvenient to constantly check your pulse, but this need not hinder your exercise program. Once you compute your target heart rate zone and check your pulse a few times while exercising, you will begin to get a "feel" for whether you are exercising in that zone and will need to take your pulse only occasionally as a spot check. As you become more and more conditioned, periodic checking will suffice to tell you when to increase your workload if further conditioning is desired. People with heart disease or hypertension need to monitor their heart rates more carefully and frequently for safety's sake, and competitive athletes may want to do so to maximize the improvement yield of each session.

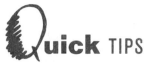

How to Take Your Pulse While Jumping Rope

1. You may not *want* to interrupt your workout to take your pulse. Don't. Take it at the end.
2. Use this rule of thumb: If you can't talk, you're going too fast; slow down. If you can sing, you're not going fast enough; speed up.

‹‹‹‹‹‹‹‹‹ How to Calculate Your Target Heart Rate Zone*

Follow along with David Williams, age 25, as he calculates his target heart rate zone.

1. *Find your resting heart rate (pulse) as described in Figure 6–2.*

   Example: David takes his resting pulse and finds it is 62.

2. *Estimate your maximum heart rate.* Subtract your age from 220 (205 if you are using swimming as your form of aerobic exercise). This provides an estimate of the absolute maximum heart rate possible for a person your age. Never exercise at this rate.

   Example: David's maximum heart rate is 220 − 25 = 195.

3. *Subtract your resting rate (1) from your maximum rate (2).*

   Example: 195 − 62 = 133.

4. *Find 60 percent of this figure.*

   Example: 0.60 × 133 = 80 (rounded off).

5. *Add the resulting number (4) to your resting heart rate (1).*

   Example: 80 + 62 = 142.

This number defines the bottom end of your target heart rate zone. Your heart should beat at least this fast when you work aerobically.

6. *Now repeat steps 4 and 5, but use 85 percent.*

   Example: 0.85 × 133 = 113 (rounded off). 113 + 62 = 175.

This number defines the top end of your target heart rate zone. Your heart should not beat faster than this when you work aerobically.

   Example (conclusion): David's target zone is between 142 and 175 beats per minute.

*All calculations are in beats per minute.

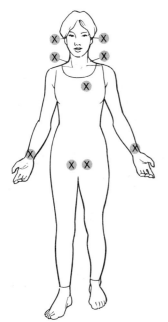

Get a watch or clock with a second hand. Rest a few minutes for a resting pulse. Place your hand over your heart or your finger firmly over an artery in any pulse location that gives a clear rhythm. Start counting your pulse at a convenient second and continue counting for 10 seconds. If a heartbeat occurs exactly on the tenth second, count it as one-half beat. Multiply by 6 to obtain the beats per minute. To ensure a true count:

- Use only fingers, not your thumb, on the pulse point (the thumb has a pulse of its own).
- Press just firmly enough to feel the pulse. Too much pressure can interfere with the pulse rhythm.

FIGURE 6–2 How to Take Your Pulse

PRINCIPLES OF CARDIOVASCULAR CONDITIONING

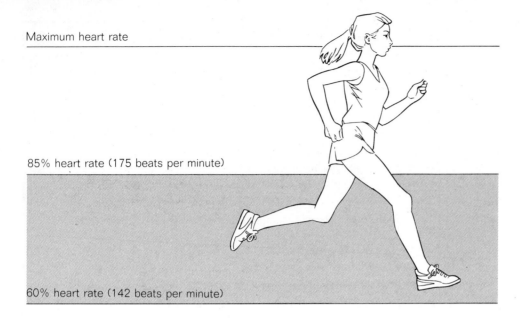

Maximum heart rate

85% heart rate (175 beats per minute)

60% heart rate (142 beats per minute)

▢ Target heart rate

FIGURE 6–3 Target Heart Rate Zone for an Example Person

---

3. For most people, 30 minutes of vigorous exercise every day is the minimum necessary to gain cardiovascular endurance.

False.

To gain cardiovascular endurance, 15 to 60 minutes, three to five days a week is recommended.

interval training: a pattern for aerobic training that alternates periods of intense and less intense activity: each session the person spends longer times in intense activity and shortens the periods of less intense activity.

Duration of Training

When you can work out within your target zone for 20 to 30 minutes, you have reached an important fitness milestone. The American College of Sports Medicine recommends exercising aerobically for 15 to 60 minutes, three to five days a week.[2] (Don't include your warm-up and cool-down in this time.) Within this time frame, the more intense the activity is, the shorter it can be. The less intense it is, the longer it should be. For sedentary people, a slow start is recommended during the first few weeks of conditioning: Aerobic exercise that is low to moderate in intensity (heart rate between 60 and 70 percent of maximum) and of moderate duration (20 to 30 minutes).

In building up cardiovascular condition, a pattern used to make progress is called **interval training.** To use it, a jogger might run at the lower end of the target zone for two minutes before tiring, rest by walking for about the same length of time, run another two minutes, then rest by walking, and so on for 20 minutes. At each session, the jogger should make the running periods longer and the resting periods shorter. Even-

TABLE 6-1 • Example Interval Training Schedule for a Beginning Running Program

Session	Program Run (in minutes)	Walk (in minutes)	Repeat (number of times)	Total Time (minutes)
1*	1	1	5	10
2	1	1	6	12
3	1	1	7	14
4	1	1	8	16
5	1	.5	8	12
6	1	.5	10	15
7	1	.5	12	18
8	1.5	.5	8	16
9	1.5	.5	10	20
10	1.5	.5	12	24
11	2	.5	8	20
12	2	.5	10	25
13	3	.5	6	21
14	4	.5	6	30
15	6	1	4	28
16	8	1	3	27
17	15	1	2	32
18	20 (continuous)			20
19	25			25
20	30			30

*Repeat session 1 every other day (or so) until you feel ready to progress. Do the same with each of the following sessions.

4. Interval training can improve aerobic condition in professional athletes, but it is not recommended for beginners.

False.

Interval training is a good way to begin building up aerobic condition.

tually, in about two months or so, the rest periods will no longer be needed at all. An example of a schedule for a beginner is provided in Table 6–1.

Frequency of Training

If you are just beginning a cardiovascular program, an every-other-day schedule (three or four days a week) stimulates adaptation, minimizes muscle soreness, and promotes conditioning. Once the body has had time to adapt, you can, if you wish, enhance conditioning by exercising more frequently, although three days a week will maintain the level of condition you have reached.

TABLE 6-2 • Schedule of Hydration Before, During and After Exercise

When to Drink	Amount of Fluid
2 hours before exercise	About 3 cups
10 to 15 minutes before exercise	About 2 cups
Every 10 to 20 minutes during exercise	About ½ cup or more
After exercise	Replace each pound of body weight lost with 2 cups fluid

Source: Adapted from J. B. Marcus, ed., *Sports Nutrition* (Chicago: American Dietetic Association, 1986), p. 57.

Comfort and Safety

Two more reminders are needed before you get into an aerobic program. First, make it safe. Many forms of aerobic work involve **high impact.** If your chosen activity includes jumping or running, your body may hit the ground with a force of several times its weight. This can injure body parts. Many people hesitate to spend money on sports equipment, and we endorse frugality, but don't injure yourself for the sake of your purse. If your chosen activity involves high impact, invest in:

- High-quality shoes and absorbent socks.
- High-quality supportive underwear (a running or sports bra, or an athletic supporter). You don't need high-fashion outerwear, but you do need high-tech underwear.

Second, remember to drink water before, during, and after your workout. Even casual exercisers must tend carefully to their fluid needs. Exercise blunts the thirst mechanism. During heavy exercise, thirst is unreliable as an indicator of how much to drink—it signals too late, after fluid stores are depleted. During exercise, don't wait to feel thirsty before drinking. Table 6–2 presents one schedule of hydration for exercise. To find out how much water you need to replenish losses after a workout, weigh yourself before and after—the difference is all water. One pound equals roughly two cups fluid (a quart equals two pounds).

What is the best fluid for an exercising body? Surprisingly, cold water, especially in warm weather, is the optimal beverage for replacing fluids. It rapidly leaves the digestive tract to replenish the tissues and cool the body.

Fitting Aerobic Activity into Your Lifestyle

A wondrous variety of aerobic activities is available. You can run, swim, dance, jump rope, stair climb, row, ski, bicycle—whatever you like. You

high impact: with great force; in exercise, activities that involve jumping, running, or bouncing in which the legs and feet have to absorb several times the body's weight.

can choose one of these and stick with it for years, or engage in all of them at various times, or choose different ones at different times of your life. Whatever you do, hopefully you will engage in some form of aerobic activity every week of your life, all your life. To make this happen, be sure to choose activities that fit your circumstances and preferences.

Elements to Weigh

Enjoying the activity is of utmost importance. If you don't enjoy it, you won't pursue it. Accessibility is important, too. If you have to drive across town in rush-hour traffic to get to your aerobic dance class, you might consider a more convenient activity. Here are a few other considerations:

- Economics. If your budget is limited, an activity such as running or walking that requires a periodic investment in a good pair of shoes is more practical for you than joining a fitness center that requires monthly dues.
- Fitness benefits. Some activities offer more in the way of strength or flexibility development than others do. For example, swimming is not only an excellent cardiovascular exercise, but it also develops overall muscle strength and endurance as well.
- Personal physical condition. Some activities are less likely to cause injury or are less physically stressful than others. For example, cycling or swimming is less likely to aggravate knee or back problems than is running.

From a physiological standpoint, any exercise that provides uninterrupted exertion to work the heart builds cardiovascular endurance. In other words, many different activities accomplish the same end.

Sticking to It

After committing yourself to building your aerobic fitness, the next task is to stick with it. Until you experience the personal health benefits of being aerobically fit, you have only your own determination to drive you to sustain your activity program. Chapter 2 offered general ways to get yourself motivated and to keep yourself going when pursuing fitness. Here are some suggestions to help you keep going, specifically for cardiovascular conditioning.

Begin your program at the level appropriate for you. If you have been sedentary for a while, do not set yourself up for discouragement or injury by exercising too hard, too fast, too soon. Use your target heart rate zone as a guide to your intensity level.

Choose the time of day that is best for you. Some people prefer to exercise first thing in the morning, to feel energized for the rest of the day. Other people find that a workout at lunchtime is just what they need to get them through the afternoon and to prevent them from eating too much lunch. Still other people walk, run, or cycle after a day's work to relieve stress before enjoying the evening's activities.

5. Aerobic training is hard on the knees.

False.

A person can choose aerobic activities that are not hard on the knees.

6. Only a few activities build cardiovascular endurance.

False.

Any exercise that provides uninterrupted exertion to work the heart will build cardiovascular endurance.

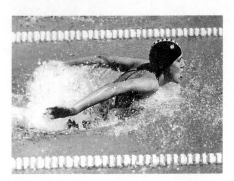

Swimming improves cardiovascular endurance and develops overall muscle strength and endurance as well.

7. Overexercising can lead to exhaustion, but it is otherwise harmless.

False.

Excessive fatigue, injuries, irritability, sleep disturbances, menstrual irregularities, and loss of interest in other activities are all signs of overexercising.

Change your exercise routine from time to time. Walk or run different routes. Alternate intense and moderate workouts. Try cross-country skiing in the winter and swimming in the summer.

Consider exercising with a friend or a group of friends. You will be less inclined to make excuses for not exercising if you have to make them to friends as well as to yourself. The camaraderie of exercising with a friend is added motivation to keep going.

If your chosen activity involves distance, don't let that be your only focus. Set your goals in time. You may not always know when you have covered a certain distance, unless you are in familiar territory; but you can time yourself anywhere.

Keep track of your progress to show where you started and how far you have come. Seeing your own progress will motivate you to keep going.

Emphasize the positive. Instead of saying "I'm too busy to exercise today," say, "I have to budget my time skillfully to plan for exercise today." The more positive thoughts you include, the better your chances of stamping out the negatives. The accompanying Quick Tips sum up these pointers.

When you begin to feel the positive physical and psychological changes that come to people who exercise vigorously on a regular basis, going without exercise can feel as unacceptable to you as going without food or sleep. Be careful about overexercising, however. Excessive fatigue and injuries are signs of overexercising. Irritability, sleep disturbances, menstrual irregularity, and loss of interest in other activities may also indicate that you are overexercising. Be flexible with yourself and with your schedule. Remember, you are exercising for health and enjoyment.

It takes less effort to maintain aerobic fitness than to acquire it, and some of the benefits persist for six weeks or longer during periods of inactivity.[3] The benefits persist longest in long-time exercisers. Runners,

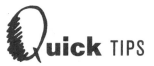

uick TIPS

Sticking to Your Fitness Plan

To help you keep going with your chosen activity:

- Begin your program at the level appropriate for you.
- Choose the time of day that is best for you.
- Change your exercise routine from time to time.
- Consider exercising with a friend or a group of friends.
- If your chosen activity involves distance, don't let that be your only focus.
- Keep track of your progress.
- Emphasize the positive.

cyclists, and swimmers who have worked out regularly and intensely for years and then abstain from all activity still retain some of their conditioning gains after twelve weeks. However, when sedentary people initiate an aerobic training program for eight weeks and then abstain, they lose *all* of their conditioning gains in just eight weeks.[4] A worthwhile goal is to develop a lifetime plan—not just a plan to get fit, but one to stay that way.

Choosing Activities

Some activities that will allow you to reach and sustain your target heart rate are:

Cross-country skiing

Swimming

Fast walking

Marching

Jogging

Bicycling

Ice skating

Stair walking

Rope jumping

Aerobic dancing

Rowing

These sports also help:

Racquetball

Soccer

Hockey

Basketball

Water polo

Lacrosse

Rugby

Once you have decided to commit yourself to regular aerobic activity, how can you be sure that the exercises or sports you have selected will help you meet your goal? First, be sure to choose activities that:

- Are steady and constant.
- Use large muscle groups, such as legs, buttocks, and abdomen. If you move 50 percent of your muscle mass continuously, the activity is aerobic.
- Are uninterrupted and last for more than twenty minutes.

The next sections offer information about some of the most effective and popular aerobic activities. Chapter 11 revisits each of these activities with an emphasis on proper form and injury prevention.

Walking

Walking is the number one form of exercise in the United States and shows little sign of losing favor. Anyone can walk, any time. Walking is especially appropriate for elderly people, pregnant women, and those in need of rehabilitation. More and more people of all ages and all fitness levels are reaping the benefits of walking. Experts classify walking styles as follows:

8. Walking is the most popular form of exercise in the United States.

True.

- Strolling. Leisurely walking at a pace of 1 to 2 miles per hour. Strolling can help you warm up, but it is too slow to build aerobic condition.
- Functional walking or brisk walking. Walking at a pace of 2 to 3.5 miles per hour. Functional walking is the most common style of walking and is a good way to ease into an exercise program.
- Fitness walking or striding. Walking at a pace of 3.5 to 5 miles per hour (or about 1 to 1.25 miles per quarter hour); the legs are thrust forward and the arms swing to exaggerate the effort. Walking this way can raise the pulse and provide aerobic conditioning.
- Race walking. Walking at a pace of 5 to 9 miles per hour using the entire body so that the cardiovascular effort involved resembles that of running.

Walking promotes aerobic conditioning if it is done at a fast enough pace. One study found that 90 percent of the women and 66 percent of the men

9. Using ankle weights when you walk is a safe and effective technique of overloading.

False.

Walking with ankle weights is hard on the back and knees.

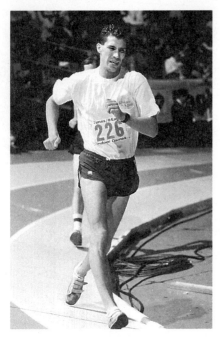

Race walking uses the entire body.

involved in a walking program achieved heart rates in their target zones by walking.[5]

Once you are walking as fast as you want to, you can progressively apply overload by carrying two hand weights (2 to 3 pounds each) and swinging your arms.[6] Don't put weights on your ankles; pulling the extra weight is hard on the back and knees and can injure them. Walking uphill or on rough terrain will also increase the workload of walking.

Walking is the easiest of all exercises to do—everyone knows how to walk—so finding a walking companion is seldom a problem. Walking clubs are popping up all over, and many cities now offer walking tours of special interest areas. People who just begin a walking program are sometimes amazed at the sights, smells, and sounds they can enjoy while walking (in contrast to driving). Walking is easy to incorporate into a busy workday or schoolday by following the Quick Tips suggestions.

Not everyone can, or wants to, walk long routes out-of-doors or in shopping malls. An ingenious piece of equipment makes stationary walking possible: The treadmill. Because it has rails and variable speeds and slopes, this machine can be adapted for use by people with special needs.

The only special equipment you need in order to begin a walking program is the protective garments mentioned earlier—especially, a good pair of comfortable shoes. What's more, injuries from walking are few and far between because it is minimally stressful to the joints. Remember to pay attention to traffic, however.

Because walking is so popular and available to everyone, Appendix B offers a program to guide the person who chooses it as an activity to develop aerobic condition. It starts with the *Rockport Fitness Walking Test,* which evaluates your fitness level based on age, gender, time to walk one mile, and heart rate after walking the mile. Based on your results, the Rockport program then offers walking routines specific to your fitness level.

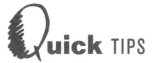

How to Walk When You're Busy

- Park the car a block away and walk.
- Walk an extra lap at the mall.
- Walk to lunch.
- Take the long way to class.
- Take walk breaks instead of coffee breaks.
- Walk with children while babysitting.
- Walk instead of waiting.
- Make talk-and-walk dates instead of talk-and-sit dates.

Aerobic Dancing

For those who enjoy dancing, aerobic dancing is a challenging and vigorous way to improve cardiovascular endurance. Aerobic dance classes combine dancing, calisthenics, rhythmic movement, and stretching against a background of music and camaraderie. Aerobic dancing provides a total body workout. For those who prefer aerobics in the comfort of their homes, an abundance of aerobic dance videocassettes are available. Guidelines for injury prevention in aerobic dance programs are available from the American College of Sports Medicine and are presented in Chapter 11.

As with walking, the only special equipment required for aerobic dance is suitable garments. Again, a good pair of shoes is critical. As the popularity of aerobic dance has grown, so has the number of injuries, especially injuries to the feet and legs. Shoes designed specifically for aerobic dance are superior to any other kind of athletic shoe for this kind of exercise. Floors that absorb some of the shock of impact are superior to those that do not. Wood floors with an air cushion underneath are the best (most good dance studios have these). Concrete floors are the worst. You can improve the cushioning effect of any floor you dance on by covering it with a thick rubber mat.

low-impact aerobic dance: a form of aerobic dance in which one foot is on the ground at all times.

Unless otherwise labeled, an aerobic dance class is likely to be a high-impact class. An alternative is **low-impact aerobic dance,** in which one foot always remains in contact with the floor. People concerned about injuring themselves while doing traditional aerobic dance find low-impact aerobics to be more accommodating. For some people, though, low-impact aerobic dance may not raise the heart rate to the target zone. A study that compared the energy expenditures and heart rates of women performing different aerobic dance routines found that both energy expenditure and heart rate were significantly lower during the low-impact routines.[7] However, other researchers compared high-impact and low-impact aerobic dance and found that the key to achieving equal cardiovascular benefits is proper performance. Specifically, the researchers recommended using what they called "multidirectional, full-body movements."[8] These movements are based on three principles:

- Move around the room as much as possible, using sliding and stepping motions and change direction (multidirectional) frequently. This is a point against overcrowded, confining classes that prevent you from moving freely.
- Use your large muscle groups. Emphasize movement of your legs, back, and hips—bend far, lift your legs high, and take long strides (full-body movements).
- Keep in control of your movements—avoid fast, jerky movements that are likely to lead to injury.

Other research supports the advice to use your large muscle groups. Researchers found that low-impact aerobic dancers who emphasized leg

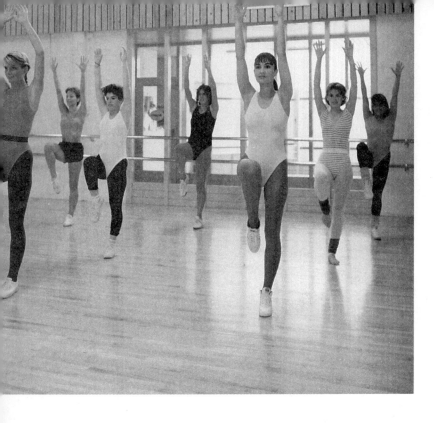

Aerobic dance is a challenging and vigorous way to gain cardiovascular endurance.

movements used similar amounts of energy and oxygen regardless of whether they moved their arms vigorously, moderately, or not at all.[9] If cardiovascular endurance is your goal and you choose low-impact aerobic dancing, check frequently to be sure you are working in your target heart rate zone.

If you choose aerobic dance, be sure to choose a safe routine. Include warm-up and cool-down exercises. Don't use ankle weights. Use proper form; choose an instructor with an established reputation for safe and effective classes, or a tried and true video workout. Instructor credentials you can trust are listed in Chapter 11. Performed safely, aerobic dance can give you years of enjoyment and fun.

Running

For some people, running is a passion; for all runners, it is a fast and effective way to build cardiovascular endurance, improve body composition, and burn energy. The challenge, simplicity, freedom, and mental and physical well-being that come with running make it the activity of choice for many people.

As for walking and aerobic dance, you need a good pair of shoes for running. The shoes are critical, however, since you hit the ground with a force of about two to three times your body weight hundreds of times per mile while running. Improper or ill-fitting shoes can greatly increase your chance of injury or discomfort. Running shoes are designed to stabilize your foot and provide a cushion against the tremendous impact of each stride. Chapter 11 tells you what to look for in a good running shoe.

Running injuries result from pushing too hard, too fast. (Chapter 11 describes preventive measures.) When you begin a running program, use interval training and start slow and easy. Increase your total running time each week by no more than 10 percent. Thus, if you are running ten minutes a day, four days a week, make it eleven minutes each day the next week.

Enjoy your time running. If you run alone, use this private time to think about the day ahead of or behind you, or simply to daydream and let your mind wander. (If you are a woman running alone, be sure to read the rape prevention cautions in Chapter 11.) One of the joys of running (and walking) is the beauty you can experience being outdoors and going practically anywhere your feet can take you. Running is an excellent way to discover new things about your neighborhood. By varying your route, listening to music, letting your mind wander, or inviting a friend to join you, you can keep your interest and motivation high.

For people who cannot run out-of-doors, some comparable activities are available—indoor tracks, trampolines, or jumping rope. Once you get into the rhythm of it, you can gain many of the same benefits.

Swimming

Swimming is one of the most effective conditioning exercises and is not hard to learn, even for adults. The buoyancy of the water reduces the stress on joints, ligaments, and tendons. For this reason, swimming is excellent for those who would be hurt by weight-bearing exercise—that is, people who are injured, have arthritis, are pregnant, or are overweight. Unlike running, swimming strengthens the upper body.

Public pools, available all over the United States, make swimming a reasonable exercise option. Many people find the convenience of their own private pool to be a motivation to exercise. Of course, pools are not the only place to swim; swimming in lakes or the ocean adds variety to a swimming program. You can even swim in a ten-foot-long lane, thanks to some ingenious devices available in some fitness centers; they either push water past you so that you can swim in place or harness you so that you can push the water yourself. Chapter 11 provides water safety tips.

Research shows that the heart beats slower when you swim than when you engage in other endurance exercises, perhaps because the water supports the body's weight.[10] Body temperature remains more stable during swimming than when exercising on land, so the circulatory system does not have to work as hard to regulate temperature. Swimmers should subtract their age from 205, rather than 220, when calculating their target zone for swimming.

Swimming ranks high as an activity to develop cardiovascular endurance and upper body muscle strength and endurance, but it may rank lower in its capacity to promote weight loss. Researchers found that swimming, walking, and cycling all produced cardiovascular gains in moderately overweight women.[11] When they looked at weight loss, however, the walkers and the cyclists lost weight (10 to 12 percent), while the swimmers gained weight (3 percent). The walkers and the cyclists reduced their percentages of body fat; the swimmers maintained their body fat and gained lean tissue. The researchers speculate that swimmers need body fat to maintain buoyancy in the water, to tolerate the cold, and to store energy for distance swimming. (The wisdom of the body is astounding.)

Keep in mind, though, that one study does not prove that swimming is a less effective exercise than land activities for fat loss. More research is needed before any firm conclusions can be drawn. However, if your main goal in exercising is to lose weight in the form of body fat, then you might prefer an activity other than swimming. If your goal is to develop cardiovascular endurance and upper body muscles and to have fun along the way, then swimming may be the perfect activity for you.

Cycling

Cycling, like walking and running, offers an opportunity to explore the outdoors while improving cardiovascular endurance. Even more than by walking and running, you can go places by cycling. The bicycle was originally developed as a mode of transportation, and you can see substantial sections of the country from a bicycle. And especially today, it has the added advantage over cars of being pollution-free. Cycling is an activity for people of all ages. Even families with small children can cycle together, thanks to the convenience of child-carrier seats that attach to bicycles. (Children should always wear helmets when riding in these seats.)

Cycling is equal to running in its cardiovascular conditioning effect.[12] An added benefit of cycling is that it is easier on the bones and joints because the feet do not repeatedly strike the ground as in running.

As with any exercise, so it is with biking: If you want to gain cardiovascular endurance, you have to cycle vigorously enough to reach your target heart rate zone. If you are just beginning a cycling program, ride on smooth terrain and pedal at a rate of about 55 to 60 revolutions per minute (rpm). Some bikes come equipped with a tachometer (the same kind found on indoor cycling machines) that tells you your rpm. To calculate it, count your pedal turns for 10 seconds and multiply by 6. Most people need to cycle twice as fast (in miles per hour) as they run to achieve cardiovascular conditioning. As you become more conditioned, try hilly terrain, or increase your rpm to between 70 and 80, but make sure you are still within your target zone. Cycling in a hilly or mountainous area may be too stressful for someone just beginning.

Cycling is not without some disadvantages. The initial investment in cycling gear is considerably higher than for walking, aerobic dancing, running, or swimming. The cost of a good 10- or 12-speed bicycle and a

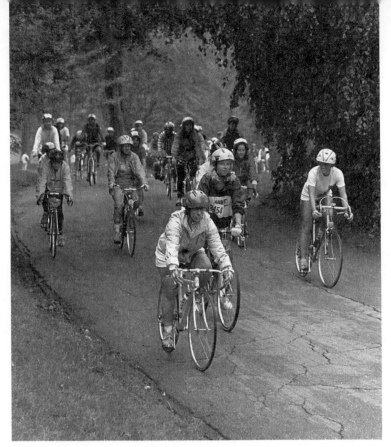

Cycling offers an opportunity to explore the outdoors while improving cardiovascular endurance.

hard-shell cycling helmet is substantial. Traffic is the cyclist's greatest hazard; cyclists should choose routes for traffic safety; a bike path is preferable. Automobile drivers can easily fail to see people on bicycles, and bicycles can be difficult to maneuver in an emergency. Before you get on your bicycle, turn to Chapter 11 and take the measures it recommends to prevent accidents and injuries.

Some people prefer to do their cycling indoors. Stationary bicycles offer an alternative to outdoor cycling, and they can promote cardiovascular endurance equally well. People can cycle while reading, watching TV, listening to their favorite music, or talking on the phone. For many people, the advantage of being able to do something else while exercising tips the scale in favor of this choice over others.

The activities just described are but a few of the many that people can enjoy while gaining cardiovascular endurance. Don't limit yourself to these; use your imagination—the choices are almost endless. Ski. Go kayaking. Jump rope. Roller skate. Go folk dancing. Have fun.

PERSONAL FOCUS 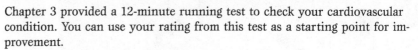   How to Improve Your Cardiovascular Endurance

Chapter 3 provided a 12-minute running test to check your cardiovascular condition. You can use your rating from this test as a starting point for improvement.

1. Choose an activity. It should consist of at least 20 minutes of aerobic work in your target heart rate zone, and you should engage in it at least three to four times a week. Describe and log your activity on the Lab Report.
2. Each month, for as many months as possible, retake the Cooper's test and record your results on the Lab Report.
3. Also take your resting pulse each month. When you take your resting pulse, it is important to take it at the same time of day each time. Record your resting pulse measures on the Lab Report. As you gain cardiovascular condition, your pulse should slow down.
4. Before you turn in the Lab Report, record any comments you want to make. Do you feel better? Do you see any improvement in your body condition? Do you sleep better? Do you have more energy? Do you have higher self-esteem? (Do not confine yourself to these impressions; convey your own experience.)

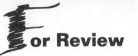

or Review

1. List some of the changes in the body that cardiovascular conditioning brings on (page 113).
2. Explain what the target heart rate zone is and how it relates to cardiovascular endurance training. Calculate your target heart rate zone (page 115–117).
3. How frequently should you exercise to develop cardiovascular endurance if you are just beginning? How should you progress (page 118)?
4. List some ways you use to keep going on your exercise program (page 122).
5. List some things to consider when deciding what kind of cardiovascular endurance exercise to pursue (page 121).

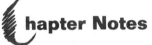

hapter Notes

1. H. Hoppeler and coauthors, Endurance training in humans: Aerobic capacity and structure of skeletal muscle, *Journal of Applied Physiology* 59 (1985): 320–327.
2. American College of Sports Medicine, Principles of Exercise Prescription, in *Guidelines for Exercise Testing and Prescription* (Philadelphia, Pa.: Lea and Febiger, 1986), pp. 31–52.
3. C. E. Thompson and coauthors, Response of HDL cholesterol, apoprotein A-1, and LCAT to exercise withdrawal, *Athersclerosis* 54 (1985): 65–73.
4. What is the detraining effect? *Berkeley Wellness Letter,* December 1988, p. 8.
5. J. Porcari and coauthors, Is fast walking an adequate aerobic training stimulus? (abstract), *Medicine and Science in Sports and Exercise,* April (supplement) 1986, p. 81.
6. J. M. Rippe and coauthors, Walking for fitness, *Physician and Sportsmedicine,* October 1986, pp. 145–159.
7. H. N. Williford and coauthors, Is low-impact aerobic dance an effective cardiovascular workout? *Physician and Sportsmedicine* 17 (1989): 95–109.
8. O. Anderson, The lowdown on low-impact aerobics, *Women's Sports and Fitness,* December 1988, pp. 26–29.
9. Anderson, 1988.
10. R. G. McMurray and coauthors, Exercise hemodynamics in water and on land in patients with coronary artery disease, *Journal of Cardiopulmonary Rehabilitation* 8 (1988): 69–75.
11. G. Gwinup, Weight loss without dietary restriction: Efficacy of different forms of aerobic exercise, *American Journal of Sports Medicine* 15 (1987): 275–279.
12. Gwinup, 1987; L. H. E. H. Snoeckx and coauthors, Cardiac dimensions in athletes in relation to variations in their training program, *European Journal of Applied Physiology* 52 (1983): 20–28.

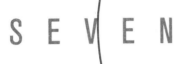

S E V E N

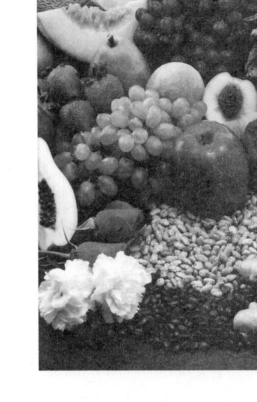

Contents

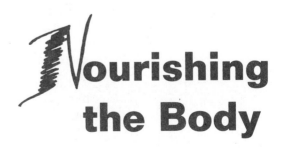

Nourishing the Body

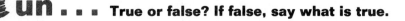

JUST FOR

un ∎ ∎ ∎ **True or false? If false, say what is true.**

1. You can rely on your appetite to tell you when you are hungry (page 136).

2. Too much protein can make you fat (page 138).

3. It is virtually impossible to eat a diet too high in fiber (page 140).

4. Honey and sugar are more similar than different (page 142).

5. Of all the things in foods that cause diseases, sugar is probably the biggest culprit (page 143).

6. Once the body has assembled its proteins into body structures, it never lets go of them (page 144).

7. Women need to be more concerned about iron than do men (page 150).

8. As far as nutrients are concerned, the more, the better (page 152).

9. Fast foods can be nutritious (page 157).

You choose to eat a meal about 1,000 times a year. Eating is so habitual that people hardly give it any thought, yet it is a voluntary activity. You can choose when to eat, what to eat, and how much to eat— 70,000 times in a lifetime. While each day's intakes of nutrients may have only tiny effects on body organs and their functions, repeated over years and decades, they accumulate to have major impacts. You may recall from Chapter 1 that your lifestyle choices can add years to, or subtract them from, your physiological age. Nutrition is one of the most influential of these lifestyle choices. By age 65, or even earlier, the nutrition choices you have made will have affected your physiological age by 15 to 30 years.[1] Sound nutrition throughout life does not ensure good health and long life, but careful attention to your day-to-day intakes of food and beverages can certainly help to weigh things in their favor.

Benefits of Nutrition

The list of diseases that are at least partially responsive to diet continues to grow as researchers delve deeper into the role of nutrition in disease prevention. The following relationships are known:

- *Infectious diseases.* Nutrients support the immune system, and deficiencies undermine it.
- *Obesity.* Overeating, as well as underactivity, helps to cause it.
- *Cardiovascular disease, including both atherosclerosis (hardening of the arteries) and high blood pressure.* Sound nutrition supports a healthy cardiovascular system, and poor nutrition hastens cardiovascular disease.
- *Diabetes.* Obesity predisposes people to diabetes; diet is important in diabetes management; and diabetes increases the risk of cardiovascular disease.
- *Ulcer and stress-related disease.* Adequate nutrition helps to protect against the effects of stress.
- *Cancer.* Many links with nutrition are known, especially for its prevention.
- *Adult bone loss.* Nutrition contributes to both its prevention and its management.
- *Dental caries.* Foods can supply the materials that enable oral bacteria to grow and cause caries.[2]

Because nutrition affects disease risks so profoundly, it warrants careful attention throughout life. Table 7–1 summarizes the U.S. government's recommendations to its citizens; most nations have similar sets of recommendations.

To manage your nutrition in your own best interest, you have to learn how to eat, because not all foods you can choose from today supply the nutrients needed for health. Some people, especially those with low incomes, suffer from **undernutrition.** Some pregnant women suffer nutrient deficiencies that retard their infants' growth. Among migratory workers and certain rural populations, more than 1 in every 10 children suffers stunted growth caused by a poor diet.[3] Iron deficiencies affect one to five percent of people severely enough to cause the deficiency symptom of anemia. Many more are affected in subtly damaging ways.

At the same time, **overnutrition** also threatens people's health. About 30 percent of men and 40 percent of women are overweight.[4] People's average daily intakes of salt are too high for the health of their hearts. People are choosing to eat foods high in fat, cholesterol, and sugar, and high incidences of several degenerative diseases are attributed to these habits.[5]

undernutrition: underconsumption of food energy or nutrients severe enough to cause disease or increased susceptibility to disease; a form of malnutrition.

overnutrition: overconsumption of food energy or nutrients sufficient to cause disease or susceptibility to disease; a form of malnutrition.

hunger: the physiological need to eat; a negative, unpleasant sensation.

Food Choices

Because your accumulated choices profoundly influence your health, it is worth questioning why you eat when you do, why you choose the foods you do—and, most important, whether they supply the nutrients you need.

To the question of what prompts you to eat, you may reply that it is **hunger.** That is often true, but hunger, the physiological need for food,

TABLE 7-1 • Dietary Recommendations to the Public

Reduce total *fat* intake to 30 percent or less of calories. Reduce saturated fatty acid intake to less than 10 percent of calories and the intake of cholesterol to less than 300 milligrams daily.	Reduce the intake of fat and cholesterol by substituting fish, poultry without skin, lean meats, and low-fat or nonfat dairy products for fatty meats and whole-milk products; by choosing more vegetables, fruits, cereals, and legumes; and by limiting fats, oils, egg yolks, and fried and other fatty foods.
Increase intake of starches and other *complex carbohydrates*.	Every day eat five or more servings of a combination of vegetables and fruits, especially green and yellow vegetables and citrus fruits and six or more daily servings of a combination of breads, cereals, and legumes. The committee does not recommend increasing the intake of added sugars because their consumption is strongly associated with dental caries.
Maintain *protein* intake at moderate levels.	Meet at least the Recommended Dietary Allowances (RDA) for protein; do not exceed twice the RDA.
Balance food intake and physical activity to maintain appropriate *body weight*.	
For those who drink *alcoholic beverages,* the committee recommends limiting consumption to the equivalent of less than 1 ounce of pure alcohol in a single day. Pregnant women should avoid alcoholic beverages.	The committee does not recommend alcohol consumption. One ounce of pure alcohol is the equivalent of two cans of beer, two small glasses of wine, or two average cocktails.
Limit total daily intake of *salt* (sodium chloride) to 6 grams or less.	Limit the use of salt in cooking and avoid adding it to food at the table. Salty, highly processed salty, salt-preserved, and salt-pickled foods should be consumed sparingly.

Source: Adapted from the National Academy of Sciences report, *Diet and Health: Implications for Reducing Chronic Disease Risk* which was produced by the Committee on Diet and Health of the Food and Nutrition Board of the National Research Council and partially reprinted verbatim in *Nutrition Reviews* 47 (1989): 142–149.

---

appetite: the psychological desire to eat, that normally accompanies hunger; by itself a pleasant sensation.

1. You can rely on your appetite to tell you when you are hungry.

   False.

   You may have an appetite when you are not hungry.

is not the only stimulus that triggers eating behavior. Another cue is **appetite**, the psychological desire for food, which may arise in response to the sight, smell, or thought of food even when you do not need to eat. You may have an appetite when you are not hungry—or the reverse. Hunger, appetite, obesity, and underweight are the subjects of Chapter 8.

As for the question of why you choose the particular foods you do, several answers come to mind:

- Personal preference (you like them).
- Habit or tradition (they are familiar; you always eat them).
- Social pressure (they are offered; you feel you can't refuse).
- Availability (they are there and ready to eat).
- Convenience (you are too rushed to prepare anything else).
- Economy (you can afford them).
- Nutritional value (you think they are good for you).

Of these seven reasons to choose foods, only one involves making a choice that puts health first. Yet the foods you eat profoundly influence how you feel right now, today, and also how well you withstand the onslaught of the years.

The Makeup of Foods

Food supplies **nutrients, fiber,** and other materials. The nutrients consist of six classes (see the accompanying box entitled *Nutrient Terms*): **Carbohydrate, fat, protein, vitamins, minerals,** and **water.**

Three classes of nutrients provide **energy** the body can use: Carbohydrate, lipid, and protein. Carbohydrate supplies the body with one of its two major fuels, the sugar **glucose.** The brain and nervous system can normally use only this fuel as their energy source. Lipid supplies the body's other major fuel, **fatty acids.** The muscles, including the heart muscle, rely heavily on this fuel. Protein is the major structural and working material of cells, but it, too, is broken down for energy to some extent. In adverse conditions such as undernutrition or severe stress, body protein may become a major fuel.

The energy from these nutrients is used by the body to do work or generate heat. The units of measure of energy are **calories** (or **kilojoules**), familiar to everyone as a reflection of how "fattening" a food is. (Indeed, both protein and carbohydrate—as well as fat—if taken in excess of need, are converted to body fat and stored, so the calorie count of

nutrients: substances obtained from food and used in the body to promote growth, maintenance, and repair. The *essential nutrients* are those the body cannot make for itself in sufficient quantity to meet physiological need, and which, therefore, must be obtained from food.

fiber: indigestible carbohydrates and other compounds in food that provide bulk in the digestive tract.

energy: the capacity to do work or produce heat.

glucose: one of the body's two major fuels; derived from carbohydrate.

fatty acids: simple forms of fat that supply fuel for most of the body's cells.

calories or **kilojoules:** units used to measure energy; determined from the heat food releases when burned. Calories reflect the extent to which a food's energy can be stored in body fat.

Energy-yielding nutrients:

> Carbohydrate—provides energy as glucose.
>
> Lipid—provides energy as fatty acids.
>
> Protein—provides working cell parts, but can be transformed into glucose or fatty acids under some conditions.

〰〰〰〰〰〰 Nutrient Terms

carbohydrate: nutrients, most of which yield energy the human body can use. The *complex carbohydrates* include starch (energy-yielding) and some fibers (primarily not energy-yielding); the *simple carbohydrates* are the sugars.

fat (technically, **lipid**): nutrients that include the energy-yielding fats and oils as well as cholesterol and other compounds.

protein: nutrients that can serve as working parts of cells, or can yield energy.

vitamins: essential nutrients synthesized by living things, required in minute amounts to help do the body's work (not energy-yielding).

minerals: a group of the earth's basic elements, some of which are essential nutrients required in small amounts to help do the body's work (not energy-yielding).

water: a substance necessary for life that provides a medium for, participates in, and results as a waste product from, life processes.

---

a food does reflect its fattening power.) One other compound people ingest provides energy: The alcohol of alcoholic beverages. Alcohol is not a nutrient because it does not promote growth, maintenance, or repair of the body, but it has to be counted as an energy source.

An important point is apparent here. People tend to think of carbohydrate as "bad for you" and "fattening," but it has been given an undeserved bad reputation by the peddlers of health-threatening low-carbohydrate diets. In fact, carbohydrate should contribute half or more of all the calories you ingest. A related point has to do with protein. Protein is thought of as "good" and as promoting thinness. But protein taken in excess loads you down with extra calories that are stored as fat. Also, protein goes hand in hand with large amounts of fat in many foods; meats are high in both calories and fat, for example, and so they are high in calories. Carbohydrate should be the source of most of the energy in the diet.

2. Too much protein can make you fat.
True.

The first set of color photos in the Food Feature (see Figure I–1 in the color insert) shows which nutrients are in which foods. (The Food Feature also presents a comparison of fat in common foods and the Four Food Group Plan. The fat in foods and the Four Food Group Plan are discussed later in this chapter.)

The other nutrients, vitamins and minerals, do not provide energy themselves, but help to regulate its release and other body processes. As for water, it is the medium in which all of the body's processes take place. Probably about 60 percent of your body's weight is water. It transports materials to and from cells and provides them with an environment much like that of the ocean. When fuel nutrients break down to release energy, they break down to water and other simple compounds. Since you lose water from your body daily, you must replace it daily. Second only to oxygen, water is the most vital substance you require; you can live only a few days without it.

Vitamins—play regulatory roles.
Minerals—play regulatory roles.
Water—provides the medium for life processes.

Energy from Food

The body derives its energy chiefly from two fuels: Glucose and fatty acids. The supply of glucose is temporary, and you must eat to maintain it. The brain's hypothalamus sends out a hunger signal when blood glucose gets too low. If you don't eat, the body turns to its four or so hours' worth of **glycogen** (a concentrated storage form of glucose) in your liver to generate glucose. And if you still do not eat after most of the glycogen has been used, your muscles and other lean body tissues begin to break down, releasing protein fragments, which your liver converts to glucose. (Energy must be obtained from lean tissue, because although the muscles and other organs can use fat as fuel, the brain ordinarily cannot. The brain needs glucose, which fat can supply only in tiny amounts.) But the wise eater turns to food before incurring tissue protein losses. Why dismantle your house for firewood when the woodpile is nearby?

glycogen: the form in which the body stores glucose.

When you eat, you replenish your fuels. Blood glucose rises within seconds when you eat carbohydrate. Your liver and muscle cells store

Liver glycogen is for the whole body's use. Muscle glycogen is normally used within the muscles only. For people who exercise intensely, the glycogen in their muscles is vital to performance. The more they can store, the longer their muscles can work. See Chapter 9.

balanced meal: a meal containing sufficient, but not excessive, amounts of foods from each food group and therefore sufficient, but not excessive, carbohydrate, fat, protein, vitamins, and minerals.

some extra glucose as glycogen; the fat cells store some as fat, creating a reserve supply of the two fuels to draw on the next time you have to postpone eating.*

When you get hungry, what should you eat? The obvious choice might seem to be a candy bar "for quick energy," and it is true that the body can quickly raise its blood glucose from a concentrated sugar source such as candy. The only trouble is that a dose of sugar by itself lasts only a short time; you'll soon be hungry again, and possibly shaky besides. You may remember how cranky and irritable you became as a child when you were hungry; a candy bar seemed to help for a while but may have made you feel worse in the end.

A better choice than pure sugar is a **balanced meal**— that is, a meal that contains several different kinds of food that offer protein, fat, and carbohydrate all together. Here's why it works:

- The carbohydrate in the meal provides an immediate source of glucose energy.
- The fat in the meal slows down the digestive system so that the glucose is not absorbed too fast. It also provides fatty acids that cells can use for energy.
- The protein in the meal prompts the body to regulate its use of the glucose, keeping it available in the bloodstream longer.

Figure 7–1 provides an example of a balanced meal.

*The liver cells convert excess glucose to fat and release it as needed; the fat cells pick it up and store it.

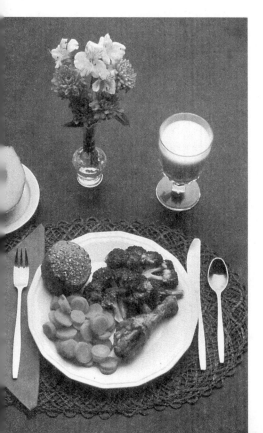

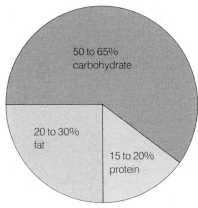

50 to 65% carbohydrate

20 to 30% fat

15 to 20% protein

FIGURE 7–1 A Balanced Meal
The meal supplies foods from every food group, as well as a recommended balance of energy sources: Less than 30 percent of its calories are from fat, and about 60 percent are from carbohydrate. Note the moderate portion of meat and the generous portions of vegetables and fruit. The bread is without butter, and the beverage is nonfat milk. Total calories: About 500.

A mistake people commonly make is to think that if fat should contribute 30 percent of the calories, then it should take up a third of the plate. On the contrary: Fat is much more calorie-dense than the other constituents of food, and much of it is invisible. In this 500-calorie meal, the only visible fat is in the chicken skin, and yet fat contributes almost 30 percent of the calories.

Carbohydrate

Complex carbohydrates (long chains of glucose):

   Glycogen—the body's storage form of glucose

   Starch—people's main food energy source

   Fibers—indigestible carbohydrates

starch: a complex carbohydrate, the predominant food energy source for human beings.

The terms *complex carbohydrate* and *simple carbohydrate* refer to one important distinction among carbohydrates—simply stated, the distinction between starch and fiber versus sugars. Another important distinction is that the simple carbohydrates come in both natural (dilute) and processed (concentrated) form—simply stated, fruit versus candy.

The complex carbohydrates are composed of long chains of glucose units. (The complex carbohydrate glycogen has already been mentioned as the form in which glucose is stored in the human liver and muscle cells.) **Starch** is the principal complex carbohydrate in grains and vegetables and the chief energy source for human beings throughout the world. Other complex carbohydrates in foods—fibers—are mostly indigestible by human beings and so yield no calories, but they help to maintain the health of the digestive tract.

Most fibers in foods are not digestible. They move through the digestive tract essentially unchanged. They hold water and so provide bulk inside the intestines, enabling the muscles of the digestive tract walls to push their contents along (see Figure 7–2). The more fibers there are in the foods you eat, the more water they hold, and the softer the stools they form. The subject may be unglamorous, but it intensely interests anyone who suffers from the consequences of a lack of fiber: Constipation, hemorrhoids, or a host of other intestinal ills.

Fiber serves the body well. It helps to prevent constipation; it helps to prevent and relieve hemorrhoids (swollen, painful rectal veins that bulge out from straining to pass hard stools). It may also, by keeping the intestinal contents moving, help to prevent infection of the appendix (appendicitis).

Fiber performs other services, too. It helps to control the blood cholesterol concentration, a risk factor for heart disease. (Certain fibers bind cholesterol and keep it from being absorbed into the body; it is excreted with the feces instead.) Fiber also moderates the blood glucose concentration and so helps to prevent diabetes. Some fibers bind cancer-causing agents in the digestive tract and keep them from coming in contact with the intestinal walls or from being absorbed.

Fiber may also help to prevent obesity. The person who eats fiber-rich foods chews longer and fills up sooner on fewer calories. Quite consistently, foods that are high in fiber are low in calories and vice versa. It is not true that fibers contribute no calories of their own to a person's intake; some fibers are digested by the bacterial inhabitants of the lower intestines, and they yield some fuel that the body can use. Still, it is hard to eat a diet high in fiber and also gain weight.

3. It is virtually impossible to eat a diet too high in fiber.

   False.

   Negative effects of fiber overdoses are known.

Is there such a thing as too much fiber? There certainly is. Some years ago, many college students overdid the high-fiber diet, much to their intestinal distress. The consequence was diarrhea, prolonged and severe enough to cause dangerous dehydration in some instances. Too much of anything, in nutrition as in all areas of life, is as harmful as too little.

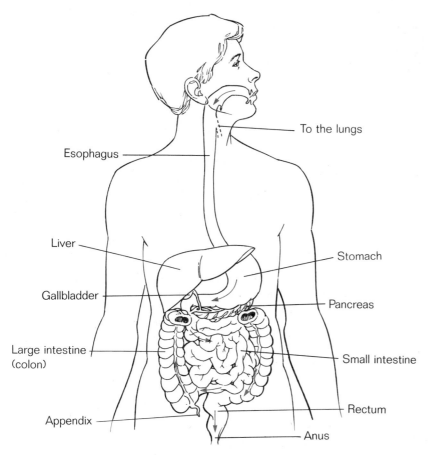

Esophagus

To the lungs

Liver

Stomach

Gallbladder

Pancreas

Large intestine
(colon)

Small intestine

Appendix

Rectum

Anus

FIGURE 7-2 The Digestive System
The system is a continuous tube of muscle that starts at the throat, and includes the esophagus, stomach, small intestine, large intestine, rectum, and anus. Two organs contribute digestive juices from outside this tube. One is the liver, which makes bile and stores it in the gallbladder; the bile is released through a duct into the small intestine when needed to help digest fat. The other organ is the pancreas, which contributes digestive fluids through another duct.

sugars: simple carbohydrates; examples are glucose, fructose, sucrose, and lactose.

The four sugars important in nutrition:

    Glucose

    Fructose

    Sucrose

    Lactose

Plant foods are high in fiber—particularly those with their skins and seeds intact. Fiber breaks down when foods are refined or cooked. Apples have more fiber than applesauce; apple juice has none. Baked potatoes with the skin have more fiber than mashed potatoes; potato chips have almost none. If you want to eat a diet high enough in fiber to benefit your health, choose whole grains, whole fruits, and whole vegetables most of the time. Cook these foods sparingly, and eat some raw.

The simple carbohydrates are the **sugars.** All sugars are chemically similar to glucose and can be converted into glucose in the body. All their names end in *ose*, which makes them easy to recognize as carbohydrates. The four sugars most important in human nutrition are glucose (the body's fuel), fructose (the sweet sugar of fruits, honey, and maple syrup), sucrose (table sugar), and lactose (milk sugar). Simple carbohydrates come mostly from fruits and milk or in concentrated form as sugar, honey, and other sweets.

Nutritionists recommend that you consume abundant quantities of fruits and vegetables that contain sugars, but they urge you in the same breath to avoid consuming "too much sugar." What's the difference?

THE MAKEUP OF FOODS

141

4. Honey and sugar are more similar than different.

True.

Snacks dentists recommend:

Milk, cheese, and yogurt (not fruit and flavored yogurts, though, which are as sugary as ice cream).

Fresh fruits (not dried fruits, jams, and jellies).

Vegetables (but not candied or glazed).

Grains (but not granola bars, which are as sticky as candy bars).

In terms of nutrition, there is no significant difference between honey and sugar.

Part of the answer lies in the phrase **empty calories.** When you eat an apple, you receive about 100 calories from the sugars in it, together with a little vitamin A, a bit of thiamin, some vitamin C, a moderate dose of fiber, a healthy bit of potassium, and several dozen other nutrients. By contrast, a 12-ounce cola beverage gives you about 150 calories from sugar without any nutrients. In fact, it creates a sort of debt: To avoid overconsuming calories, you now have to derive the nutrients you need in a day from food containing 150 calories less.

Honey is considered by some people to be the ideal substitute for sugar because, they say, it offers sweetness *and* nutrients; it is not empty calories. True, honey does contain traces of a few vitamins and minerals, but relative to a person's daily need, these nutrients don't add up to much. A tablespoon of honey (65 calories) offers one-tenth milligram of iron, for example, but an adult's daily need for iron can be as high as 15 milligrams or more. Consequently an adult would need 150 tablespoons in a day—almost 10,000 calories of honey! (Most people can eat only 2,000 to 3,000 calories a day without getting fat.) The nutrients just do not add up as fast as the calories do; so honey, like sugar, is a relatively empty-calorie food. Honey is almost identical to sugar chemically, too.

Also, the bacteria that cause dental caries thrive on sugar. They can double their numbers when carbohydrate sticks to tooth surfaces for twenty minutes or more at a time—and sugar tends to stick. Caries form when three factors are present: A susceptible tooth, a carbohydrate supply, and bacteria to consume the carbohydrate and produce acid from it that decays the tooth enamel. A few people are born with decay-resistant teeth, but most people need to protect their teeth to prevent decay. An obvious preventive measure is to avoid exposing the teeth to carbohydrate for long periods and, after exposure, to brush and floss them promptly. If you drink a cola beverage, finish it quickly and follow with a vigorous water rinse.

Fat

Nearly all the body's tissues (except the brain and nervous system) can use fat as an energy source. It is the major fuel for muscles, as long as they have enough oxygen to break it down.

Fat is stored in a layer of cells beneath the skin and also in many pads surrounding and underlying vital organs. As well as providing an energy reserve, it helps to insulate the body from the cold, from changes in temperature, and from mechanical shock. Whenever you eat, you store some fat, and within a few hours after a meal, you start taking it out of storage and using it for energy until the next meal. Thus, both glucose and fat are stored after meals, and both are released later when needed as fuel for the cells' work.

The body has scanty reserves of carbohydrate and not much protein to spare, but it can store fat in practically unlimited amounts. A pound of body fat is worth 3,500 calories, and a person's body can easily carry 30 to 50 pounds of fat without looking fat at all. In fact, a man of normal

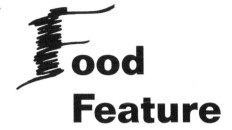

Food Feature

Choosing a Healthy Diet

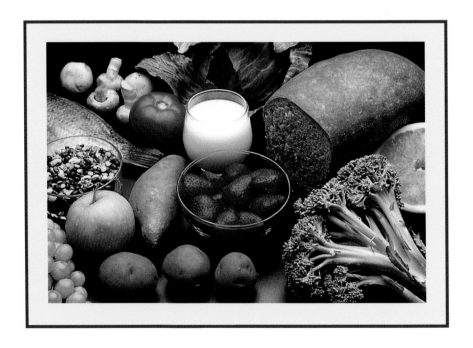

To succeed in choosing a nutritionally sound diet, you need to eat the right amounts of foods, watch your fat intake, and select a variety of foods to ensure that you receive all the nutrients you need. The following color portfolio is designed to help you achieve your goals. Figure I–1 shows portion sizes of various foods to guide you in serving yourself appropriate amounts—portions that are neither too large, nor too small.

Figure I–2 reveals the impact of fat on the calorie content of foods—an impact that should motivate you to control your fat intake. Finally, Figure I–3 shows you how many servings of each type of food to include in the foundation of a food plan that balances the diet and provides needed nutrients. Taken together, portion control, fat moderation, and nutrient adequacy are the cornerstones of a diet that supports health.

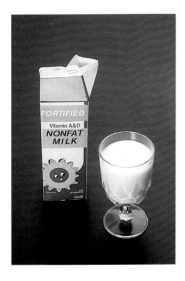

FIGURE I–1 Portion Sizes of Foods
Five categories of foods contain vitamins, minerals, and energy. The sixth contains essentially pure energy. The portion sizes shown are useful for diet planning. The meat portion (moderate—3 ounces) and the vegetable portion (ample—1 cup) are consistent with recommended guidelines.

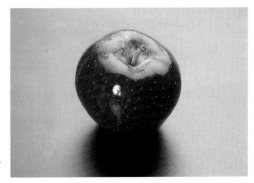

Milk
Carbohydrate
Protein
plus vitamins, minerals, and water

Fruit
Carbohydrate
plus vitamins, minerals, and water

Meat
Protein
Fat
plus vitamins, minerals, and water

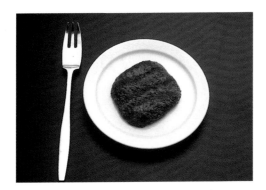

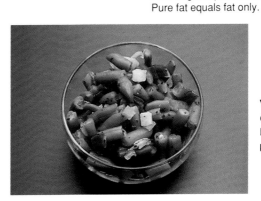

Sugar and Fat
Pure sugar equals carbohydrate only.
Pure fat equals fat only.

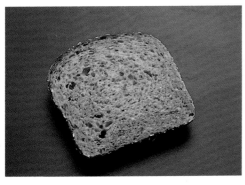

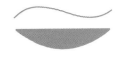

Vegetable
Carbohydrate
Protein
plus vitamins, minerals, and water

Bread
Carbohydrate
Protein
plus vitamins and minerals

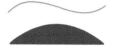

FIGURE I–2 Impact of Fat on Calorie Content of Foods

When fat is trimmed from food, calories are drastically reduced.

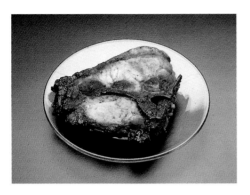

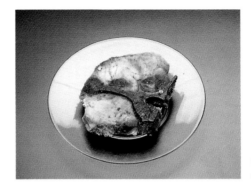

Pork chop with fat trimmed off = 165 calories.

Pork chop with a half-inch of fat = 275 calories.

Potato with 1 tablespoon sour cream = 350 calories.

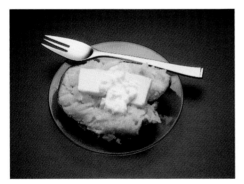

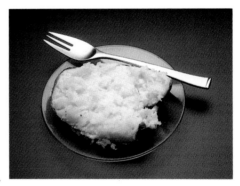

Plain potato = 220 calories.

Whole milk; 1 cup = 150 calories.

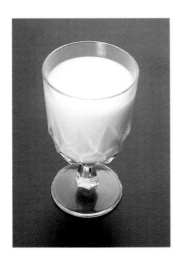

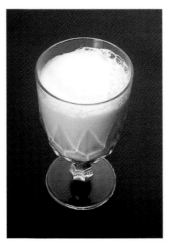

Nonfat milk; 1 cup = 90 calories.

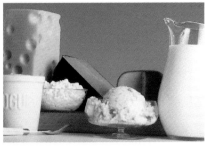

Milk and Milk Products

Calcium, riboflavin, protein, vitamin B₁₂. (vitamin D and vitamin A, when fortified).

Serving = 1 c milk or yogurt; ¼ c Parmesan cheese or process cheese spread; 2 c cottage cheese; 1½ c ice cream or ice milk; 2 oz process cheese food; 1⅓ oz cheese.
2 servings per day for adults.
3 servings per day for children.
4 servings per day for teenagers, pregnant and lactating women, women past menopause.
5 servings per day for pregnant and lactating teenagers.

- Nonfat milk, buttermilk, low-fat milk, plain yogurt.
- Whole milk, cheese, fruit-flavored yogurt, cottage cheese.
- Custard, milk shakes, pudding, ice cream.

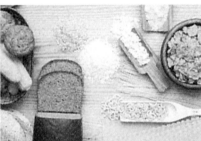

Breads and Cereals

Riboflavin, thiamin, niacin, iron, protein, magnesium, folate, fiber.

Serving = 1 slice bread; ½ to ¾ c cooked cereals, rice, or pastas; 1 oz ready-to-eat cereals.
4 servings per day.

- Whole grains (wheat, oats, barley, millet, rye, bulgur) enriched breads, rolls, tortillas.
- Rice, cereals, pastas (macaroni, spaghetti), bagels.
- Pancakes, muffins, cornbread, biscuits, presweetened cereals.

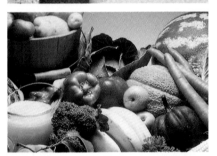

Vegetables and Fruits

Vitamin A, vitamin C, riboflavin, folate, iron, magnesium, low in fat, no cholesterol.

Serving = ½ c or typical portion (such as 1 medium apple, ½ grapefruit, or 1 wedge lettuce).
4 servings per day.

- Apricots, bean sprouts, broccoli, brussels sprouts, cabbage, cantaloupe, carrots, cauliflower, cucumbers, grapefruit, green beans, green peas, leafy greens (spinach, mustard, and collard greens), lettuce, mush-rooms, oranges, orange juice, peaches, strawberries, tomatoes, winter squash.
- Apples, bananas, canned fruit, corn, pears, potatoes.
- Avocados, dried fruit, sweet potatoes.

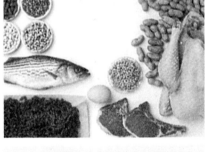

Meat and Meat Alternates

Protein, phosphorus, vitamin B₆, vitamin B₁₂, zinc, magnesium, iron, niacin, thiamin.

Serving = 2 to 3 oz lean, cooked meat, poultry, or fish; 1 oz meat, poultry, or fish = 1 egg, ½ to ¾ c legumes, 2 tbsp peanut butter, ¼ to ½ c nuts or seeds.
2 servings per day for adults, children, teenagers.
3 servings per day for pregnant and lactating women and teenagers.

- Poultry, fish, lean meat (beef, lamb, pork), dried peas and beans, eggs.
- Beef, lamb, pork, refried beans.
- Hotdogs, luncheon meats, peanut butter, nuts.

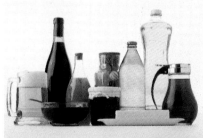

Miscellaneous Group

Sugar, fat (vitamin E), salt, alcohol, calories.

No serving sizes are provided because servings of these foods are not recommended. Concentrate on the four food groups that provide nutrients; the foods in the miscellaneous group will find their way into your diet as ingredients in prepared foods, or added at the table, or just as "extras". Note that some of the following items could be placed in more than one group or in a combination group. For example, potato chips are high in both salt and fat; doughnuts are high in both sugar and fat.

- Miscellaneous foods, not high in calories, include spices, herbs, coffee, tea, and diet soft drinks.
- Foods high in fat include margarine, salad dressing, oils, mayonnaise, cream, cream cheese, butter, gravy, and sauces.
- Foods high in salt include potato chips, corn chips, pretzels, pickels, olives, bouillon, prepared mustard, soy sauce, steak sauce, salt, and seasoned salt.
- Foods high in sugar include cake, pie, cookies, doughnuts, sweet rolls, candy, soft drinks, fruit drinks, jelly, syrup, gelatin desserts, sugar, and honey.
- Alcoholic beverages include wine, beer, and liquor.

**FIGURE I-3
The Four Food Group Plan**

Note which foods are
- highest in calories
- moderate in calories
- and lowest in calories.

5. Of all the things in foods that cause diseases, sugar is probably the biggest culprit.

False.

Of all the things in foods that cause diseases, fat is by far the biggest culprit.

weight might have about 15 percent, and a woman about 20 percent, of the body weight as fat.

Fat comes in different forms. In foods, most of it comes as fats and oils—that is, **triglycerides**—and it is stored in the body's fat cells in the same form. The triglycerides you eat come in two forms—saturated and unsaturated (includes polyunsaturated). People who are at risk for heart and artery disease are encouraged to reduce their total fat, and especially their saturated fat, intakes. (Saturated fats come primarily from animal-derived foods such as meats, butter, and cream; unsaturated fats come primarily from vegetable oils, including olive oil, corn oil, and canola oil.)

Another form of fat is **cholesterol.** Some cholesterol is made and used in the body, but in excess it is associated with heart and artery disease. Cholesterol forms a major part of the deposits that accumulate along arteries and increase the risk of heart attacks and strokes. For people trying to lower blood cholesterol, however, it is not effective to limit only cholesterol intake; it is necessary to limit total fat intake, including both saturated fat and cholesterol.

Reducing fat intake offers a fringe benefit to people who wish to cut calories. A spoon of fat contains more than twice as many calories as a spoon of sugar or pure protein. By removing the fat from a food, you can drastically reduce the calorie count. The second set of color photos in the Food Feature (see Figure I–2) shows that the single most effective step you can take to reduce the energy value of a food is to eat it with less fat.

Of all the dietary factors related to diseases prevalent in developed countries, high fat intake is by far the most significant. Heart disease and many forms of cancer are linked to high fat intake; probably many other diseases are, too, including arthritis, gallbladder disease, diabetes, and all diseases aggravated by obesity. The most important dietary steps you can take to prevent these diseases are to control your fat intake and to control your weight.

Protein

Protein is well-known as the body-building nutrient, the material of strong muscles, and rightly so. No new living tissue can be built without it, for protein is part of every cell, every bone, the blood, and every other tissue. Proteins constitute the cells' machinery—they do the cells' work. The energy to fuel that work comes from carbohydrate and fat as they break down.

Among the cells' working parts are a multitude of proteins called **enzymes.** Each enzyme performs a specific chemical step in the building or breakdown of cellular materials. A single human cell may contain several thousand kinds of enzymes, each triggering a different chemical reaction.

The instructions that tell cells how to make their proteins are inherited. When geneticists talk about hereditary differences among people, they are really talking about differences in the codes people inherit for their proteins, most of which are enzymes. Among other proteins that

amino acids: building blocks, 20 in all, from which proteins are made. The *essential amino acids* are a group of nine of these that cannot be made by the body and thus must be obtained in food.

6. Once the body has assembled its proteins into body structures, it never lets go of them.

False.

Your body loses protein every day.

vegetarians: people who omit meat, fish, and poultry from their diets. *Lacto-ovo vegetarians* use milk and milk products and eggs as well as plant foods; *strict vegetarians* eat only plant foods.

Examples of protein-rich plant food combinations:

Beans and rice

Peanut butter and bread

Soy bean curd (tofu) and rice

Any grain and legume

confer individuality on people are the antibodies, which confer resistance to disease and facilitate the body's rejection of foreign materials.

Proteins are made of building blocks called **amino acids.** A set of 20 distinct amino acids form proteins (much as letters form sentences), but your body can make only 11 of them. The nine amino acids the body cannot make are the essential amino acids, which you must obtain from food.

Your body loses protein every day. Digestive tract cells wear out and are excreted in the feces. Skin cells flake off or are rubbed off. Hair and nails (made of protein) grow longer daily and are shed or cut away. An adult loses about one-quarter cup of pure protein a day. People need to eat protein-containing foods every day to replace the protein they lose.

You know you are eating protein when you eat meats, fish, poultry, eggs, cheese, and milk. Plant foods such as grains, legumes (chile beans, lima beans, and the like), and other vegetables eaten in quantity also provide protein. It is easy to consume more than enough protein from these foods. An adult can obtain enough protein from one egg, two cups of milk, and an assortment of grains and vegetables—without a single serving of meat. Yet many people eat two or three eggs for breakfast, hamburgers for lunch, and 12-ounce steaks for dinner.

Protein-rich foods from animal sources are often high in fat and calories, and all are low in fiber, so they can pose a triple problem. It is beneficial to health for people to obtain at least half of their protein from plants, and it is possible to get enough protein from plant foods alone, as **vegetarians** do.

Thus far, this chapter has dealt with the calorie-bearing nutrients—carbohydrate, fat, and protein. The next section deals with the nutrients everyone thinks of when they think about nutrition—the vitamins and minerals.

Vitamins and Minerals

Vitamins and minerals occur in foods in much smaller quantities than do the energy-yielding nutrients, and they make no contribution of energy themselves. Nor do they contribute building material, except for the minerals of bone. Instead they serve mostly as helpers, or facilitators, of body processes. They are, nonetheless, a powerful group of substances, as their absence attests. Vitamin A deficiency can cause blindness; a lack of niacin causes mental illness; a lack of vitamin D causes growth retardation; a lack of iron causes anemia. The consequences of deficiencies are so dire and the effects of restoring the needed nutrients so dramatic that they make wonderful stories for faddists to tell: Are you bald? Impotent? Do you have pimples? Are you nearsighted? The right vitamin will cure whatever ails you.

Actually, a vitamin or mineral can cure only the disease caused by a deficiency of that vitamin or mineral. Also, an overdose of any vitamin or mineral can make people as sick as a deficiency, and can even cause death. It is remarkable and fortunate for people who haven't studied nutrition that a balanced diet of ordinary foods supplies enough, but not too much, of each of the vitamins and minerals.

The vitamins and minerals are listed and some of their more important roles in the body are shown in Table 7–2. This section discusses only a few vitamins and minerals that exemplify the importance of meeting your body's needs for all of them. It refers frequently to foods; the end of the chapter puts the foods together into an eating plan that will meet your needs for all nutrients.

Thiamin.   Thiamin is a typical vitamin in that its presence is not felt, but its absence makes itself known all over the body. A severe thiamin deficiency causes a paralysis that begins at the fingers and toes and works its way inward toward the spine, with extreme wasting and loss of muscle tissue, swelling all over the body, and enlargement of the heart and irregular heartbeat. Ultimately, the victim dies from heart failure. You probably have never witnessed such an extreme deficiency, but consider how a mild lack manifests its presence: Stomachaches, headaches, fatigue, restlessness, disturbances of sleep, chest pains, fevers, personality changes (aggressiveness and hostility), and a whole string of symptoms often classed as neurosis. Mild thiamin deficiencies are likely to be seen in consumers of "junk" diets—that is, diets that emphasize foods low in nutrients and high in calories, sugar, fat, and salt.

Proof that thiamin was deficient in some people who snacked heavily on empty-calorie foods came from research that showed below-normal activity of a thiamin-containing enzyme in their blood.[6] They also had the symptoms of neurosis just mentioned. When they took thiamin supplements for a month or more, the symptoms disappeared as the blood enzyme activity returned to normal.

On hearing stories like this, people tend to want to rush out to the drugstore and buy bottles of vitamin pills. There's a problem, though: Although you might get the amount of thiamin you need this way, more than 40 other essential nutrients are all equally vital to your well-being. Foods are far more effective than pills in supplying the assortment of nutrients you need because they contain such rich mixtures of nutrients in forms the body is adapted to use.

What foods in particular supply thiamin, then? Almost no one food you can eat will supply your daily need in a single serving. In fact, thiamin is delivered in adequate amounts only to people who eat *ten or more servings of nutritious foods each day,* as the Four Food Group Plan advises (see the third set of color photos—Figure I–3—in the Food Feature).

Folate.   Folate deficiency is probably more widespread than most people realize. It distorts the red blood cells and impairs their ability to carry sufficient oxygen to all the body's other cells, causing a kind of **anemia.** Folate deficiency causes a generalized misery with many symptoms, including fatigue, diarrhea, irritability, forgetfulness, lack of appetite, headache, and many more.

anemia: reduced size or number or altered shape of the red blood cells; a symptom of any of a number of different disease conditions, including several nutrient deficiencies.

TABLE 7-2 • Major Roles of the Vitamins and Minerals

Fat-Soluble Vitamins[a]

Vitamin A	Contributes a pigment of the eye important in vision, especially night vision.
	Participates in the modeling of bones during growth and in the mending of breaks.
	Helps maintain the body's many surfaces (skin and linings of lungs, digestive tract, urinary tract, vagina, eyelids).
Vitamin D	Regulates the calcium concentration in the blood.
Vitamin E	Protects compounds that are susceptible to destruction by oxidation. Important in protecting red blood cells from bursting as they pass through the lungs.
Vitamin K	Assists in normal clotting of blood.

Water-Soluble Vitamins[a]

Thiamin Riboflavin Niacin Biotin Pantothenic acid	Help enzymes to facilitate the release of energy from nutrients needed in every cell of the body.
Vitamin B_6	Assists in the metabolism of protein.
Vitamin B_{12} Folate	Help cells to divide, especially blood cells and cells of the intestinal lining.
Vitamin C	Maintains the body's connective tissue. Important to the healing of wounds.

continued

NOTE: The vitamin names given here are the official names as of 1979. Other names still commonly used and seen on labels are *alpha-tocopherol* for vitamin E, *vitamin B_1* for thiamin, *vitamin B_2* for riboflavin, *pyridoxine* for vitamin B_6, *folic acid* for folate, and *ascorbic acid* for vitamin C.

[a]The fat-soluble and water-soluble vitamins were originally separated on the basis of their solubility. The fat-soluble vitamins tend to be stored in the body and so can be eaten in large quantities at intervals, whereas the water-soluble vitamins tend to be excreted daily in urine and not to accumulate, and so must be eaten daily. Of the water-soluble vitamins, the first eight are B vitamins.

The term *anemia*, which means literally "without blood," is a symptom, not a disease, it is a shortage or abnormality of the red blood cells. Many nutrient deficiencies and diseases can cause it.

Why is folate deficiency so widespread? For one thing, the vitamin is predominantly found in *fresh* foods, the kind that do not store well, primarily vegetables. It is easily destroyed when foods are canned, dehydrated, or otherwise processed, or even overcooked. Finally, some people need more folate than others. For example, anyone who is growing new cells needs extra folate: Children, pregnant women, and people recovering from illness or surgery.

Vitamin B_6.   As for vitamin B_6, it, too, is an indispensable cog in the body's machinery, and the price of a deficiency is a multitude of symp-

TABLE 7–2 • Continued

Major Minerals

Calcium Phosphorus	Serve as principal minerals of bones and teeth. Calcium is involved with muscle contraction, nerve transmission, immune function, and blood clotting. Phosphorus is important in the genetic material and in energy transfer.
Magnesium	Helps with bone mineralization, protein synthesis, muscle contraction, and transmission of nerve impulses.
Sodium Chlorine Potassium	Serve as electrolytes that maintain fluid balance and the balance of acids and bases inside and outside cells. Chlorine is also part of the hydrochloric acid of the stomach, necessary for digestion. Potassium also facilitates protein synthesis and the maintenance of nerves and muscles.
Sulfur	Serves as a component of certain amino acids and as part of the vitamins biotin and thiamin and the hormone insulin.

Trace Minerals

Iodine	As part of the thyroid hormone, helps to regulate growth, development, and metabolic rate in the body.
Fluoride	Helps form bones and teeth, making them resistant to loss of their minerals.
Selenium	Along with vitamin E, protects body compounds from oxidation.
Iron	Serves as part of the red blood cell protein hemoglobin, which carries oxygen from place to place in the body, and of the muscle protein myoglobin, which makes oxygen available for muscle work.
Zinc	Serves as a working part of many enzymes and of the hormone insulin.

toms. Vitamin B_6 illustrates another nutrition principle—excesses are also toxic. Whenever people start overusing a nutrient, no matter how nontoxic the nutrient may seem at first, it is only a matter of time before toxic effects appear. This happened in the 1970s with vitamin C after the publication of the popular book *Vitamin C and the Common Cold*.[7] In the 1980s, it happened with vitamin B_6. People were "diagnosing" vitamin B_6 deficiencies on grossly inadequate evidence and "prescribing" large doses.

The first major report of toxic effects of high doses of vitamin B_6 described people who had numb feet, then lost sensation in their hands, then became unable to work. Later, their mouths became numb.[8] Since then, other reports have followed, showing nervous system damage from more moderate doses of vitamin B_6.[9]

Not everyone is likely to suffer toxicity symptoms with high doses of vitamin B_6. Because it is easily excreted in the urine, vitamin B_6 is a relatively nontoxic nutrient, but individual tolerances vary, and we cannot say that supplements are "safe" for anyone. The same fact holds true for every vitamin.

Calcium.   Calcium bears the distinction of being the most abundant mineral in the human body. It is the major mineral of bones and teeth, and everyone is aware that children, therefore, need milk daily to support their growth. Calcium is not abundant in the diet, and low intakes are common. A deficit of calcium during childhood and adulthood threatens the integrity of the bones and contributes to gradual bone loss, **osteoporosis,** that can totally cripple a person in later life.

Many people, even as young as 30, are gradually losing calcium, but the body sends no detectable signals saying that the bones are growing weak. The deficiency becomes apparent only when an older person breaks a hip or pelvic bone or suffers collapse of a spinal bone. Osteoporosis strikes at least one out of every three people over age 65. Adult bone loss is eight times more prevalent in women than in men after age 50. One reason is that women's estrogen levels fall abruptly at menopause, accelerating bone loss and reducing calcium absorption. Figure 7–3 shows the effect of the loss of spinal bone on a woman's height and posture. It is not inevitable that people "grow shorter" as they age, but it does happen if they experience bone loss.

Bone strength depends not only on nutrients but on physical activity. Bones respond to activity just as muscles do, by becoming stronger. If you lie in bed all day, you cannot build bone, no matter how much milk you drink; and the converse may also be true: If you exercise regularly, you cannot help but build bone. The body adapts both its absorption rate and its bone-building activity to its needs, so a major part of the preventive prescription is exercise.

The cornerstones of prevention, then, are regular exercise, adequate calcium intakes throughout life, and for women, estrogen replacement after menopause. Also recommended are adequate fluoride and vitamin D intakes, abstinence from alcohol and other drugs, moderation in caffeine use, minimal prescription drug use, and control of stress.

For people who can tolerate milk and milk products, the obvious way to meet calcium needs is to include them in the diet daily, because they are almost the only foods that contain significant quantities. Table 7–3 shows the amounts of milk recommended for children and adults. People who cannot tolerate fresh milk can try cheese or fermented dairy products as substitutes for fluid milk, but they need to use large quantities to obtain enough calcium. A few plant foods make significant contributions to those who plan their diets carefully: They use selected nuts, greens, legumes, and calcium-fortified beverages to meet their needs. Calcium supplements may be of some value.

osteoporosis: reduced density of the bones.

TABLE 7–3 • Recommended Fluid Milk Intakes

The Four Food Group Plan recommends daily milk servings (1 c):

- Children under 9: 2 to 3
- Children 9 to 12: 3 or more
- Teenagers: 4 or more
- Adults: 2
- Pregnant women: 3 or more
- Lactating women: 4 or more
- Older women: 3

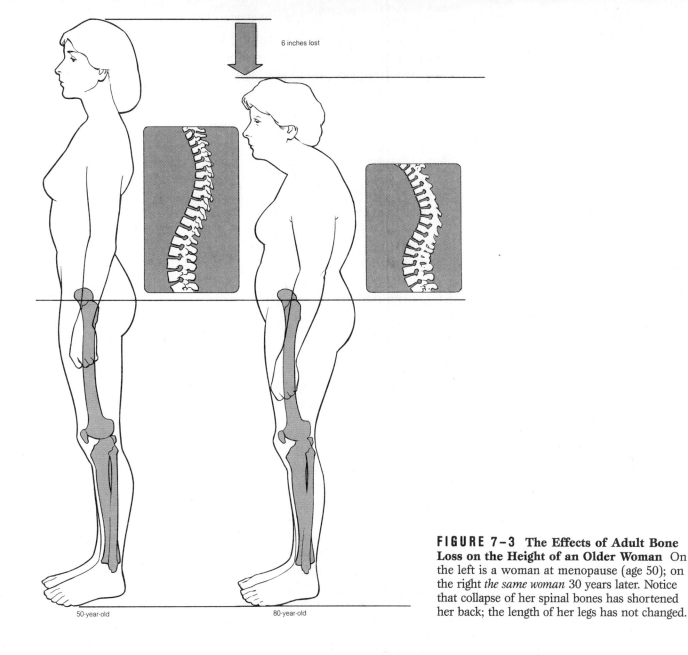

6 inches lost

50-year-old

80-year-old

FIGURE 7–3 The Effects of Adult Bone Loss on the Height of an Older Woman On the left is a woman at menopause (age 50); on the right *the same woman* 30 years later. Notice that collapse of her spinal bones has shortened her back; the length of her legs has not changed.

hemoglobin: the oxygen-carrying protein of the red blood cells.

Iron.   Iron's presence in every living cell testifies to its enormous importance in the body. Iron is part of the protein **hemoglobin,** the body's oxygen carrier. Bound into hemoglobin in the red blood cells, iron enables them to ferry oxygen from lungs to tissues, thus permitting the release of energy from fuels to do the cells' work. Iron-deficiency anemia is characterized by weakness, tiredness, apathy, headaches, and a paleness that reflects a reduction in number and size of red blood cells. (In dark-skinned people, this paleness can be seen in the corner of the eye.) A person with this anemia can do very little muscular work without experiencing disabling fatigue but will feel more energetic after a few weeks of eating the needed iron-rich foods.

Women may often have their blood iron concentration pronounced normal, and yet they may need more iron because their body stores may be depleted. This condition is not detected by standard tests. Because most women eat less food than men, their iron intakes are lower. And because women menstruate, their iron losses are greater. These two factors predispose women to iron deficiencies.

Iron is one of the **trace minerals,** so called because only tiny amounts are needed in the diet. Despite this, iron deficiency occurs in as many as half of all persons, even in developed countries—most predictably, in inner-city and rural families of limited means. People begin to lose energy long before iron deficiency anemia is diagnosed. They have no obvious disease, they appear unmotivated and apathetic, they work and play less, and they are less physically fit. Incidence rates for iron deficiency anemia in developed countries range from 10 to 20 percent; rates are higher in the developing countries. Therefore, the incidence of iron deficiency not severe enough to cause anemia may be higher still.[10] If this one worldwide malnutrition problem could be alleviated, millions of people's lives would brighten.

The cause of iron deficiency is usually poor nutrition—that is, inadequate intake, either from sheer lack of food or from high consumption of empty-calorie foods. Among non-nutritional causes, blood loss, usually caused by infection, is the primary one. Meats, fish, poultry, and legumes are iron-rich, and an easy way to obtain the needed iron is to eat them regularly. But foods that are rich in iron are poor in calcium and vice versa. Thus, it is important to use enough, but not too much, of each.

Sodium.   Some minerals serve as **electrolytes,** dissolved substances in blood and body fluid that carry electrical charges. Fluids and electrolytes provide the environment in which the cells' work takes place—work such as nerve-to-nerve communication, heartbeats, contraction of muscles, and so forth. When people lose fluid—whether it is sweat, blood, or urine—they also lose electrolytes. When too much body fluid is lost, as in heat stroke, diarrhea, or injury, its replacement is essential and may require medical assistance.

Sodium is an example of an electrolyte. It is best known as part of sodium chloride, ordinary table **salt,** a highly prized food seasoning and preservative. No recommendation need be made for a minimum intake of sodium, because it is so abundant in the diet. For some people, however, a ceiling is suggested, because excesses can contribute to high blood pressure (**hypertension**) in those who are genetically susceptible. Foods high in salt are not always easy to recognize, so people wishing to avoid salt must rely on reading labels.

Zinc.   Zinc plays roles of major importance in association with the cellular machinery in every body organ. It is lost from the body daily, in much the same way as protein is, and so it must be replenished daily to

---

7. Women need to be more concerned about iron than do men.

True.

trace minerals: minerals essential in nutrition, needed in small quantities (traces) daily. Iron and zinc are examples.

electrolytes: minerals that carry electrical charges when dissolved in fluid.

Fluid replacement for sweat losses in heavy exercise or work is discussed in Chapter 9.

salt: a compound that, in water, separates into electrolytes.

hypertension: high blood pressure.

ward off deficiencies. Zinc is highest in foods of high protein content, such as shellfish, meats, and liver.

At one time, zinc deficiencies were unheard of, but they are now known to be present in many of the world's people. In the Middle East, for example, zinc deficiencies have caused severe growth retardation and arrested sexual maturation in adolescent boys. In the United States and Canada, zinc deficiencies occur in the most vulnerable population groups—pregnant women, young children, the elderly, and people with low incomes. Cases of zinc deficiency have been reported in U.S. and Canadian schoolchildren.[11] A number of Denver schoolchildren had poor growth, poor appetite, and decreased taste sensitivity due to zinc deficiency. The children were described as "picky eaters" and ate less than an ounce of meat per day. This is another indication that a balanced diet is important, especially in growing children.

This section has described all of the classes of nutrients and given thumbnail sketches of a few of them. It has emphasized foods as the sources of these nutrients. The last section of the chapter shows you how to arrange foods into patterns that provide the full spectrum of nutrients you need. However, some people are still not sure that they are meeting their nutrient needs using foods alone; consequently, many people rely on vitamin-mineral supplements.

Vitamin-Mineral Supplements

Fully half of the population uses nutrient supplements regularly, collectively spending billions of dollars on them each year.[12] You may be wondering if you might benefit from supplements. This discussion is intended to help you make that decision.

Even if people's food choices are poor, taking supplements does not guarantee that they will get the particular nutrients they need. It is just as likely that they will duplicate the nutrients their food supplies and still lack the ones they need. The only way to be sure to get the needed assortment of nutrients is to construct a balanced diet from a variety of foods.

No supplement supplies all the nutrients that foods do. There is no way you can package in a single pill the bulk nutrients you need— protein, fiber, carbohydrate, calcium, and others—because you need such large amounts that a single pill would be too large to swallow. No one supplement can match a balanced diet, and no combination of supplements can, either. No one knows enough, yet, to construct a synthetic substitute for food. Even in the hospital, "complete" synthetic formulas given to patients for months enable those patients only to survive. They won't thrive until they are back on food.[13]

Nutrient supplements, however, are useful at times. A person may need a specific nutrient to counteract a specific deficiency—iron for iron-deficiency anemia, for example. But it takes medical training and tests to make a correct diagnosis; vitamin salespeople cannot do it, and buyers too, would be foolish to try.

The purveyors of supplements like to make the claim that people under stress (alcohol users, cigarette smokers, and athletes) need their products—of course, because they can sell more products that way. The claim works; lots of people buy nutrient supplements because they identify with the ads. Stresses, including smoking and moderate alcohol use, do deplete people's nutrient stores somewhat, but the composition of the supplements for those people is just guesswork on the part of the manufacturer. The way to counteract nutrient losses is still to eat well, not to take supplements. People who drink to excess have major nutrition problems and need to stop drinking. As for athletes, they need supplements *less* than other people, because they are able to eat more food.

Some special circumstances warrant the taking of nutrient supplements.[14] The following are examples:

- People with low energy intakes (below about 1,500 calories), such as habitual dieters.
- People who know that, for whatever reason, they are going to be eating irregularly for a limited time.
- People with illnesses that take away the appetite.
- People with illnesses that impair nutrient absorption—including diseases of the liver and digestive system.
- People taking medications that interfere with the body's use of specific nutrients.
- People who have diseases, injuries, or infections, or who have undergone surgery resulting in increased needs.
- Pregnant or lactating women.
- Vegetarians who exclude all animal-derived foods from their diets.
- Women who bleed excessively during menstruation.

Health care providers can make judgments on these and other special circumstances.

When you do need a supplement, do not be taken in by claims that organic, natural supplements are preferable to synthetic ones. *Organic* and *natural* are terms that have no meaning in relation to the contents of supplements. All vitamins are organic, no matter where they come from. *Natural* has no legal meaning at all. These terms mean only that the product will be expensive. Do not let these labels fool you. Read the ingredient lists, and buy the product that contains the nutrients you are looking for, at the lowest price. Remember that if vitamins are needed, minerals are needed, too, and a vitamin pill is not enough. A vitamin-mineral supplement is called for.

Whenever a health care provider recommends a supplement, carefully follow directions as to the type and dose to take. When you are selecting one yourself, a single, balanced vitamin-mineral supplement should suffice. Look for one in which the nutrient levels are at or slightly below the RDA. (The RDA, or Recommended Dietary Allowances, are shown in Appendix C.) Avoid preparations that exceed the RDA. Re-

8. As far as nutrients are concerned, the more, the better.

False.

All of the vitamins and minerals can be toxic when excessive amounts are taken.

member, you will still be getting some nutrients from foods. It is a myth that vitamins and minerals are nontoxic. All of the vitamins, not only the well-known vitamins A and D, but also the B vitamins and vitamin C, have been shown to have toxic effects, at least in some people, when taken in large doses.[15] As for the minerals, many are toxic, and often in quantities not far above normal intakes. Clearly, then, supplements are useful in some limited circumstances, but they cannot serve as a shortcut to good nutrition. You need foods, with all the multitude of nutrients and related compounds they contain, if you really want good health.

How to Choose Nutritious Foods

About 40 vitamins and minerals are needed altogether. How can people meet their needs for all of these nutrients?

Each nutrient has its own unique pattern of distribution in foods. It might seem like quite a tricky business, then, to work them all into the meals you eat, and yet you probably do well, nutritionally, without even trying. People all over the world obtain fine nutrition from an astonishing variety of diets.

People sometimes think that to eat wisely requires giving up all their favorite foods and all the pleasures they derive from them. This is not true. In almost every case, all a person's diet needs to become nutritionally superb is just a little fine-tuning. Eat this food more often, eat that food a little less often—that's all. For many people, whether they know it or not, the Four Food Group Plan serves as the basis for planning adequate, balanced diets.

The third set of color photos in the Food Feature (see Figure I–3) shows the Four Food Group Plan. The number of servings recommended daily from each group (milk and milk products, meats and meat alternates, vegetables and fruits, and breads and cereals) for an adult is two, two, four, and four, respectively. The table shows some of the major nutrients each food group supplies and offers specific examples of foods in each group. This information can help a diet planner design an adequate and balanced diet.

The plan also helps with calorie control. The foods color-coded with green boxes are lowest in calories within the group; those with yellow boxes are intermediate; and those with red boxes are highest in calories. A person who makes the minimum selections from the Four Food Group Plan need eat no more than 1200 to 1400 calories a day to achieve diet adequacy. For more calories, additions should be mostly from the plant food groups.

The beauty of the Four Food Group Plan lies in its simplicity and ease in learning. It may appear quite rigid but it can be used with great flexibility. For example, cheese can be substituted for milk because both supply the same nutrients (protein, calcium, and riboflavin) in about the same amounts. Legumes and nuts are alternatives for meats. The plan can also be adapted to casseroles and other mixed dishes and to different

Diet planning principles:

Adequacy—enough of each type of food

Balance—not too much of any type of food

Calorie control—not too many calories

Economy—not too expensive

Moderation—not too much fat or sugar

Variety—as many different foods as possible

The more nutrients and the fewer calories a food offers relative to a person's needs, the greater that food's **nutrient density.**

nutrient density: the amount of nutrients a food contains relative to the calories it contains. The higher the nutrients and lower the calories, the more nutrient dense the food.

national and cultural cuisines. A study of the plan and some thought about the questions asked in this chapter's Personal Focus should provide the information you need to obtain a virtual guarantee of diet adequacy.

What if you are not the person who buys and prepares the food you eat? You can still exercise sound nutrition judgment in the choices you make. First of all, when you are hungry, eat; and eat a balanced meal. Second, learn to identify the more nutritious foods. Figure 7–4 and the box entitled *Terms on Food Labels* show how you can use food labels to make informed choices.

Here are some pointers to help you choose nutritious foods:

- Given the choice between whole foods and refined, processed foods, choose the former (apples rather than apple pie; potatoes rather than french fries). The whole foods are more nutrient dense; fewer nutrients have been refined out of them; less fat, salt, and sugar have been added.
- Fill your plate with vegetables and unrefined starchy foods. A small portion of meat or milk is all you need for protein.
- Use both raw and cooked vegetables and fruits. Cooking foods affects them for the better in some ways, but for the worse in others. It destroys some vitamins and some fiber, but makes some vitamins and minerals more available, and makes food easier to digest.
- When choosing meats, choose the lean ones. Select fish or poultry often, beef seldom. Ask for broiled, not fried foods, to control your fat intake.
- Include milk or milk products daily—two cups or more—for the calcium you need; or make wise substitutions. Use low-fat or non-fat items to save calories to spend on other foods.
- When choosing breads and cereals, choose the whole-grain varieties.
- Learn to use margarine, butter, and oils sparingly; only a little gives flavor; a lot overloads you with fat and calories.
- Vary your choices. Eat broccoli today, carrots tomorrow, and corn the next day. Eat Chinese today, Italian tomorrow, and hot dogs and beans on Saturday.

The Quick Tips on page 157 sum up these pointers for choosing nutritious foods.

When you go to a fast-food place, choose the more nutrient dense items:

- The plain broiled sandwich with lettuce, tomatoes, and other goodies—and hold the mayo—rather than the patties or nuggets coated with breadcrumbs and cooked in fat.
- The salad bar—and use more plain raw vegetables than those mixed with oily or mayonnaise-based dressings.
- Chili, with more beans than meat.
- Milk or orange juice rather than a cola beverage.

FIGURE 7-4 • How to Read a Food Label

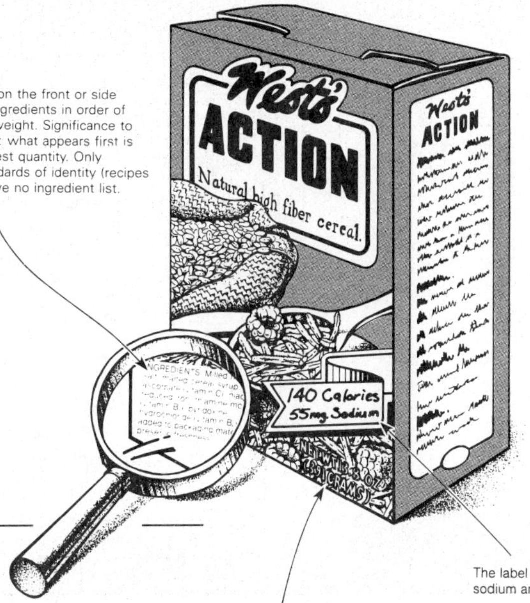

The ingredient list on the front or side panel names the ingredients in order of predominance by weight. Significance to you, the consumer: what appears first is present in the largest quantity. Only products with standards of identity (recipes defined by law) have no ingredient list.

The label may also state information about sodium and kcalories.

The front of the package must always tell you the product name, the name and address of the company, and the weight or measure; and it may list the ingredients.

Nutrition Information (per serving)[a]
Serving Size = ½ c
Servings per Container = 10

	Cereal	With ½ c nonfat milk (Vitamins A- and D-fortified)[b]
Calories	140	180
Protein (g)[c]	4	8
Total carbohydrates (g)[d]	32	38
Simple sugars (g)	11	17
Complex carbohydrates (g)	17	17
Fiber (g)	4	4
Fat (g)[e]	1	1
Cholesterol (mg)	0	0
Sodium (mg)[f]	55	120

Percentage of U.S. Recommended Daily Allowances (U.S. RDA)[g]

	Cereal	With milk
Protein	6	15
Vitamin A	4	10
Vitamin C	*	2
Thiamin	25	30
Riboflavin	25	35
Niacin	25	25
Calcium	2	15
Iron	25	25

*Contains less than 2% of the U.S. RDA of this nutrient.

[a]The nutrition information panel tells you the nutrients in a serving. The serving size may or may not be the same as the amount you eat. Check the servings per container to get an idea if it is.

[b]The nutrient contents are listed in the food and as served (after adding milk, in this example).

[c]The energy-yielding nutrients are given in grams (units of weight). This is especially meaningful with respect to protein, because you need 40 to 80 g/day, depending on your size and other factors. Protein is also given in percentage of U.S. RDA in the list below.

[d]The carbohydrate breakdown tells you how much simple sugar, starch, and dietary fiber is in the product.

[e]A fat breakdown may also be listed, including saturated fat, unsaturated fat, and cholesterol.

[f]Sodium is listed in milligrams. A safe minimum intake is 500 mg sodium/day; recommendations limit salt intake to 6,000 mg salt/day (2,400 mg sodium/day). A teaspoon of salt contains just over 2,000 mg sodium.

[g]Protein, vitamins, and minerals are given in percentages of U.S. RDA. Significance to you, the consumer: If it meets 10% of the U.S. RDA, it almost undoubtedly meets at least 10% of your daily needs.

Cholesterol terms:

cholesterol-free: less than 2 mg per serving.

low-cholesterol: less than 20 mg per serving.

reduced cholesterol: processed to reduce the cholesterol by at least 75 percent compared with the original.

Energy terms:

diet, dietetic: terms used to indicate that a food is either *low in calories* or a *reduced calorie* food.

light, lite: for alcoholic beverages, 20 percent fewer calories than regular products; for meat products, 33 percent fewer. For other foods, the terms have no definition, but can mean light in color, texture, or taste, or it can mean reduced in some component.[a]

low-calorie: no more than 40 calories per serving or 0.9 calories per gram.

reduced-calorie: containing at least a third fewer calories than the food it most closely resembles.

Fat terms (these apply only to meat and poultry products):

extra lean: 95 percent fat free.

lean or lowfat[b]: not more than 10 percent fat by weight.

leaner, lower fat: reduced in fat by 25 percent when compared to the company's regular product.

Sodium terms:

low-sodium: 140 mg or less per serving.

reduced-sodium: processed to reduce the usual level of sodium by 75 percent.

sodium-free: less than 5 mg per serving.

unsalted, no added salt, salt-free: no salt added during processing, but not necessarily low in sodium.

very-low-sodium: 35 mg or less per serving.

Sugar terms:

sugar-free, sugarless, no added sugar: does not contain sucrose, but may contain other sweeteners.

Weight terms:

gram: a unit of weight. A teaspoon of any dry powder (such as salt) weighs about 5 grams. A half-cup of food (such as vegetables) or liquid (such as milk or juice) weighs about 100 grams.

milligram: 1/1000 of a gram.

continued

9. Fast foods can be nutritious.

True.

When you get home, add the fruit and the dark green vegetables that were missing earlier. Even the best fast foods pack more calories, fat, and more sodium than a whole day's worth of home-cooked foods, but a fast-food meal once in a while is not inconsistent with a nutritionally healthy lifestyle.

Even if you have to eat food from a vending machine, there are more and less nutritious choices:

- Choose cracker sandwiches over chips and pork rinds (which are virtually pure fat).
- Choose peanuts, pretzels, and popcorn over cookies and candy.
- Choose milks and juices over cola beverages.

No doubt you can create other ideas from the facts in this chapter. Apply them. And keep on learning about nutrition; it is worth a lot to your wellness.

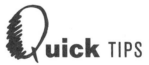

Quick TIPS

Choosing Nutritious Foods

- Choose whole foods rather than refined, processed foods.
- Fill your plate with vegetables.
- Choose both raw and cooked vegetables and fruits.
- Choose lean meats.
- Include milk or milk products every day.
- Choose whole-grain breads and cereals.
- Use margarine, butter, and oils sparingly.
- Vary your choices.

PERSONAL FOCUS

How Is Your Nutrition?

This Personal Focus and Lab Report 7 enable you to evaluate your own eating habits. The more points you get (see Lab Report 7 for scoring), the better your nutritional health is likely to be.

Part 1 — Milk and Milk Products	Response
1. I have two or more cups of milk or the equivalent in milk products every day.	Yes/No
2. I drink low-fat (2 percent or less butterfat) or nonfat milk rather than whole milk.	Yes/No
3. I eat ice cream or ice milk twice a week at the most.	Yes/No
4. I seldom have more than about three teaspoons of margarine or butter per day.	Yes/No

Part 2 — Meats and Meat Alternates	Response
5. I usually limit my meat, fish, poultry, or egg servings to one or two a day.	Yes/No
6. I eat red meats (beef, ham, lamb, or pork) not more than about three times a week.	Yes/No
7. I remove fat or ask that fat be trimmed from meat before cooking.	Yes/No
8. I eat about three or four eggs per week, including those cooked with other foods.	Yes/No
9. I sometimes have meatless days and eat such protein-rich foods as legumes and nuts.	Yes/No
10. I usually broil, boil, bake, or roast meat, fish, or poultry; I usually don't fry it.	Yes/No

Part 3 — Vegetables and Fruits	Response
11. I usually have one serving (½ cup) of citrus fruit or juice (oranges, grapefruit, and so forth) each day.	Yes/No
12. I have at least one serving of dark green or deep orange vegetables each day.	Yes/No
13. I eat fresh fruits and vegetables when I can get them.	Yes/No
14. I cook vegetables without fat (if I use margarine, I add it after cooking).	Yes/No
15. I eat fresh fruit at the end of a meal more often than desserts.	Yes/No

continued

Part 4 — Breads and Cereals	Response
16. I generally eat whole-grain breads and cereals.	Yes/No
17. Most of the breads and cereals I eat are high in fiber.	Yes/No
18. The breads and cereals I eat have little or no sugar added.	Yes/No
19. I generally eat brown rice in preference to white rice.	Yes/No
20. I generally have at least four servings of bread or cereal grains each day.	Yes/No

Part 5 — Extra Foods and Calories	Response
21. I am usually within 5 to 10 pounds of the weight considered appropriate for my height.	Yes/No
22. I drink no more than two drinks of alcoholic beverages a day.	Yes/No
23. I do not add salt to food after preparation and generally use foods salted lightly or not salted at all.	Yes/No
24. I try to avoid foods high in sugar and use sugar sparingly.	Yes/No
25. I usually eat a breakfast of at least cereal and milk, egg and toast, or other protein-carbohydrate combination with fruit or fruit juice.	Yes/No

Source: Adapted with permission from Roger Sargent, *Have a Good Life* series (Greenville, S.C.: Liberty Life).

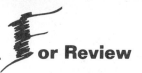

For Review

1. Describe what is meant by a *balanced meal* (page 139).
2. Explain why, although starch and sugar are both carbohydrates, starchy foods confer greater benefits on the body (page 142).
3. Identify foods high in fiber (page 141).
4. Identify some symptoms of deficiencies of several vitamins and minerals (page 144).
5. Describe strategies for putting diet planning principles into practice (page 154).

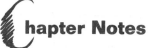

Chapter Notes

1. N. B. Belloc and L. Breslow, Relationship of physical health status and health practices, *Preventive Medicine* 1 (1972): 409–421.
2. U.S. Department of Health and Human Services, Public Health Service, *Promoting Health, Preventing Disease: Objectives for the Nation* (Washington, D.C.: Government Printing Office, 1980), as cited in M. Nestle, Promoting health and preventing disease: National nutrition objectives for 1990 and 2000, *Nutrition Today* June, 1988, pp. 26–30.
3. Improved nutrition, *Public Health Reports Supplement,* September/October 1983, p. 132.
4. T. B. Van Itallie, Health implications of overweight and obesity in the United States, *Annals of Internal Medicine* 103 (1985): 983–988, as cited in M. R. C. Greenwood and V. A. Pittman-Waller, Weight control: A complex, various, and controversial problem, in R. T. Frankle and M. U. Yang, *Obesity and Weight Control: The Health Professional's Guide to Understanding and Treatment:* (Rockville, Md.: Aspen Publication, 1988), pp. 3–15.
5. U.S. Department of Health and Human Services, 1980, as cited in Nestle, 1988.
6. D. Lonsdale and R. J. Shamberger, Red cell transketolase as an indicator of nutritional deficiency, *American Journal of Clinical Nutrition* 33 (1980): 205–211.
7. L. C. Pauling, *Vitamin C and the Common Cold* (San Francisco: W. H. Freeman, 1970).
8. H. Schaumberg and coauthors, Sensory neuropathy from pyridoxine abuse, *New England Journal of Medicine* 309 (1983): 445–448.
9. More B_6 toxicity reported, *Nutrition Forum,* November 1985, p. 84.
10. N. S. Scrimshaw, Functional consequences of iron deficiency in human populations, *Journal of Nutrition Science and Vitaminology* 30 (1984): 47–63.
11. R. S. Gibson and coauthors, A growth limiting, mild zinc-deficiency syndrome in some southern Ontario boys with low height percentiles, *American Journal of Clinical Nutrition* 49 (1989): 1266–1273.
12. $2.9 billion for vitamins, *FDA Consumer*, April 1987, p. 4.
13. R. L. Koretz and J. H. Meyer, Elemental diets: Facts and fantasies, *Gastroenterology* 78 (1980): 393–410.
14. E. N. Whitney, E. M. N. Hamilton, and S. R. Rolfes, *Understanding Nutrition,* 5th ed. (St. Paul, Minn.: West, 1990), pp. 267–270.
15. L. Alhadeff, T. Gualtieri, and M. Lipton, Toxic effects of water-soluble vitamins, *Nutrition Reviews* 42 (1984): 33–40.

E I G H T

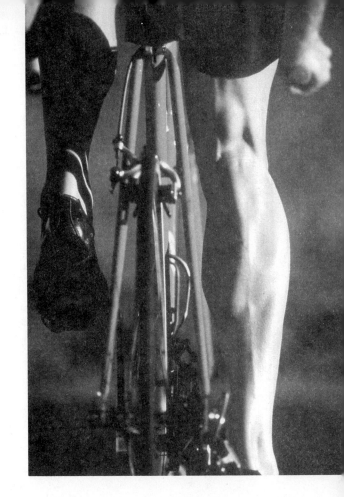

Contents

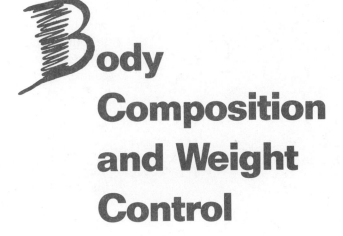

Body Composition and Weight Control

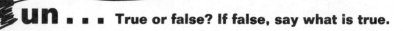
1. People can control their weight if they try (page 162).

2. Most of the energy you normally spend in a day is for breathing and other involuntary activities (page 163).

3. When you eat excess fat or carbohydrate, you store it as body fat; when you eat excess protein, you store it as muscle (page 167).

4. The fastest way to lose body *fat* is to stop eating (page 169).

5. If you're overweight on the scale, then face it: You're too fat (page 170).

6. If an inactive person begins exercising each day, the person will end up spending more calories all day, even during sleep (page 175).

7. Gaining weight is easier for underweight people than losing weight is for overweight people (page 180).

8. Dancers can never be too thin (page 182).

9. Binging and purging are rare and pathological behaviors (page 185).

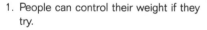

1. People can control their weight if they try.

False.

People can control only their behavior, but this may affect their weight in the way they hope it will.

Are you pleased with your body weight? If your answer is yes, you are a rare individual. Nearly all people in our society think they should weigh more or less (mostly less) than they do. People also think they can control their weight. A pair of misconceptions makes their task difficult. The first focuses on *weight;* the second focuses on *controlling* weight. To put it simply, it isn't body *weight* you need to control; it's the amount of *fat* on your body in proportion to the amount of lean tissue, and it isn't possible to control that directly. You can control only your *behavior.* This chapter, therefore, dedicates most of its space to behaviors that achieve weight control.

The Energy Budget: A Balancing Act

Your body's weight reflects its composition—the total mass of its bone, muscles, fat, fluids, and other tissues. The more of any of these you have, the more you weigh. All of your body components can vary in quantity and quality—the bones can be dense or porous; the muscles can be well developed or underdeveloped, fat, abundant or scarce, and so on. One tissue, though, stands out as by far the most variable: Your body fat. Fat is the material in which the body can store the most food energy; it is fat that responds most to changes in food intake and exercise; and it is fat that is usually the target of efforts at weight control.

If a person's weight is within the appropriate range for height, the person has a balanced energy budget. Deposits of fat made at one time have been compensated for by withdrawals made at another: Food energy intake has equaled energy expenditure. In other words, your body fat is similar to a savings account; it differs from money only in that more is not better; there is an optimum. A day's energy balance can be stated like this:

Change in body fat stores (calories) = Food energy taken in (calories) − Energy spent on metabolic and other activities (calories).

More simply:

Change in fat stores (calories) = Energy in (calories) − Energy out (calories).

You know about the "energy in" side of this equation. An apple gives you about 100 calories; a candy bar contains about 300 calories. (Calorie amounts for several hundred foods are listed in Appendix D.) On the "energy out" side, if you are physically active for an hour, you may spend 100, 300, or even 500 calories or more. For each 3,500 calories you eat in excess of expenditures, you store one pound of body fat.*

The body spends energy in two major ways: To fuel its **basal metabolism** and to fuel its **voluntary activities.** You can change your voluntary activities to spend more or less energy in a day, and over time you can also change your basal metabolism, as explained later.

The basal metabolism supports the work that goes on all the time without conscious awareness. The beating of the heart, the inhaling and exhaling of air, the maintenance of body temperature, and the sending of nerve and hormonal messages to direct these activities are the basal processes that maintain life. Basal metabolic needs are surprisingly large. A person whose total energy needs are 2,000 calories a day spends 1,200 to 1,400 of them to support basal metabolism. The box entitled "Estimation of Energy Output" shows you how to estimate your energy expenditure for basal metabolism.

The number of calories spent on voluntary activities depends on three factors. The larger the muscle mass required, the heavier the weight of the body part being moved, and the longer the activity takes, the more calories are spent. Table 8−1 shows the approximate number of calories required for various activities. How much energy an activity costs also depends on several other things. One is the intensity of the activity: The more intense, the more calories are spent per minute. Another is the person's style: The streamlined moves of an expert swimmer, for example, cost less than the movements of the untrained swimmer.

basal metabolism: the sum total of all the involuntary chemical activities of the cells necessary to sustain life. Basal metabolism, sometimes called *basal metabolic rate (BMR)*, is normally the largest component of a person's daily energy expenditure.

voluntary activities: the component of a person's daily energy expenditure that involves conscious and deliberate muscular work—walking, lifting, climbing, and other physical activities. Voluntary activities normally account for a smaller component of daily energy expenditure than basal metabolism does.

2. Most of the energy you normally spend in a day is for breathing and other involuntary activities.

True.

*Pure fat is worth 9 calories per gram. A pound of it (450 grams), then, would store 4,050 calories. A pound of body fat is not pure fat, though; it contains water, protein, and other materials, and thus has a lower calorie value.

Basal Metabolism. Convert your body weight from pounds to kilograms and then use the factor 1.0 calorie per kilogram of body weight per hour for men, or 0.9 for women.* Example (for a 150-pound man):

1. Change pounds to kilograms:

   Example: 150 lb ÷ 2.2 lb/kg = 68 kg.

2. Multiply weight in kilograms by the BMR factor:

   Example: 68 kg × 1 cal/kg/hour = 68 cal/hour.

3. Multiply calories used in one hour by the hours in a day:

   Example: 68 cal/hour × 24 hours/day = 1,632 cal/day.

Energy for BMR equals 1,632 cal/day.

   Voluntary Muscular Activity. The following figures are crude approximations based on the amounts of muscular work people typically perform in a day. To select the category appropriate for you, remember to think in terms of the amount of *muscular* work performed; don't confuse being *busy* with being *active.* Calculate your energy need for activities using both percentages given for your gender and activity level. This will give you the range of energy needs appropriate for people similar to you.**

For sedentary (mostly sitting) activity (a typist), add 25 to 40% (*Men*) or 25-35% (*Women*) of the BMR.

For light activity (a teacher), add 50-70% (*Men*) or 40-60% (*Women*).

For moderate activity (a nurse), add 65 to 80% (*Men*) or 50-70% (*Women*).

For heavy work (a roofer), add 90 to 120% (*Men*) or 80-100% (*Women*) or more.

For exceptional activity (a football player), add 130–145% (*Men*) or 110–130% (*Women*).

Suppose the man we are using as an example is a student who bikes about 10 minutes a day, and walks to classes but otherwise sits and studies. To estimate the energy he needs for physical activities (light), first multiply his BMR calories per day by 50% and then by 70%:

   Example: 1,632 cal/day × 50% = 816 cal/day.
   1,632 cal/day × 70% = 1,142 cal/day.

   Energy for activities equals 816 cal/day to 1,142 cal/day.

   Total: The man in our example spends, in a day: 1,632 cal/day + 816 cal/day = 2,448 cal/day. *or* 1,632 cal/day + 1,142 cal/day = 2,774 cal/day.

Because the exact figure is based on several estimates, express the man's expenditure as falling within a range:

   Total energy spent equals about 2,448 to 2,774 cal/day.

*Men's metabolic energy needs are assumed to be higher than women's because their hormones induce them to develop more lean tissue than do most women, and lean tissue burns more energy per hour.
**Percentages derived from the RDA (1990) formula for energy expenditure within about twenty percent of total calories.

TABLE 8-1 • Energy Demands of Activities

Activity	Cal/lb/min[a]	Body Weight (lb) 110	125	150	175	200
		Calories per minute				
Aerobic dance (vigorous)	.062	6.8	7.8	9.3	10.9	12.4
Basketball (vigorous, full court)	.097	10.7	12.1	14.6	17.0	19.4
Bicycling						
13 miles-per-hour	.045	5.0	5.6	6.8	7.9	9.0
15 miles-per-hour	.049	5.4	6.1	7.4	8.6	9.8
17 miles-per-hour	.057	6.3	7.1	8.6	10.0	11.4
19 miles-per-hour	.076	8.4	9.5	11.4	13.3	15.2
21 miles-per-hour	.090	9.9	11.3	13.5	15.8	18.0
23 miles-per-hour	.109	12.0	13.6	16.4	19.0	21.8
25 miles-per-hour	.139	15.3	17.4	20.9	24.3	27.8
Cross-country skiing (8 miles-per-hour)	.104	11.4	13.0	15.6	18.2	20.8
Golf (carrying clubs)	.045	5.0	5.6	6.8	7.9	9.0
Handball	.078	8.6	9.8	11.7	13.7	15.6
Horseback riding (trot)	.052	5.7	6.5	7.8	9.1	10.4
Rowing (vigorous)	.097	10.7	12.1	14.6	17.0	19.4
Running						
5 miles-per-hour	.061	6.7	7.6	9.2	10.7	12.2
6 miles-per-hour	.074	8.1	9.2	11.1	13.0	14.8
7.5 miles-per-hour	.094	10.3	11.8	14.1	16.4	18.8
9 miles-per-hour	.103	11.3	12.9	15.5	18.0	20.6
10 miles-per-hour	.114	12.5	14.3	17.1	20.0	22.9
11 miles-per-hour	.131	14.4	16.4	19.7	22.9	26.2
Studying	.011	1.2	1.4	1.7	1.9	2.2
Soccer (vigorous)	.097	10.7	12.1	14.6	17.0	19.4
Swimming						
20 yards-per-minute	.032	3.5	4.0	4.8	5.6	6.4
45 yard-per-minute	.058	6.4	7.3	8.7	10.2	11.6
50 yards-per-minute	.070	7.7	8.8	10.5	12.3	14.0
Table tennis (skilled)	.045	5.0	5.6	6.8	7.9	9.0
Tennis (beginner)	.032	3.5	4.0	4.8	5.6	6.4
Walking (brisk pace)						
3.5 miles-per-hour	.035	3.9	4.4	5.2	6.1	7.0
4.5 miles-per-hour	.048	5.3	6.0	7.2	8.4	9.6

[a]To calculate calories spent per minute of activity for your own body weight, multiply cal/lb/min by your exact weight and then multiply that number by the number of minutes spent in the activity. For example, if you weigh 142 pounds, and you want to know how many calories you spent doing 30 minutes of vigorous aerobic dance: .062 × 142 = 8.8 calories per minute. 8.8 × 30 (minutes) = 264 total calories spent.

© 1983 by Consumers Union of United States, Inc., Mount Vernon, NY. Adapted by permission: Consumer Reports Books, 1983. *Physical Fitness for Practically Everybody: The Consumer's Union Report on Exercise*. Reprinted with permission of Ross Laboratories, Columbus, OH: from G.P. Town and K.B. Wheeler, Nutritional Concerns for the Endurance Athlete, *Dietetic Currents* 13 (1986): 7–12.

A typical breakdown of the total energy spent by a lightly active person (for example, a student who walks from class to class) might look like this:

a. Energy for basal metabolism: 1,400 calories
b. Energy for voluntary activities: 840 calories
            Total energy needs: 2,240 calories

You can obtain an estimate of the energy you spend on voluntary activities by using the rules of thumb shown in the "Estimation of Energy Output" box.*

As you can see, even for a somewhat active person, the larger component of the energy spent in a day is for basal metabolism. This surprises most people; they are not aware that they are spending any energy on these unconscious functions.

In summary, the energy you spend in a day is the sum of two components—your basal metabolic energy and your activity energy. The second of these, the activity energy, falls within a range of two values. To compute the range of total energy you spend in a day, calculate your metabolic energy, and the range of activity energy, and add them together as shown in the box. This expenditure represents your approximate energy need, which you meet by eating food. If you eat more than this, you will store the extra energy in your body, mostly as fat. If you eat less than this, you will use up body tissue as fuel to make up the deficit.

Weight Gain and Loss

When you step on the scale and note that you weigh a pound more or less than you did the last time you weighed, this usually means you have gained or lost body fat. However, it can reflect changes in other tissues such as body fluids or muscles. It is important for people concerned with weight control to realize this, because those who want to lose weight generally want to lose mostly fat, while those who want to gain want to gain muscle and fat.

Some people are unaware of the distinction between gains or losses of body fat and those of other tissues; all they see is a change in their weight on the scales. Overweight people may welcome any weight loss; underweight people may welcome any gain. However, weight gains that are gains of body fat alone are unhealthy; gains should be balanced among all tissues. Similarly, losses of body tissues should be balanced, but should certainly be mostly fat. Large losses of tissues other than fat are usually undesirable even though they may produce the most rapid changes on the scale. To lose fluid, for example, one can take a "water pill" (diuretic), causing the kidneys to siphon extra water from the blood

---

*A third component of energy expenditure is that the presence of food stimulates the general metabolism. This diet-induced thermogenesis, or the specific dynamic effect of food, is thought to represent about 6 to 10 percent of the total food energy taken in. For rough estimates, it can be ignored.

into the urine. Or one can exercise heavily in the heat, losing abundant fluid in sweat. However, both practices are dangerous. Most quick-weight-loss diets promote large fluid losses that register temporary, dramatic changes on the scale but accomplish little loss of body fat. The rest of this chapter underscores this distinction, and a later section on strategy stresses physical activity as a means of maintaining lean tissue during weight loss and gain.

Weight Gain

When you eat more food than you need, the energy-yielding nutrients in the food contribute to body stores as follows (see Figure 8–1):

- Carbohydrate is broken down to small units (sugars) for absorption. Inside the body, these may be built up to glycogen or converted to fat and stored.
- Fat is broken down to its component parts (including fatty acids) for absorption. Inside the body, these may be built up to fat for storage.
- Protein, too, is broken down to its basic units (amino acids) for absorption. Inside the body, these may be used to replace lost body protein. Any extra amino acids lose their nitrogen and are converted to fat.

3. When you eat excess fat or carbohydrate, you store it as body fat; when you eat excess protein, you store it as muscle.

False.

When you eat excess fat, carbohydrate, or protein, you store it as fat.

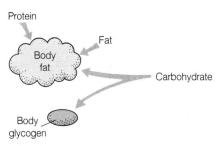

FIGURE 8-1 **Feasting and Fasting**

Excess energy nutrients from food are mainly stored as fat; a little carbohydrate is stored as glycogen.

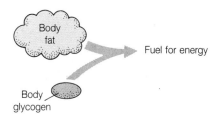

In times of little food, the body draws on its stored fat and glycogen for the fuel it needs; note that body stores cannot supply needed protein, even though food protein contributes to body fat.

Any food can make you fat. The total amount of calories is what makes the difference, and protein foods have calories, too.

Protein is not stored in the body to any great extent; it is present only as working tissue. Working protein tissue is lost each day and so it is desirable to eat protein each day.

RDA stands for Recommended Dietary Allowances, but they are amounts of nutrients recommended for *daily* consumption and so are often called daily allowances. See Appendix C.

The nervous system cannot use fat as fuel, only glucose.

Body fat cannot be converted to glucose.

Body protein can be converted to glucose.

Notice that although three kinds of energy nutrients enter the body, they are stored there in only two forms: Glycogen and fat. Also notice that when excess protein is converted to fat, it cannot be recovered later as protein. The amino acids "lose" their nitrogen—it is actually excreted in the urine. Whether you are eating steak, brownies, or baked beans, then, if you eat enough of them, the excess is turned to storage forms of energy within hours. And no matter how much protein you may eat today, you still need some more tomorrow (hence the RDA, Recommended *Daily* Allowances, for protein).

Weight Loss and Fasting

When the tables are turned and you eat less than you need, the body draws on its stored nutrients to keep going. Nothing is wrong with this; in fact, it is a great advantage to us that we can eat periodically, store fuel, and then use it up between meals. (Some animals, such as cattle, must spend virtually all their waking hours eating—a necessity that leaves them little time for self-improvement.) The between-meal interval is ideally about four to six daytime hours, or 12 to 14 nighttime hours. (Energy use slows down at night.) This is the length of time it takes to use up most of the glycogen that was stored at the last meal and to complete metabolism of the protein from that meal. At the end of that time, carbohydrate is again needed to replenish glycogen stores, and protein is again needed because all of the previous meal's amino acids have been either incorporated into body proteins or converted to fat.

If a person doesn't eat for, say, three whole days or a week, the body makes one adjustment after another. After about a day, the liver's glycogen is essentially exhausted. The body needs glucose to keep its nervous system going and can't obtain it from the muscles' glycogen because that is reserved for the muscles' own use. Nor can it use the body's fat, at first, because the nervous system cannot use fat as fuel. The body's fat cannot be converted to glucose either because the body possesses no enzymes to perform this chemical reaction.* It does, however, possess enzymes to convert protein to glucose.

The body, therefore, turns to its own lean tissues to keep up the supply of glucose for its brain and nervous system. The reason why people who fast lose weight so dramatically within the first three days is that they are devouring their own protein tissues as fuel; since protein contains only half as many calories per pound as fat, it disappears twice as fast; and with each pound of body protein, three or four pounds of associated water are also lost.

If the body were to continue to consume itself at this rate, death would ensue within about ten days. Fasting or starving people remain alive only until their body fat is gone or until half their lean tissue is gone, whichever comes first. But now the body plays its last ace: It begins converting fat stores into a form it can use to help feed the nervous system and so forestall the end. This is **ketosis.**

*Glycerol, 5 percent of fat, can yield glucose but it is a negligible source.

ketosis (kee-TOE-sis): an adaptation of the body to prolonged (several days) fasting or carbohydrate restriction: Body fat is converted to ketone bodies, which can be used as fuel for some brain cells.

ketone bodies: products of the incomplete breakdown of fat when carbohydrate is not available.

4. The fastest way to lose body *fat* is to stop eating.

False.

A low-calorie diet can promote the same rate of *weight* loss, and a faster rate of *fat* loss, than a total fast.

In ketosis, the body combines partially broken-down fat fragments into **ketone bodies** (compounds that are normally rare in the blood), and lets them circulate in the bloodstream. About half of the brain's cells can use these compounds for energy. Thus, indirectly, the nervous system begins to feed on the body's fat stores. This reduces the need for glucose, spares lean tissue from being devoured so quickly, and prolongs the starving person's life. Thanks to ketosis, an initially healthy person deprived of food can live for as long as six to eight weeks.

Fasting has been practiced as a periodic discipline by respected, wise people in many cultures. However, ketosis may be harmful to the body. Some ketone bodies are acids, and when they are circulating in the blood, they can make the body fluids acidic, which is a dangerous condition. Besides, even in ketosis, the body's lean tissue continues to be lost at a rapid rate to supply glucose to those nervous system cells that cannot use ketones as fuel. Moreover, the body slows its metabolism during a fast to conserve energy. For the person who merely wants to lose weight, then, fasting is usually not the best way. A low-calorie diet has actually been observed to promote the same rate of *weight* loss, and a faster rate of *fat* loss, than a total fast.[1] Just how to design a low-calorie diet is the subject of a later section, and the hazards of low-carbohydrate diets are further described in Chapter 12.

Appropriate Weight

Both deficient and excessive body fat carry health risks. It has long been known that thin people will die first during a siege, in a famine, or in a concentration camp. Underweight also increases the risk for any person fighting a wasting disease. And while no serious hazards accompany *mild* degrees of underweight, underweight does pose hazards when it is accompanied by undernutrition. Thus, underweight people are urged to learn how to nourish themselves optimally—to gain lean tissue, to gain body fat as an energy reserve, and to acquire protective amounts of all the nutrients that can be stored.

As for overfatness, for one thing, it aggravates high blood pressure (hypertension). Often weight loss alone can normalize the blood pressure of an overfat person. Some people can tell exactly at what weight their blood pressure begins to rise. Weight gain can also precipitate diabetes in genetically susceptible people. If hypertension or diabetes runs in your family, you urgently need a sensible program to keep from getting too fat.

Excess body fatness also increases the risk of heart disease. Excess fat pads crowd the heart muscle within the body cavity, and excess blood fat leads to fat deposits in the arteries (atherosclerosis). Excess fat demands to be fed by miles of extra capillaries, increasing the heart's workload to the point of damaging it. Other conditions brought on or made worse by overfatness include abdominal hernias, breast and colon cancer, varicose veins, gout, gallbladder disease, arthritis, respiratory problems, complications in pregnancy, and even a high accident rate. The health risks of overfatness are so many that it has been declared a disease: **Obesity.** If you are obese, you are urged to reduce. You can expect your health risks to diminish as you do.[2]

Obesity makes people vulnerable to still another health hazard: Fad diets, many of which are more hazardous to health than obesity itself. One survey of 29,000 weight-loss strategies found fewer than 6 percent of them effective—and 13 percent were dangerous.[3] Before making your diet plan, read the "Diet" section of this chapter, and to learn to evaluate fad diets, turn to Chapter 12.

A few obese people can escape these health problems for genetic reasons, but no one who is fat in our society quite escapes the social and economic handicaps. Fat people are less sought after for romance, they pay higher insurance premiums, they pay more for clothes, and they suffer job discrimination. Psychologically, too, a body size that embarrasses a person diminishes self-esteem.

All of these liabilities make clear the disadvantages of being too thin or too fat. How thin, then, is too thin—and how fat is too fat?

The traditional way of assigning desirable weights to people is to use one of the insurance company tables of weights for height, which used to be called the "ideal weight tables" (see Table 8–2). You find your height in the table; decide whether you have a small, medium, or large frame (see Table 8–3); and then find your weight range. That weight range is consistent with good health for most people, and you can narrow it down further, based on your own personal preferences. Traditionally, a weight 20 percent or more above the table weight defines obesity—that is, too much body fat for health; a weight 10 percent or more below the table weight defines **underweight** (too little body fat).

The use of body weight as an indicator of overfatness is unsatisfactory for some purposes. For one thing, as mentioned, weight and fatness do not always coincide: A healthy person with dense bones and muscles may seem overweight on the scale, while a person whose scale weight seems reasonable may have too much body fat for health.

A standard derived from height and weight measures that is useful for estimating the risk to health associated with obesity is the **body mass index (BMI),** which can be obtained from Figure 8–2. A body mass index of greater than 27.8 in men or 27.3 in women indicates the need for weight reduction. This chapter's Personal Focus shows you how to use both the traditional tables and the body mass index (see Figure 8–2) to arrive at a tentative answer to the question of what weight is appropriate for you. (BMI tables are on the inside back cover.)

When a person decides to lose or gain weight, that person would do well to examine the motive behind the decision. Is overweight or underweight truly a problem? Much precious effort is wasted when people chase a wild goose by dieting to attain a "perfect" body as seen in magazines or on television. That effort would be much better spent on things that actually need attention, such as stopping smoking, gaining physical fitness, or developing spiritual perspectives. Once a person decides that overweight or underweight is a real problem that demands attention,

underweight: weight too low for health.

Obesity is traditionally defined as weight 20 percent or more above the appropriate weight for height.

Underweight is traditionally defined as 10 percent below the appropriate weight for height.

body mass index (BMI): an index of a person's weight in relation to height.

The equation for BMI is weight (in kilograms) divided by height (in meters) squared.

5. If you're overweight on the scale, then face it: You're too fat.

   False.

   Weight and fatness do not always coincide: A person who seems overweight on the scale may have a healthy body.

TABLE 8-2 • The Weight Tables*

Men

Height

Feet	Inches	Small Frame	Medium Frame	Large Frame
5	2	128–134	131–141	138–150
5	3	130–136	133–143	140–153
5	4	132–138	135–145	142–156
5	5	134–140	137–148	144–160
5	6	136–142	139–151	146–164
5	7	138–145	142–154	149–168
5	8	140–148	145–157	152–172
5	9	142–151	148–160	155–176
5	10	144–154	151–163	158–180
5	11	146–157	154–166	161–184
6	0	149–160	157–170	164–188
6	1	152–164	160–174	168–192
6	2	155–168	164–178	172–197
6	3	158–172	167–182	176–202
6	4	162–176	171–187	181–207

Women

Height

Feet	Inches	Small Frame	Medium Frame	Large Frame
4	10	102–111	109–121	118–131
4	11	103–113	113–123	120–134
5	0	104–115	113–126	122–137
5	1	106–118	115–129	125–140
5	2	108–121	118–132	128–143
5	3	111–124	121–135	131–147
5	4	114–127	124–138	134–151
5	5	117–130	127–141	137–155
5	6	120–133	130–144	140–159
5	7	123–136	133–147	143–163
5	8	126–139	136–150	146–167
5	9	129–142	139–153	149–170
5	10	132–145	142–156	152–173
5	11	135–148	145–159	155–176
6	0	138–151	148–162	158–179

*Weights at ages 25 to 29 based on lowest mortality. Weights in pounds according to frame (in indoor clothing weighing 5 lb for men or 3 lb for women; shoes with 1-inch heels). For frame size standards, see Table 8–3.

Source: Reproduced with permission of Metropolitan Life Insurance Company. Source of basic data: Society of Actuaries and Association of Life Insurance Medical Directors of America, *1979 Build Study,* 1980.

TABLE 8–3 • Frame Size

To make a simple approximation of your frame size: Extend your arm, and bend the forearm upward at 90-degree angle. Keep the fingers straight, and turn the inside of your wrist away from the body. Place the thumb and index finger of your other hand on the two prominent bones on *either side* of your elbow. Measure the space between your fingers against a ruler or a tape measure.[a] Compare the measurements with the following standards.[b]

Men

Height in 1-Inch Heels	Elbow Breadth
5 ft. 2 inches to 5 ft. 3 inches	2 ½ to 2 ⅞ inches
5 ft. 4 inches to 5 ft. 7 inches	2 ⅝ to 2 ⅞ inches
5 ft. 8 inches to 5 ft. 11 inches	2 ¾ to 3 inches
6 ft. 0 inches to 6 ft. 3 inches	2 ¾ to 3 ⅛ inches
6 ft. 4 inches and over	2 ⅞ to 3 ¼

Women

Height in 1-Inch Heels	Elbow Breadth
4 ft. 10 inches to 4 ft. 11 inches	2 ¼ to 2 ½ inches
5 ft. 0 inches to 5 ft. 3 inches	2 ¼ to 2 ½ inches
5 ft. 4 inches to 5 ft. 7 inches	2 ⅜ to 2 ⅝ inches
5 ft. 8 inches to 5 ft. 11 inches	2 ⅜ to 2 ⅝ inches
6 ft. 0 inches and over	2 ½ to 2 ¾ inches

[a]For the most accurate measurement, have your health care provider measure your elbow breadth with a caliper.

[b]These standards represent the elbow measurements for medium-framed men and women of various heights. Measurements smaller than those listed indicate you have a small frame and larger measurements indicate a large frame.

Source: Metropolitan Life Insurance Company.

they must get ready to make a long-term commitment. The following sections offer strategies for losing or gaining weight.

Weight-Loss Strategies

How can a person lose weight safely and permanently? The secret is a sensible approach (we didn't say *easy*) that combines diet, physical activity, and behavior modification. It takes tremendous dedication, especially at first, for a person whose habits have all promoted obesity to adopt as habits the hundred or so new behaviors that promote thinness. When people succeed, they do so because they have employed many of the techniques described in this chapter.[4]

To emphasize the personal nature of weight-loss plans, the following sections are written as advice to "you." This is intended to give you the

	Men	Women
Underweight	<20.7	<19.1
Acceptable weight	20.7 to 27.8	19.1 to 27.3
Overweight	·27.8	·27.3
Severe overweight	·31.1	·32.3
Morbid obesity	·45.4	·44.8

Source: From the 1983 Metropolitan Life Insurance Company tables, designed by B. T. Burton and W. R. Foster, Health Implications of Obesity, an NIH Consensus Development Conference, *Journal of the American Dietetic Association* 85 (1985): 1117–1121.

FIGURE 8–2 Nomogram for Body Mass Index Find and mark your height on the left scale and your weight on the right scale. Draw a straight line between them and note where the line crosses the center scale. Read off your BMI from that scale and compare with the table above. **Note:** weights and heights in the figure are without clothing.

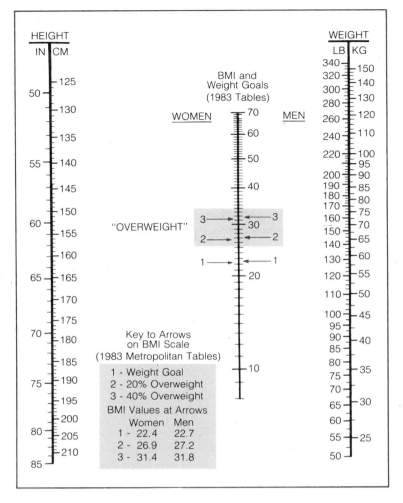

illusion of listening in on a conversation in which an obese person is being competently counseled by someone familiar with the techniques known to be effective.

Diet Planning

Strategies for diet planning:

1. Be involved in planning your own program.

The key to planning a diet for weight control *is* control: Yours. You are the one who will have to live with the meals, so you had better plan them. If you want to follow a commercial program, choose one that will help you to take responsibility, not one that takes it from you. Go to Weight Watchers or a similar program; do not get involved in a scam. (To identify scams, turn to Table 12–1 in Chapter 12.) No particular diet is magical, and no particular food must be either included or avoided. Don't think of it as a diet you are going "on", because then you may be tempted to go "off." Think of it as an eating plan that you will adopt for life. It must consist of foods that you like or can learn to like, that are available to you, and that are within your means.

2. Keep in mind that you will want to maintain your lost weight. Practice the needed behaviors as you go.

3. Adopt a realistic plan.

4. Make your meals adequate by emphasizing high-nutrient-density foods that you like.
5. Make tasty vegetables and fruits central to your weight-control plan.

6. Select complex carbohydrate-rich foods high in bulk.

7. Select low-fat foods regularly.

8. Drink plenty of water.

To be successful, people must first lose weight and then maintain the weight loss. If you adopt an "eating plan" rather than a "diet," you can be practicing maintenance behaviors all the time you are losing weight. You will be ready to succeed for the rest of your life, once you arrive at your goal weight.

Choose a calorie level you can live with. A deficit of 500 calories a day for seven days is a 3,500-calorie deficit—enough to lose a pound of body fat. It is best to do this by both increasing activity and reducing food intake. A rule of thumb is that you need to eat at least 10 calories for each pound of your current weight each day. There is no point in hurrying because you will never go off the plan—and adequate nutrient intakes can't be achieved on too few calories.

Make your meals adequate. This is a way of putting yourself first. "I like me, and I'm going to take good care of me" is the attitude to adopt. This means including low-calorie foods that are rich in valuable nutrients: Tasty vegetables and fruits; whole-grain breads and cereals; modest portions of lean protein-rich foods like poultry, fish, and eggs; nutritious meat alternates like dried beans and peas; and low-fat milk products such as nonfat milk and yogurt. A recommended pattern to follow is the Four Food Group Plan in Chapter 7. A plan that uses the minimum servings without frills and allows a teaspoon of added fat at each meal provides less than 1,200 calories; most people can lose weight at a satisfactory rate following such a plan and can meet their nutrient needs, too. Within each food group, learn what foods you like and use them often. If you plan resolutely to include a certain number of servings of food from each group each day, you may be so busy making sure you get what you need that you will have little time or appetite left for high-calorie or empty-calorie foods.

Slow down. The signal that you are full is sent after a 20-minute lag, so unless you slow down, you can eat a great deal more than you need before the signal reaches your brain.

Foods such as vegetables and whole grains (complex carbohydrate foods) require more chewing, so they can help you to slow down. Besides, crunchy, wholesome foods offer bulk and satisfy the appetite for far fewer calories than smooth, refined foods. People who eat crunchy, fibrous foods in abundance have been observed to spontaneously eat for longer times and to eat a fourth to a third fewer calories than when eating foods of high-calorie density.[5] This switch alone, consistently made, can enable you to reduce your energy intake by 500 or so calories a day. You can eat until you are full and never miss the foods you've omitted.

Measure your dietary fat with extra caution. A slip of the butter knife adds even more calories than a slip of the sugar spoon. Fat is to be avoided for another reason too. Of two diets that offer the same number of calories, the one with less fat will put less fat on the body. Dietary fat tends to add to body fat, whereas dietary carbohydrate and fiber tend not to add so much body fat.[6]

Learn to satisfy your thirst with water. Overeaters often use food to satisfy thirst (food provides water, as you may recall). Instead, drink

9. Visualize a changed future self.

10. Take well-spaced weighings to avoid discouragement.

11. Use positive reinforcement. Never blame, never punish.

12. Be honest with yourself.

13. Stress personal responsibility.
14. Maintain self-esteem.

6. If an inactive person begins exercising each day, the person will end up spending more calories all day, even during sleep.

True.

plenty of water. A generous water intake will do several things for you. It will help to fill your stomach between meals, keep your mouth happy, and keep you busy. It will meet the water need that you formerly met by eating extra food. It is a calorie-free pleasure; cultivate it enthusiastically.

At first it may seem as if you have to spend all your waking hours thinking about and planning your meals. Such a massive effort is always required when a new skill is being learned. (You spent hours practicing writing the alphabet when you were in the first grade.) Although it is hard at first, after about three weeks, planning your meals will be much easier. Use positive imaging: See yourself as a person who "eats thin." Your new eating pattern will become a habit.

Do not weigh yourself more than every week or two. Gains or losses of a pound or more in a matter of days reverse themselves quickly; a smoothed-out average is what is real. Don't expect to lose continuously as fast as you did at first. A sizable water loss is common in the first week, but it will not happen again. If you have been working out lately, occasional weighings may show no loss, or even a gain. This may reflect a welcome development: The gain of lean body mass—just what you want, if you want to be healthy.

If you slip, don't punish yourself. Positive reinforcement is effective in changing behavior, but punishment seldom works. If you ate an extra 1,000 calories yesterday, don't try to eat 1,000 fewer calories today; it will only propel you into overeating again, and this can become an endless cycle. Just go back to your plan. On the other hand, you can plan ahead and budget for special occasions. If you want to celebrate your birthday with cake and ice cream, cut a few calories from your bread and milk allowances for several days *beforehand*. Your weight loss will be as smooth as if you had stayed with the daily plan.

You may have to get tough with yourself if you stop losing weight or start gaining unexpectedly. Ask yourself honestly (no one is listening in), "What am I doing wrong?" Seldom does an unpredicted weight plateau of any duration have no explanation in the dieter's own choices.

Finally, if you stop losing weight or begin to gain, be aware that you may be choosing that course. Your behavior is under your control. Rather than feeling guilty or that you are a failure, hold your head high and take the attitude, "This is me, and this is the way I am choosing to be right now."

Physical Activity

Physical activity makes many contributions to weight control. For one thing, it directly increases energy output. Remember Table 8–1: It shows how many calories each of many activities costs.

Activity also contributes to energy output in an indirect way—by increasing basal metabolism. It does this in two ways—today, and over the long term. Today, if you exercise vigorously (for an hour, for example), your metabolism may stay speeded up for several hours afterwards, even overnight. That will make a small contribution toward the loss of the pound you are currently working to lose. Over the long term, if you keep repeating such vigorous activity daily for many weeks, your body composition will gradually change to favor more lean tissue. Your metabolic rate will rise accordingly, because lean tissue is more active metabolically than fat tissue—and that, over still more time, will make a contribution toward continued weight loss or maintenance of a healthy weight. The more lean tissue you develop, the more calories you spend, and the more you can afford to eat. Eating more brings you both pleasure and nutrients. Exercise continues to maintain your raised metabolic rate for as long as you keep your body conditioned.

Another thing activity helps with is appetite control. People think that exercising will make them hungry, but this is not entirely true. Yes, active people do have healthy appetites, but immediately after a good workout, most people do not feel like eating. They want to shower; they may be thirsty; but they are not hungry. The reason is that the body has responded to the stress of exercise by mobilizing fuels from storage—glucose and fatty acids are abundant in the blood. (A physiologist would say you are in a "fed state.") At the same time, the body has suppressed its digestive functions. Hard physical work and eating are not compatible. You must calm down, put your fuels back in storage, and relax before you can eat. Thus exercise helps curb appetite, especially the inappropriate appetite that accompanies boredom, anxiety, or depression, which might prompt you to eat when you really do not need to. (Weight-control programs encourage you to go out and exercise when you're tempted to eat, but not really hungry. It will fill your time, relieve your mood, and curb your misleading appetite. Later, when true hunger comes, it will be appropriate to eat.)

Activity also helps reduce stress, as earlier chapters have shown. Since stress, too, is a cue to inappropriate eating behavior for many people, activity can help here, too.

Activity offers still more psychological benefits. The fit person looks and feels healthy, and high self-esteem accompanies these benefits. High self-esteem tends to support a person's resolve to persist in a weight-control effort, rounding out a beneficial cycle.

Weight loss *without* exercise can have a negative effect on body composition. A person who diets without exercising loses both lean and fat tissue, as described earlier. Now suppose the person then regains weight without exercising; the gain will be mostly fat. Finally, suppose the person eats the same amount as before. Because fat tissue burns fewer calories to maintain itself, the person's weight will zoom higher than before, the so-called **ratchet effect,** or **yoyo effect,** of dieting without exercise (Figure 8–3).

Clearly, then, physical activity is a beneficial part of a weight-control program. What kind of physical activity is best? For the person seeking to *lose* weight, the activities that burn the most *fat,* not necessarily the ones that burn the most *calories,* are the ones to choose. Intense exercise burns a lot of calories, but many of them come from glycogen, not fat. In any one person, the amount of fat burned is about the same above a certain

Benefits of physical activity in a weight-control program:

- Increased expenditure of energy today (including metabolic energy)
- Long-term increase (slight) in resting metabolic rate
- Control of inappropriate eating urges
- Stress reduction
- Physical, and therefore psychological, well-being
- High self-esteem

ratchet effect or **yoyo effect:** the effect of repeated rounds of dieting without exercise; the person rebounds to a higher weight and higher body fat content at the end of each round.

Thinness is not the same as fitness.

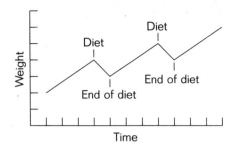

FIGURE 8-3 The Ratchet Effect of Dieting without Exercise Each round of dieting without exercise is followed by a rebound of weight to a higher level than before.

threshold of intensity—that is, you burn more and more fat per minute up to a certain threshold, but above that threshold, your fat use continues unchanged or even declines, and only your glycogen use increases. That is because above a certain intensity level, you can use only anaerobic fuel. Aerobic exercises or cardiovascular endurance exercises, therefore, are best.

This brings us to another point in favor of regular physical activity in weight control. The body that trains to do aerobic work develops greater and greater ability to use fat as an energy source, even at high intensities. (In other words, it raises the threshold, mentioned earlier, that limits fat-burning ability.) The conditioned athlete burns fat at an intensity level where the unconditioned person would be burning mostly glycogen. Therefore, training leads to the highly prized goal of being able to get the maximum fat-burning benefit of activity—to burn more calories and to burn more of them as fat.

People sometimes ask about "spot reducing." Can you lose fat in particular locations? Unfortunately, muscles do not "own" the fat that surrounds them. Fat cells release fat not into the underlying muscles, but into the blood, and the fat is shared by all the muscles. Spot-reducing exercises, therefore, do not work to take the fat from particular areas— and incidentally, neither do massage machines that claim to break up fat on trouble spots. Being moved passively by machines or pounded by massages takes off neither fat nor calories. You have to move your muscles, so choose active exercises.

Exercise can help with trouble spots in another way, though. Strengthening loose muscles in a trouble area can help to improve their condition; stretching to gain flexibility can help with associated posture problems. Thus, not only aerobic, but also strength and flexibility workouts, have their place in a weight-control routine.

This all adds up to a recommendation you might have guessed by the time you had finished reading Chapter 6. The best way to use physical activity to enhance weight control is to do it all—cultivate flexibility, strength, and endurance together with proper nutrition, and the desired body composition will follow.

Behavior Modification

The person who needs to gain control of a weight problem engages in a hundred small behaviors of overeating and underexercising every day, many of which have contributed to, and maintain, that weight problem. The person needs to learn to change all of these behaviors—and behavior modification can help. Figure 2–2 in Chapter 2 showed six strategies you could use to modify your behavior; in relation to eating and exercise, they might be phrased as follows:

1. Eliminate inappropriate eating cues.
2. Suppress the cues you cannot eliminate.
3. Strengthen cues to appropriate eating and exercise.
4. Engage in the desired eating and exercise behaviors.

1. *To eliminate inappropriate eating cues:*

   Don't buy problem foods (shop when you aren't hungry).
   Don't serve rich sauces and toppings.
   Let spouse and children buy, store, and serve their own sweets.
   Change channels or look away when the television shows food commercials.
   Shop only from a list and stay away from convenience stores.
   Carry appropriate snacks from home and avoid vending machines.

2. *To suppress the cues you cannot eliminate:*

   Eat only in one place, and in one room.
   Clear plates directly into the garbage.
   Create obstacles to the eating of problem foods (for example, make it necessary to unwrap, cook, and serve each one separately).
   Minimize contact with excessive food (serve individual plates, don't put serving dishes on the table, and leave the table when you are finished).
   Make small portions of food look large (spread food out, serve on small plates).
   Control states of deprivation (eat regular meals, don't skip meals, avoid getting tired, avoid boredom by keeping cues to fun activities in sight).

3. *To strengthen the cues to appropriate eating and exercise:*

   Encourage others to eat appropriate foods with you.
   Keep your favorite appropriate foods in the front of the refrigerator.
   Learn appropriate portion sizes.
   Save permitted foods from meals for snacks (and make these your only snacks).
   Prepare permitted foods attractively.
   Keep your ski poles (hiking boots, tennis racket) by the door.

4. *To engage in desired eating or exercise behaviors:*

   Slow down (pause for two to three minutes, put down utensils, chew slowly, swallow before reloading the fork, always use utensils).
   Leave some food on the plate.
   Move more (shake a leg, pace, fidget, flex your muscles).
   Join in and exercise with a group of active people.

5. *To arrange or emphasize negative consequences of inappropriate eating:*

   Eat your meals with other people.
   Ask that others respond neutrally to your deviations (make no comment). This is a negative consequence because it withholds attention.

   continued

6. *To arrange or emphasize positive consequences of appropriate behaviors:*

   Update records of food intake, exercise, and weight change regularly.

   Arrange for rewards for each unit of behavior change or weight loss.

   Ask for social reinforcement and encouragement.

5. Arrange or emphasize negative consequences of inappropriate eating.
6. Arrange or emphasize positive consequences of appropriate eating and exercise behaviors.

The "Behavior Modifications for Weight Loss" box shows how a person might apply each of these strategies to a weight-control program. Before you begin, establish a baseline, which is a record of your present eating behaviors against which to measure future progress. Keep a diary to learn what your particular eating stimuli, or cues, are.

More strategies for weight control:

1. Learn and practice assertiveness.

You may find it helpful to join a group such as TOPS (Take Off Pounds Sensibly), Weight Watchers, or Overeaters Anonymous. A modest expenditure for your own health is worthwhile (but avoid ripoffs, of course). Many dieters find it helpful to form their own self-help groups. If you are especially sensitive to social situations where you feel you have to eat, it will also help to have some assertiveness training. Learning to say "No, thank you" might be one of your first objectives. Learning not to "clean your plate" might be another.

2. Use small-step modification.

From all the behavior changes available to you, you can choose the ones to begin with. Don't try to master them all at once. No one who attempts too many changes at one time is successful. Set your own priorities. Pick one trouble area that you think you can handle, start with that, and practice your strategy until it is automatic. Then select another trouble area to work on, and so on.

Enjoy your new, emerging self. Inside every fat person is a thin person struggling to be freed. Get in touch with your thin self, and help that self to emerge comfortably.

Finally, be aware that it can be harder to maintain weight loss than to lose the weight. On arriving at the goal weight after months of self-discipline and new habit formation, the victorious weight loser must at all costs avoid "celebrating" by resuming old eating habits. They are gone forever—remember? Membership in an ongoing weight-control organization and regular, continued physical activity with others can give indispensable support for the formerly fat person who wants to remain trim.

Weight-Gain Strategies

It is as hard for a person who tends to be underweight to gain a pound as it is for a person who tends to be overweight to lose one. Like the weight-loser, the person who wants to gain must learn new habits and learn to like new foods.

Diet and Exercise

The person who is underweight has a special problem—deciding whether, and how, to try to gain. The first question to ask is whether the underweight represents a healthy or unhealthy state. It is well known that to be slightly under the table weight, for most people, represents a desirable state. But if the underweight is due to anorexia nervosa (see the later section, "Eating Disorders") or a wasting disease such as tuberculosis or cancer, it may be a dangerous state, and weight gain, if possible, may be indicated. The answer, then, is: If you are healthy at your present weight, stay there; if you are at risk of illness, try to gain. Medical advice can help you to make the distinction.

Some people may wish to gain weight for appearance's sake—provided that the gain is muscle and fat, not just fat. Athletes may wish, or be advised by their coaches, to gain weight to improve their performance. Such people need to be fully aware that a weight gain can be achieved only by physical conditioning combined with a high-calorie diet. A high-calorie diet alone will make a person gain fat only, and even if it makes the appearance look more acceptable in the person's own eyes, it is more likely to be detrimental than beneficial to health. Furthermore, some people are unalterably thin by reason of heredity or early environmental influences. Such people find it so difficult to gain weight that it seems not worth the trouble. In increasing food energy intake, such a person might gain some fat and become uncomfortable but would not achieve the desired change in body composition. In an athlete, a weight gain like this might impair performance.

Weight gain, like weight loss, is a highly individual matter. In deciding whether to undertake it, be as aware as you can be of what your body will permit and tolerate, and be willing to accept what you cannot change.

For the person who wants to gain weight, just as for the one who wants to lose, a combination of diet and exercise is best, but different considerations apply. For your choice of exercise, use strength training primarily, as discussed in Chapter 5. As you add exercise, you must eat additional calories to support that exercise—otherwise, you will lose weight (body fat). If you eat just enough to support the exercise, you will build muscle, but at the expense of body fat; that is, fat will be burned to support the muscle-building. If you eat more, you will gain both muscle and fat.

It takes an excess of about 2000 to 2500 calories, in theory, to support the gain of a pound of pure lean tissue.[7] The rate at which a person can build muscle tissue also depends on the person. Both men and women have a mixture of both male and female hormones; those with more male hormones build muscle more easily than others, but it is not known what

7. Gaining weight is easier for underweight people than losing weight is for overweight people.

False.

It is as hard for a person who tends to be underweight to gain a pound as it is for a person who tends to be overweight to lose one.

the limits are. (Chapter 12 provides cautions on the use of steroid hormones.) Conventional advice on diet to the bodybuilder is to eat about 700 to 1000 calories a day above normal energy needs; this is enough to support both the added exercise and the building of muscle.

If you want to gain weight, you may need to learn to eat different foods. No matter how many sticks of celery you consume, you won't gain weight very fast, because celery simply doesn't offer enough calories. The person who cannot eat much volume is encouraged to use calorie-dense foods in meals (the very ones the dieter is trying to stay away from). Use the items colored red in the Four Food Group Plan in Chapter 7. Yes, these foods are high in fat, but if they are contributing energy that will be spent sparing protein, they will not contribute to heart disease. They will help you to build a stronger body. Choose nutritious foods, but choose milkshakes instead of milk, peanut butter instead of lean meat, avocado instead of cucumber, whole-wheat muffins instead of whole-wheat bread. When you do eat celery, put cream cheese on it; add cream and sugar to coffee; use creamy dressings on salads, whipped cream on fruit, and sour cream on potatoes. (Because fat contains twice as many calories per teaspoon as sugar, it adds calories without adding much bulk.)

Eat more frequently. Make three sandwiches in the morning and eat them between classes, in addition to the day's three regular meals. Spend more time eating each meal: If you fill up fast, eat the highest calorie items first. Don't start with soup or salad; start with the main course. Drink between meals, not with them, to save space for higher calorie foods. Ask your health care provider for a liquid supplement to drink between meals — or make your own milkshakes. Always finish with dessert. Many an underweight person has simply been too busy (for months) to eat enough to gain or maintain weight. These strategies will help you to change this behavior pattern.

Expect to feel full, sometimes even uncomfortably so. Most underweight individuals are accustomed to small quantities of food. When they begin eating significantly more food, they complain of uncomfortable fullness. This is normal and it passes over time.

Behavior Modification

Behavior modification principles can work to change the behaviors of undereating as well as overeating. The person who needs to gain weight must, like the person who needs to lose weight, strengthen cues to appropriate eating and exercise (see the Box, "Behavior Modifications for Weight Loss"). The undereater might identify and select the cues that the overeater is trying to eliminate. For example, *do* snack while watching television; make large portions of food look small; relax more.

Eating Disorders

An estimated 2 million people, primarily girls and women, in the United States suffer from some form of eating disorder.[8] In developed nations such as the United States, society favors thinness. Magazines, newspapers, and television display camera-ready women, flaws concealed, unreasonably thin. The message is clear—the way you are isn't good enough. You are worthy only so long as you are lovely to look at. You should become like the cover girl who doesn't sweat; doesn't grow hair on her slender legs; has firm, small breasts, a flat stomach, a perfect face, small feet; and is always perfectly happy. If *you*, young woman or young man, are not perfectly happy, it is because your body is not beautiful enough. Acceptance of such unreasonable expectations has driven nearly everyone in our society to be engaged in the "pursuit of thinness."

Pursuing an appropriate body weight in a safe manner is healthy. An obsession with excessive thinness, however, can be dangerous. In fact, two eating disorders, **anorexia nervosa** and **bulimia,** focus on an obsession with, and an extreme pursuit of, thinness.

Anorexia Nervosa

The story of Julie illustrates a typical case of anorexia nervosa. Julie is 18 years old. She is a superachiever in school and in dance. She watches her diet with great care, and she exercises and practices ballet daily, maintaining a heroic schedule of self-discipline. She is thin, but she is not satisfied with her weight and is determined to lose more. She is 5 feet 6 inches tall and weighs 85 pounds.

She is unaware that she is undernourished, and she sees no need to obtain treatment. She stopped menstruating several months ago and has become moody. She insists that she is too fat, although her eyes lie in deep hollows in her face; she denies that she is ever tired although she is close to physical exhaustion, and she no longer sleeps easily.

Her family has characteristics that promote her obsession with thinness. Her mother is the dominant figure; her father is absent or distant; and they both value achievement and outward appearances more than an inner sense of self-worth and self-actualization. She values her parents' opinion and works hard to attain perfection for them.

Young women look to their male parent or parent substitute for important feedback on their self-worth, and when they don't receive it, they tend to be oversensitive to negative cultural influences such as the drive for thinness and the view of emaciation as beautiful.[9] Julie's father has alcoholism, and her mother left him a year ago. Anorexia, being obsessive-compulsive behavior, resembles an addiction, and often there are other addictions in the family.

As a child, when Julie cried with hunger, her parents didn't respond by feeding her. Rather, they fed her on a rigid schedule. They forced food on her at times when she didn't want it, and they withheld it when she was hungry; in short, they controlled her eating rather than letting her learn to respond to her own hunger signals. Now, she feels she has to control her eating from outside, as her parents did.

You may wonder how a person as thin as Julie could possibly continue to starve herself as she does. She is fiercely hungry, but she controls

anorexia nervosa: a disorder seen (usually) in teenage girls, characterized by self-starvation to the extreme.

bulimia (alternative spelling, **bulemia**) (byoo-LEEM-ee-uh): recurring binge eating, often associated with purging or laxative abuse after binging.

8. Dancers can never be too thin.

False.

Anyone can be dangerously thin.

her food intake with tremendous discipline. If she feels that she has slipped and eaten more than she intended, she runs or jumps rope until she is sure she has exercised it off, or takes laxatives to hasten the exit of the food from her system. (She is unaware that this doesn't work to reduce the calories.) It is her fierce determination to achieve self-control, not lack of hunger, that prevents her from eating.

The physical effects of anorexia nervosa are similar to those of starvation and can become life-threatening. They can escape notice, though, because thinness, being stylish, is often valued and even envied and encouraged rather than being recognized as a danger sign. Often the coach or dance teacher is in a position to detect the condition and point the way toward recovery.

athletic amenorrhea: cessation of menstruation associated with strenuous athletic training.

Excessive thinness and undereating combined with vigorous physical activity, even if not as extreme as that of anorexia nervosa, sets the stage for medical problems that need attention. One is **athletic amenorrhea**—cessation of menstruation associated with strenuous athletic training. Extreme depletion of body fat seems to interfere with the secretion of estrogen, a key hormone of the menstrual cycle. Since estrogen also helps maintain the bones, it seems that amenorrheic athletes may also be prone to bone loss—osteoporosis—and to **stress fractures,** bone breaks incurred by exercise.

stress fractures: bone damage or break caused by stress on bone surfaces during exercise.

As weight loss progresses to the extreme in the person with anorexia nervosa, blood pressure drops. The heart pumps less efficiently; its muscle becomes weak and thin, its chambers diminish in size, and its rhythms may change, with a characteristic abnormality appearing on the heart monitor. Sudden stopping of the heart, due to lean tissue loss or mineral deficiencies, accounts for many cases of sudden death among severely emaciated subjects. It is crucial that people with this condition be recognized and persuaded into treatment long before they reach this point. The Quick Tips suggest ways to accomplish this.

Treatment outcomes are better than they used to be. Residential treatment centers specializing in eating disorders are often especially successful. Three-quarters of those in treatment may regain weight up to within 25 percent of the desired weight. Half to three-quarters may resume normal menstrual cycles. About two-thirds fail to eat normally on follow-up, but they may eat better than they did before. About 6 percent die, 1 percent by suicide.*

Bulimia

Bulimia is a distinct eating disorder that shares some characteristics with anorexia nervosa. The case of Sophie illustrates the plight of the person with bulimia. Like the "typical" person with bulimia, Sophie is single,

*This is from a review of 19 studies of about 1,000 clients over a five-year period. Other deaths are from infection, heart disease, lung disease, and treatment-related causes including aspiration, electrolyte imbalance from intravenous therapy, and vitamin D poisoning. (M. A. Balaa and D. A. Drossman, *Anorexia Nervosa and Bulimia: The Eating Disorders, Disease-a-Month* (Chicago: Year Book Medical Publishers) June 1985, p. 34.)

Caucasian, in her early twenties, is well educated, and close to her ideal body weight. Sophie is a charming, intelligent woman who thinks constantly about food. She alternatively starves herself and binges, and when she has eaten too much, she vomits.

Her periodic binges take place in secret, usually at night, and they last an hour or more. She seldom lets binging interfere with her work or social activities, although a third of all bingers do. She is like most people with bulimia in that she starts the binge after having gone through a period of rigid dieting, so that her eating is accelerated by her hunger. Each time, she consumes thousands of calories of easy-to-eat, high-calorie food. Typically, she chooses cookies, cake, ice cream, or bread, although sometimes she binges on atypical foods, such as vegetables, when she is dieting. The binge is not like normal eating. It is a compulsion and usually occurs in several stages: "Anticipation and planning, anxiety, urgency to begin, rapid and uncontrollable consumption of food, relief and relaxation, disappointment, and finally shame or disgust."[10]

The physical cost of bulimia, like that of anorexia, is high. Immediately following a binge, Sophie pays the price of having swollen hands and feet, bloating, fatigue, headache, nausea, and pain. Repetition of this behavior causes more serious consequences. Fluid and electrolyte imbalance caused by vomiting can lead to abnormal heart rhythms and injury to the kidneys. Vomiting causes irritation and infection of the pharynx, esophagus, and salivary glands; erosion of the teeth; and dental caries. The esophagus may rupture or tear, as may the stomach. Sometimes the eyes become red from pressure on vomiting. The hands may be bruised and lacerated from scraping on the teeth while inducing vomiting.

Some people use **cathartics**—laxatives that can injure the lower intestinal tract. Others use **emetics** to induce vomiting; it was overuse of emetics that caused the death of popular singer Karen Carpenter in 1983.

cathartic: a strong laxative.

emetic (em-ETT-ic): an agent that causes vomiting.

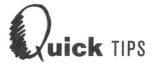

Strategies for Helping Someone Who has an Eating Disorder

If you suspect a person has an eating disorder:

- Approach the person privately and keep the person's condition confidential.
- Describe to the person nonjudgmentally the behaviors and physical findings that concern you.
- Ask if the person is having problems with weight control or food.
- Seek the person's willingness to obtain treatment or at least professional attention—this is indispensable to success.
- Arrange for contact with a knowledgeable professional. The most successful approach is a team approach involving a nutrition expert and a psychologist.[11]

The behavioral and psychological consequences of bulimia are severe. The rates of alcohol, marijuana, and cigarette use and of depression among bulimics are high.[12] For these reasons, a mental health professional should be one of the members on the treatment team.

Family dynamics suggest some clues to what makes a person bulimic. Much like Julie, who has anorexia nervosa, Sophie has been a high-achiever with a strong feeling of dependence on her parents. Her mother is a bright, well-educated woman who chose to stay at home with the children; her father is a powerful and respected but distant figure.

Her family often combined hearty eating with much socializing around the dinner table. Food was always involved in celebrations and used to console the family during periods of mourning. She felt it would be disrespectful to not celebrate or mourn by not eating; equally strong was the demand to be thin.

Sophie feels inadequate because she is unable to control her eating, and so she tends to be passive and to look to men for confirmation of her sense of worth. When she is rejected, either in reality or in her imagination, her bulimia becomes worse; in fact, many women point to male rejection as the event that led to the first binge.[13]

Both anorexia nervosa and bulimia occur only in developed nations and become more prevalent as wealth increases. The incidence of anorexia in our country and in other industrially advanced countries is steadily increasing. The disease afflicts women mostly (although men are not immune), and it now occurs in almost 1 of every 100 women.[14]

Bulimia occurs more frequently than anorexia nervosa. Although bulimia predominantly afflicts women, bulimia is more common among men than anorexia. More people are claiming to have bulimia than ever before. In a survey of 300 suburban women shoppers in Boston, over 10 percent reported a history of bulimia, and almost 5 percent were currently practicing it.[15] Among college women, the incidence may range anywhere from 5 to 20 percent.

The causes of both bulimia and anorexia nervosa are unknown, but one school of thought labels them as social problems. Perhaps they began when privileged young women internalized a message of their own low worth and adopted the ideal of some unachievable, "perfect" image.

Slowly, society is changing. Recognition of the success and desirability of a growing number of outstanding women in such traditionally male-dominated fields as athletics, science, law, and politics has raised women's collective self-esteem. Perhaps anorexia nervosa and bulimia will disappear as feminine roles and ideals change. Prevention may be most effective if begun early in children's lives. Warnings to children that the Madison Avenue female figure is simply an advertising gimmick designed to sell products, and not an ideal with which to compare one's own living body, may help. The simple concept—to respect and value your own uniqueness—may be lifesaving for a future generation.

9. Binging and purging are rare and pathological behaviors.

False.

Among college women, the incidence of binging and purging may be as high as 20 percent.

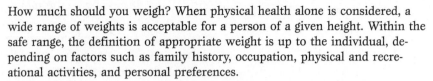

PERSONAL FOCUS What Is an Appropriate Weight for You?

How much should you weigh? When physical health alone is considered, a wide range of weights is acceptable for a person of a given height. Within the safe range, the definition of appropriate weight is up to the individual, depending on factors such as family history, occupation, physical and recreational activities, and personal preferences.

A. Determine the safe weight range for a person of your height and sex:
1. Record your height on the Lab Report, Part A. Note that the Height-Weight Table (see Table 8–2) assumes you measured your height in shoes with 1-inch heels. If you measured your barefoot height, add an inch; if you wore shoes with heels higher or lower than an inch, adjust accordingly.
2. Determine your frame size, using the Frame Size Table (see Table 8–3). Record whether you have a small, medium, or large frame on the Lab Report, Part A.
3. Look up the appropriate weight for a person of your height, sex, and frame size in the Height-Weight Table. Record the entire range on the Lab Report, Part A.

   Example: For a man 5 feet 7 inches tall (in shoes) with a small frame, the range of weights is 138 to 145 pounds.

4. Determine the bottom end of the safe range. A person who is more than 10 percent below the lowest indicated weight for height is considered underweight to a degree that might compromise health. Take 10 percent off the bottom end of your appropriate weight range to discover this limit and record it on the Lab Report, Part A.

   Example: 10 percent of 138 pounds is 13.8 pounds (rounded off to 14 pounds). The bottom end of the range is 138 minus 14, or 124 pounds.

5. Determine the top end of the safe range. A person who is more than 20 percent above the highest indicated weight for height is considered obese. Add 20 percent to the top end of your range and record it on the Lab Report, Part A.

   Example: 20 percent of 145 pounds is 29 pounds. The top end of the range is 145 plus 29, or 174 pounds.

6. The number in 4 is the bottom end of your safe range, and 5 is the top. Record your safe range on the Lab Report, Part A.

   Example: 124 to 174 pounds.

If your weight is below the bottom end of this safe range, you need to gain weight; if it is above the top end, you need to lose weight for your health's sake.

B. If your weight is above the top end of the range, determine your body mass index to obtain confirmation that you need to lose weight. (Refer to Figure 8–2. Use your weight without clothing and your height without shoes.) A body mass index greater than 27.8 in men or 27.3 in women indicates the need for weight loss.

C. Skip this question if your weight is within the safe range or your BMI is below the line indicating the need for weight loss. If your BMI indicates the need for weight loss, check your health history for further confirmation. A family or personal medical history of diabetes (noninsulin-dependent type), hypertension, or high blood cholesterol indicates the need for weight loss.

D. Choose a goal weight within the safe range. Answering the following questions should help you to determine where, within the safe range, your appropriate weight may be:

1. Does your chosen occupation demand that you have a certain body shape? Record the weight, within the safe range, that would most nearly approximate this body shape on the Lab Report, Part D.

   Example: A dancer or model might choose a weight near the bottom end of the range.

2. Do you engage in a sport or other physical activity that requires a particular body weight for optimal performance? Consult your instructor or other expert in that sport or activity, and record the weight recommended on that basis on the Lab Report.

3. Do you hope to start a pregnancy soon? If so, consult your health care provider as to the ideal weight with which to begin a pregnancy and record it on the Lab Report.

4. Undress and stand before a mirror. Do you think you need to gain or lose weight? Record your personal preferences on the Lab Report, Part D (but be sure to stay within the safe range).

E. Now choose a goal weight, giving consideration to each of the weights you just listed. No formula exists for this estimate: You decide, but don't choose a weight outside the safe range. Record your choice on the Lab Report, Part E.

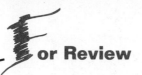

For Review

1. Explain, in terms of body composition, the various possible ways in which weight may be gained or lost (page 166).
2. Identify the major health risks associated with being overweight or underweight (page 169).
3. Describe how the body maintains itself when a person eats:
   a. Too much food (page 167).
   b. Just enough food (page 168).
   c. Not enough food (page 168).
   d. No food (page 168).
4. Outline the principles of sound diet planning as they relate to weight loss, weight gain, and weight maintenance (page 174, 181).
5. Show how diet, exercise, and behavior modification each can contribute to weight control (page 174, 176, 178).

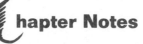

Chapter Notes

1. T. B. Van Itallie and M. U. Yang, Current concepts in nutrition and diet and weight loss, *New England Journal of Medicine* 297 (1977): 1158–1161; Evaluation of 3 weight-reducing diets, *Nutrition and the MD,* March 1978. An experiment in which fasting caused increased weight loss but decreased fat loss compared with a low-calorie mixed diet was reported in M. F. Ball, J. J. Canary, and L. H. Kyle, Comparative effects of caloric restriction and total starvation on body composition in obesity, *Annals of Internal Medicine* 67 (1967): 60–67.
2. G. Kolata, Obesity declared a disease (Research News), *Science* 227 (1985): 1019–1020.
3. M. Simonton, An overview: Advances in research and treatment of obesity, *Food and Nutrition News,* March/April 1982.
4. The section entitled Behavior Modification is adapted from Chapter 12, Energy balance and weight control, in *Understanding Nutrition,* 5th ed., by E. N. Whitney, E. M. N. Hamilton, and S. R. Rolfes (St. Paul, Minn.: West, 1990).
5. R. L. Hammer and coauthors, Calorie-restricted low-fat diet and exercise in obese women, *American Journal of Clinical Nutrition* 49 (1989): 77–85; K. H. Duncan, J. A. Bacon, and R. L. Weinsier, The effects of high and low energy density diets on satiety, energy intake, and eating time of obese and nonobese subjects, *American Journal of Clinical Nutrition* 37 (1983): 763–767.
6. D. M. Dreon and coauthors, Dietary fat: Carbohydrate ratio and obesity in middle-aged men, *American Journal of Clinical Nutrition* 47 (1988): 995–1000.
7. W. D. McArdle, F. I. Katch, and V. L. Katch, *Exercise Physiology: Energy, Nutrition, and Human Performance,* 2d. ed. (Philadelphia: Lea & Febiger, 1986), pp. 527–528.

8. D. Farley, Eating disorders: When thinness becomes an obsession, *FDA Consumer,* May 1986, pp. 20–23.

9. K. McCleary, Eating disorders: Daddy dearest, *American Health,* January/February 1986, p. 86.

10. M. A. Balaa and D. A. Drossman, *Anorexia Nervosa and Bulimia: The Eating Disorders, Disease a Month* (Chicago: Year Book Medical Publishers, June 1985), p. 38.

11. C. L. Otis, Women and sports: Preventing eating disorders, *Sportsmedicine Digest,* June 1989, p. 5.

12. J. D. Killen and coauthors, Depressive symptoms and substance use among adolescent binge eaters and purgers: A defined population study, *American Journal of Public Health* 77 (1987): 1539–1541; Health and Public Policy Committee, American College of Physicians, Eating disorders: Anorexia nervosa and bulimia, *Annals of Internal Medicine* 105 (1986): 790–794.

13. M. Baskind-Lodahl and J. Sirlin, The gorging-purging syndrome: Bulimarexia, *Psychology Today,* March 1977, pp. 50–52, 82, 85.

14. Balaa and Drossman, 1985, pp. 1–52.

15. H. G. Pope, Jr., J. I. Hudson, and D. Yurgelun-Todd, Anorexia nervosa and bulimia among 300 suburban women shoppers, *American Journal of Psychiatry* 141 (1984): 2, as cited by Balaa and Drossman, 1985.

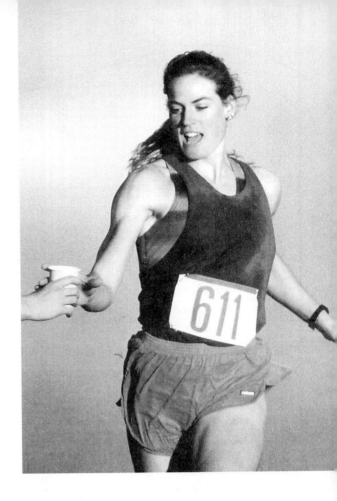

N I N E

Contents

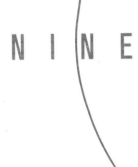

Nutrition
and
Physical
Activity

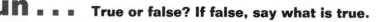

un . . . True or false? If false, say what is true.

1. Of the three energy fuels—carbohydrate, fat, and protein—protein will keep you going longest in an endurance contest (page 194).

2. Burning pain caused by lactic acid in muscles during intense contraction can be relieved simply by relaxing them (page 195).

3. A dose of sugar taken just before a physical activity can enhance the performance of that activity (page 195).

4. To burn fat as fast as possible, you should run as fast as possible (page 196).

5. Active people use more energy and so they need more vitamins (page 199).

6. Active people need more vitamins, and so they need vitamin supplements (page 200).

7. Candy has no place in the diet of a healthy person (page 203).

8. People who exercise vigorously on a regular basis need to take protein supplements (page 206).

9. A good way to warm up before exercise is to consume a little caffeine (page 208).

10. The best time to eat the pregame meal is just before your event (page 209).

In the body, nutrition and physical activity go hand in hand. It is when the body is working that the energy-yielding nutrients are most in demand. The body also needs vitamins and minerals for physical activity because they help to release energy from fuels and to transport oxygen, functions crucial to physical performance. This chapter is about how the body uses energy for movement, how it adapts to use nutrients efficiently to support physical activity, and how a person can best choose foods for that purpose. To both serious athletes and casual exercisers, control of nutrient intake, and thus available fuels, can help make the difference between performance sessions that are difficult and those that seem like a breeze.

The Active Body's Use of Fuels

The more active a person is, the more the person's body alters its nutrient use. The body at rest relies on about equal portions of its fat and carbohydrate, along with a small percentage of protein, for energy. How much of which fuels the muscles use during physical activity depends on an interplay between the fuels available, the intensity of the exercise, and the duration of the exercise; and on the degree to which the body is conditioned to perform that activity. Later sections explain these relationships in detail. First, though, let us take a look at how nutrients support the moving body when a person decides to get up and go.

Quick-Energy Fuels

Have you ever noticed how fast muscles can contract? When a muscle is called upon, it responds instantaneously, without taking time to break down fat or carbohydrate for energy. In the first fractions of seconds of exercise, muscles depend on their supplies of quick-energy compounds for fuel. Whatever you do with your muscles—whether you just blink your eyes or lift a heavy weight—at that moment you are using **ATP**.

ATP (adenosine triphosphate): the body's quick-energy compound, containing energy derived from carbohydrate, fat, and protein.

ATP is present in small amounts in all the tissues all the time, and it can deliver energy instantaneously. It can be made from any energy nutrient, and in muscles, it supplies the chemical driving force for muscle contraction. When ATP is split, its energy is released, and the muscle cells channel most of that energy into mechanical movement and some into heat—heat you can feel building up during muscle work. Muscles always maintain a tiny but essential pool of this quick-energy compound ready to meet sudden demands for movement. All fuels—carbohydrate, fat, and protein—drive muscle contractions by way of ATP.

ATP is a quick-energy compound that drives muscle contraction.

Unlike a single reflexive muscle jerk, prolonged activity involves sustained or repeated muscle contractions that demand a continuous supply of ATP. The muscles' ongoing use of ATP creates a demand that more be made. If the demand for fuel continues beyond about a minute or so, the muscles begin to generate ATP from the more abundant fuels: Carbohydrate, fat, and protein.* The next sections look at each of these fuels and their roles in supporting physical activity.

Carbohydrate and Performance

The body's carbohydrate glucose, stored in the liver and muscles as glycogen, is vital to physical activity. During exertion, the liver releases its glucose into the bloodstream and the muscles pick it up and use it, in addition to glucose from their own glycogen stores. Compared with ATP, glycogen supplies are abundant; compared with fat, though, the glycogen stores are limited.

Body glycogen is constantly being used and replenished, and the extent of glycogen storage is closely related to the carbohydrate content of the diet. How much carbohydrate you eat affects how much glycogen you store, which in turn influences how much you will use during

---

*Another source of quick energy, interconvertible with ATP and stored in small amounts in muscle, is used within the first minute after onset of demand: The intermediate compound phosphocreatine (PC).

activity.[1] Thus, diet bears on performance because the more glycogen you store, the longer the stores will last as you work.

A classic study compared fuel use during exercise among three groups of runners, each on a different diet. For several days before testing, one of the groups consumed a normal mixed diet (55 percent of the calories from carbohydrate), the second group consumed a high-carbohydrate diet (83 percent carbohydrate), and the third group consumed a high-fat diet (94 percent fat). The results of the study are shown in Figure 9–1: The high-carbohydrate group was able to keep going longest before exhaustion. This study and many others that followed suggest that a high-carbohydrate diet enhances endurance by promoting the storage of ample glycogen. The last section of this chapter describes how to choose a performance diet with special attention paid to carbohydrate.

How long an exercising person's glycogen lasts depends not only on diet, but also partly on the intensity of the exercise. The most intense activities—the kind, such as sprinting, that make it difficult for you to "catch your breath"—quickly use up glycogen.[2] Other, less intense activities, such as jogging, during which breathing is steady and easy, use glycogen more slowly. But joggers still use it, and if they run long enough, eventually they run out of it. Glycogen depletion usually occurs within less than two hours from the onset of moderately intense exercise.

The reason why muscles use glycogen especially rapidly during high-intensity exercise is that they can derive glucose from it—and glucose from glycogen can serve as a fuel even when you are out of breath. Glucose can "burn" without oxygen; it can serve as an anaerobic fuel. Thus, whenever you are exerting yourself at a rate that exceeds the rate at which your heart and lungs can supply oxygen to your muscles, the

1. Of the three energy fuels—carbohydrate, fat, and protein—protein will keep you going longest in an endurance contest.

False.

Carbohydrate best supports endurance.

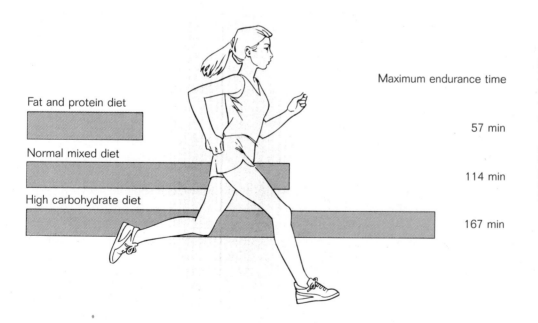

Maximum endurance time

Fat and protein diet

57 min

Normal mixed diet

114 min

High carbohydrate diet

167 min

FIGURE 9–1 The Effect of Diet on Physical Endurance A high-carbohydrate diet can triple a person's endurance.

Source: Data from P. Astrand. Something old and something new . . . very new. *Nutrition Today*, June 1968; pp.9–11.

2. Burning pain caused by lactic acid in muscles during intense contraction can be relieved simply by relaxing them.

   True.

These factors affect glucose use in exercise:

- Dietary and stored carbohydrate
- Intensity of the exercise
- Duration of the exercise

3. A dose of sugar taken just before a physical activity can enhance the performance of that activity.

   False.

   A dose of sugar taken before an activity can hinder performance.

muscles obtain their energy from glucose that they take from their stored glycogen supply. This supply is limited; hence the concern about eating sufficient carbohydrate to make the supply as large as possible before endurance events.

The way that muscles use glucose anaerobically is to break it down only partway to a compound you may have heard of: **Lactic acid.** This acid builds up and causes burning pain in the muscles. Lactic acid accumulation can lead to muscle exhaustion within seconds if it is not cleared away. A strategy for dealing with lactic acid buildup is to relax the muscles at every opportunity so that the circulating blood can carry it away to the liver, which can reconvert it to glucose. You can rise to physical challenges that you might never have thought you could conquer by using this technique: Tired mountain climbers can ascend the final peak by relaxing their leg muscles at each step (the "mountain rest step").

Glycogen use during exercise depends not only on the *intensity,* but also on the *duration,* of the exercise—how long it continues. Within the first 20 minutes or so of moderate exercise, a person uses mostly glycogen for fuel. A person who continues exercising moderately for longer than 20 minutes begins to use less and less glycogen and more and more fat. Still, glycogen use continues, and if the activity is long and hard enough, glycogen stores run out almost completely. Exercise can continue for a short time thereafter only because the liver scrambles to produce from available lactic acid and amino acids the minimum amount of glucose needed to briefly forestall total depletion. When glycogen and glucose depletion hits, it brings nervous system function almost to a halt, making continued exertion almost impossible.*

Since glucose depletion brings on fatigue, people who compete try to maintain their blood glucose concentrations. Some eat sugary foods or drink liquids that provide glucose. This extra glucose may indeed be of value to endurance athletes who often run short of glucose at the end of competition. Taken at such times, glucose can slowly make its way from the digestive tract to the muscles. The glucose in dilute drinks can augment the body's supply just enough to forestall exhaustion.

Before concluding that sugar might be good for your own performance, though, consider whether you engage in *endurance* activity. Do you run, swim, bike, or ski nonstop at a steady pace for more than an hour and a half at a time? If not, the sugar picture changes. For an everyday jog, swim, or game match, sugar will not help performance, and, unless the timing is right, it may actually hinder it. Whenever a person takes sugar calories before they are needed, the body responds by packing them away as fat. If you take a dose of sugar three hours or less before exertion, your body will be busy storing it away right at the time

*Exhaustion from glycogen depletion is different from the sudden fatigue that a weight-lifter feels after only a few seconds of lifting heavy weights. The weight-lifter works at such a high intensity that the muscles' energy needs outstrip their quick-energy supply. Their fatigue reflects diminishing ATP and accumulating lactic acid within each muscle cell. A moment's relaxation relieves this and permits another pump of the weights.

Another factor also affects glucose use:
The extent of the person's training to perform the exercise.

when you want to be drawing it forth from storage. Research on runners shows that a sugar drink taken directly before an event can shorten endurance by 25 percent.[3]

One more factor affects carbohydrate use during exercise—the degree of training. Overall, when you first attempt an activity, you use much more glucose than a person who is trained to perform it. Trained muscles require a lower percentage of their fuel to be glucose because they have developed more equipment that permits them to burn fat, even if their work is strenuous. Thanks to this adaptation, a body well trained for a specific activity can stretch its glycogen stores longer and so can keep going at high intensity somewhat longer than a less-trained body.

Fat and Performance

Unlike glycogen stores, which are limited, body fat stores can fuel hours of activity without running out, as long as the activity is not too intense. Fat is a virtually unlimited source of energy. Early in an activity, the muscles draw on and use the fatty acids already available to them from the blood. If the activity continues for more than a few minutes, the fat cells get the message that more fat is needed for energy, and they begin rapidly breaking down their stored fat to keep the supply going. After about 20 minutes of sustained, moderate exercise, the fat cells are significantly shrinking in size as they empty out their lipid stores.

In addition to duration, intensity also affects fat use. As intensity increases, fat makes less and less of a contribution to the total fuel used. Fat can be broken down for energy in one way only—aerobically. Thus, for fat to fuel exercise, oxygen is indispensable. (Remember, if you are breathing easily during exercise, your muscles are getting all the oxygen they need and are able to burn fat.)

4. To burn fat as fast as possible, you should run as fast as possible.

False.

To burn fat as fast as possible, you should run (or otherwise exercise aerobically) steadily and easily.

The body adapts in response to aerobic activity. For one thing, the trained person's heart and lungs become stronger and better able to deliver oxygen at high exercise intensities. For another, as already mentioned, the muscles cells develop greater capacity to use fat as fuel. For still another, the trained person's hormones slow glucose release from the liver and encourage fat use instead. The person who wishes to burn fat by exercising can conclude that patient, persistent training is worthwhile, and that steady, long-duration activity works best. The intensity to choose depends on your present conditioning level: Work so that you breathe faster than usual but not so fast as to feel out of breath.

The key to burning fat is that steady, long-duration exercise works best.

The body adapted to aerobic exercise burns more fat all day long, not just during exercise. This is because the hormones called forth by exercise favor the continued liberation of stored fat after the activity ceases.[4]

Unlike carbohydrate, fat is not recommended in large quantities in the diets of active people. Your body can supply your fat for you, and it will make more when it needs to as long as you eat enough calories. High-fat diets do promote fat use during exercise, but at the expense of performance, and at the risk of heart disease.

TABLE 9-1 • Carbohydrate and Fat Use during Activity

Fuel Used[a]	Performance Time	Oxygen Needed	Exercise Intensity	Activity Examples
Carbohydrate	30 seconds to 3 minutes	No	Very high	¼ mile sprint, a football play
Mostly carbohydrate (and some fat)	3 minutes to 20 minutes	Yes	High	Distance swimming or running
Mostly fat (and some carbohydrate)	More than 20 minutes	Yes	Moderate	Distance running or jogging, cross-country skiing

[a]All of these fuels are converted to ATP for use as energy. The ATP pool already available donates the first 30 seconds of energy.

Source: Adapted in part from M. H. Williams, Human Energy, in *Nutritional Aspects of Human Physical Performance,* 2d ed. (Springfield, Ill.: Charles C. Thomas, 1985), pp. 21–57; E. L. Fox, Sports Activities and the Energy Continuum, in *Sports Physiology,* 2d ed. (New York: W. B. Saunders Company, 1984), pp. 26–39.

Table 9-1 provides a summary of fuel use during exercise as discussed so far. You may wonder why the third energy-yielding nutrient, protein, is not listed in the table. The reason is that protein is not a major donor of energy to exercise. However, it does donate some energy, and it provides the structural material of muscle tissue, so it is still important to active people.

Protein and Physical Activity

The body handles protein differently during activity than at rest. Synthesis of body proteins is suppressed during exercise and for several hours afterwards. In the hours following this period, though, protein synthesis rebounds beyond normal resting levels.[5] The body must adapt and build the tissues it needs for the next period of exercise. Whenever the body remodels a part of itself, it must tear down old structures to make way for new ones. Repeated exercise, with just a slight overload, triggers the equipment of each muscle cell to do so—that is, they adapt.

The physical work of each muscle cell acts as a signal to its protein-building systems to begin producing the kinds of proteins that best support that work.[6] Take jogging, for example. In the first difficult sessions, the body is not yet fully equipped to perform—the muscle fibers have not adapted to producing the energy needed for aerobic work. But with each session, the cells get the message that an overhaul is needed. In the hours that follow the session, muscle cells get busy breaking down any un-needed protein structures and begin producing the needed new structures. This does not appreciably affect the muscles in just one or two exercise sessions, but within a few weeks, remodeling occurs and jogging becomes easier.[7]

Such remodeling requires protein. Studies show that during active muscle-building phases of training, a weight-lifter might add to existing muscle mass between a third of an ounce and an ounce of protein each day.[8] This happens only during periods of *building,* by exercising at high intensities, and not during periods of maintenance exercise.

Not only do exercisers retain more protein in their muscles, but they also burn some as fuel. Studies show that muscles speed up their use of amino acids as fuel during exercise, just as they speed up their use of fat and carbohydrate.[9] Protein is not a major source of energy; it is estimated to contribute an average of about 10 percent of the total fuel used.[10] Endurance athletes use up enormous amounts of total energy fuels during performance, though, and so use up considerable amounts of protein, too.

The factors that modify how much protein is used during an activity seem to be the same ones that modify the use of fat and carbohydrate. Among them are the intensity and duration of the activity.[11] Another factor is the degree of training. As you might expect, the better trained a person is, the less protein the person uses during an activity.

You might also guess, correctly, that diet modifies the amount of protein used as fuel. People who consume diets rich in *carbohydrate* burn less protein than those who eat protein- and fat-rich diets.[12] This could be related to the protein-sparing effect of carbohydrate first discussed in Chapter 7.

All athletes, as well as those who work like athletes, probably need a little more protein than do sedentary people. How much protein should an active person consume? The American Dietetic Association (ADA) recommends about 25 percent over the recommendation for sedentary people.[13]* Other experts recommend more than this for power athletes and up to twice as much for such athletes early in training.** How all of these recommendations translate into diet is a question answered in a later section. As you will see, no one needs protein supplements, or even large servings of meat, to obtain the highest recommended protein intakes.

---

*The ADA recommends for an active person 1 gram protein per kilogram of body weight per day, or about 60 grams for a 135-pound (60-kilogram) person. (Compare the regular recommendation of 0.8 grams per kilogram, or 45 grams, for a sedentary 135-pound person.)

**One expert recommends 1.0 to 1.2 grams per kilogram for endurance athletes and 1.3 to 1.6 for power athletes (J. R. Brotherhood, Nutrition and Sports Performance, *Sports Medicine* 1 (1984): 350–389). Another expert recommends 2.0 grams per kilogram for early training (H. Yoshimura and coauthors, Anaemia During Hard Physical Training (Sports Anaemia) and Its Causal Mechanism with Special Reference to Protein Nutrition, *World Review of Nutrition and Dietetics* 35 (1980): 1–86, as cited by Brotherhood, 1984).

Vitamins and Performance

Popular belief has it that vitamin supplements have something to offer those who work out, both in health benefits and in physical performance. According to one survey, 84 percent of world-class athletes use vitamin supplements.[14] It goes without saying that athletes need adequate vitamins and minerals to do what they do, as Table 9–2 shows. But are the amounts that are adequate for sedentary people also adequate for active people? And if not, which nutrients do active people need more of? The answers are still not certain, but science is searching for them in the workings of the muscles and in the roles that vitamins play there.

If asked which nutrients an active person might need more of, you might guess it would be the energy-related ones. Physical activity requires more energy in a day, so it might produce a demand for more of the vitamins involved in the breakdown of energy-yielding nutrients — the B vitamins. This is a logical argument, and is used to sell special supplements to athletes, but it is not the whole truth. Active people do need more energy, and they also eat more food. In the process, they get more vitamins, so they do not need supplements. In other words, active people

5. Active people use more energy and so they need more vitamins.

True.

TABLE 9–2 • **Role of Vitamins and Minerals in Exercise**

Vitamin or Mineral	Function
Thiamin, riboflavin, niacin, magnesium	Energy-releasing reactions
Vitamin B_6, zinc	Building of muscle protein
Folate, vitamin B_{12}	Building of red blood cells to carry oxygen
Vitamin C	Collagen formation for joint and other tissue integrity; hormone synthesis
Iron	Transport of oxygen in blood and in muscle tissue; energy transformation reactions
Calcium	Building of bone structure; muscle contractions; nerve transmissions
Phosphorus	ATP component
Sodium, potassium, chloride	Maintenance of fluid balance; transmission of nerve impulses for muscle contraction
Chromium	Assistance in insulin's energy-storage function
Magnesium	Cardiac and other muscle contraction

Note: This is just a sampling. Other vitamins and minerals play equally indispensable roles in exercise.

The RDA tables are in Appendix C.

need the same amount of vitamins in proportion to the energy they spend, as other people do.

The B vitamin riboflavin plays a role in energy release. Researchers have tried to answer the question whether extra riboflavin (at levels beyond the Recommended Dietary Allowances [RDA]) assists in athletic performance. They studied groups of overweight, sedentary women who began an exercise regimen as part of a weight-loss effort.[15] One group of women consumed slightly less than the RDA of riboflavin, and the other group consumed slightly more. Blood tests to evaluate riboflavin activity seemed to indicate a deficiency in the group that consumed the lesser amounts. However, the ability of both groups to exercise aerobically increased similarly. That is, extra riboflavin did not improve physical performance as would be expected if a true riboflavin deficiency had existed in the below-RDA group. To answer questions about riboflavin requirements during exercise will require more research. Riboflavin is abundant in the diets of developed countries, so deficiencies are almost nonexistent.

Unlike riboflavin, niacin may affect performance when taken as a supplement—but negatively. Niacin taken before exercise suppresses the release of fatty acids, forcing muscles to use extra glycogen for fuel. Whether this impedes physical activity is unknown, but it probably shortens the time to glycogen depletion and makes the work seem more difficult to the exerciser.[16] Exercisers need no more niacin than that supplied by a nutrient-dense diet, and people who take niacin supplements before exercise probably impair their workouts.

Some athletes take vitamin B_{12} injections or pills before competition because they believe that they can enhance endurance this way. The limited research thus far available shows that athletes do not need more vitamin B_{12}, and that injections do not stretch endurance. In fact, taking *any* vitamin directly before competition runs contrary to science. Vitamins function only as small parts of larger working units. A molecule of a vitamin floating around in the blood is simply waiting for the tissues to combine it with its appropriate other parts so that it can do its work. This takes time—hours or days. A vitamin taken right before competition is still in the blood during the event and does not improve performance, even if the person were clinically deficient in that vitamin. Vitamin B_{12} supplements are the appropriate treatment for a vitamin B_{12} deficiency. For a well-nourished exerciser, they are useless.[17]

Years ago, evidence that excretion of vitamin C was increased after exercise seemed to indicate that vitamin C in amounts two or three times the RDA might best serve the needs of physically active people. Since that time, the great bulk of work designed to explore this theory has disproved it. Most experiments show that physical performance is no better when people take vitamin C supplements than when they receive the RDA amount from food. Even so, athletes are often told by "advisors" in health food stores to ingest huge quantities of vitamin C, measured in multiples of a gram. These amounts are clearly not useful, and could be harmful.

Besides, for people who eat reasonable diets, it is almost impossible *not* to receive two or three times the RDA for vitamin C. A person who drinks a glass of orange juice and eats a baked potato and a serving of broccoli in a day receives about four times the RDA for vitamin C from these foods alone. When shown the amounts of vitamins and minerals in foods, people have been known to throw away their pills and learn to cook broccoli.

This section has mentioned only 4 of the 15 vitamins, but the story is the same about the others: Active people do not need supplements—they can get them from food. Chapter 12 explodes popular myths about other vitamins and nutrients.

Minerals and Performance

Like the vitamins, the nutrient minerals are essential to exercise—all of them. Three are of special current interest: Chromium, zinc, and copper, which people excrete in their urine in larger amounts when they exercise than when they are sedentary.[18] So far, though, it is too early to say whether these added losses increase people's nutrient needs. Studies have shown that even with low blood zinc, runners can turn in excellent physical performances.[19] In general, the minerals are probably like the vitamins in that active people do not need them in supplement form. You can get enough minerals from a balanced and adequate diet.

Iron and Performance

Iron is an exception to the rule just stated. Endurance athletes, and especially women athletes, are prone to iron deficiency. In one nutrition survey, more than a third of women runners were found to have diminished iron stores.[20] Habitually low intakes of iron-rich foods, combined with iron losses aggravated by exercise, may cause iron deficiency in young women athletes. Iron is in every cell, so growing children have high needs; the blood is especially rich in iron, so bleeding (or excessive menstrual losses) increase iron needs.

Iron deficiency impairs physical performance because iron is crucial to the body's handling of oxygen. Iron is the key ingredient of hemoglobin, the protein in the red blood cells that carries oxygen to all the tissues, including the muscles. Without adequate oxygen transport to your muscles, as you know already, you cannot combust fat as fuel; you cannot perform aerobic activity; and you will tire easily. People with iron deficiency anemia can do less work, less well, and even think less well, than people with adequate iron status. Even marginal iron deficiency without obvious symptoms of anemia is known to impair physical performance to some extent.[21]

The condition known as **sports anemia** is not a true iron-deficiency condition. Sports anemia manifests itself in a temporary decrease in hemoglobin concentration after a sudden increase in aerobic exercise.

sports anemia: a transient condition of low hemoglobin in the blood, associated with the early stages of sports training or other strenuous activity.

Strenuous aerobic exercise promotes destruction of fragile, older, red blood cells; this cleanup work reduces the blood's iron content, although it may not reduce its *effective* iron by much. Strenuous aerobic exercise also prompts the body to increase its blood volume. It does this by adding fluid to the blood supply, thereby diluting its contents and making the iron in a blood sample seem less. Again, this may not diminish the working iron much, if at all. The exact causes of sports anemia remain controversial. Marginal iron intakes may contribute to it, but most people seem to think it is just an adaptive, temporary response to endurance training. Iron-deficiency anemia requires iron-supplementation therapy; sports anemia goes away by itself.

Another term that people use to describe iron status in athletes is **runner's anemia**, which refers to an apparent or real iron-deficiency condition in high-mileage runners. Some people consider this term synonymous with sports anemia; others use it to refer to a true iron-deficiency condition. When you read *runner's anemia,* be sure to notice which meaning is ascribed to it.

Because true iron deficiency is a real possibility for all people, and especially for active people and athletes, it is important to keep track of your own iron status. (All routine physical examinations that include blood work check you for the extreme deficiency state, anemia, but you should also be aware that such tests will not tell you if your iron stores are low.) Consider your individual needs. Many young menstruating women probably border on iron deficiency even without the additional iron losses incurred through exercise. Active teens of both sexes, because they are growing, have high iron needs, too. Especially for women and teens, then, supplements may be needed to maintain iron stores or to correct a deficiency of iron. Iron supplements are available over the counter, and because the absorption of iron from them is poor, it may take a dose as high as twice the RDA or more for several weeks to deliver an amount of iron sufficient to replenish depleted stores. Taking a self-prescribed supplement may mask symptoms of a dangerous condition such as gastrointestinal bleeding from ulcers or cancer, though, so anyone considering this course of action should consult a health care professional before adopting it.

Electrolytes and Performance

Electrolytes, the charged minerals sodium, potassium, chloride, and magnesium, are lost from the body in sweat. People who are just beginning an exercise regimen lose electrolytes to a much greater extent than do trained people; as the body adapts to exercise, it becomes better at conserving most electrolytes. People normally need make no special effort to replenish lost electrolytes. A regular diet that meets their energy and nutrient needs also supplies all the electrolytes they need.

During exercise, electrolyte replacement is also not necessary, unless a person works up a drenching sweat amounting to 5 to 10 pounds or

runner's anemia: an apparent or real iron-deficiency condition in runners.

more each day (3 percent of body weight) for several consecutive days. In that case, drinking plain water and relying on food to replace lost electrolytes may not suffice, and a commercial "sweat replacer" beverage, diluted by half with water, may be drunk for fluid and electrolyte replacement. A homemade mixture of one-third teaspoon of table salt and one cup of fruit juice added to each quart of water will also serve the purpose. Avoid electrolyte or salt tablets; they can irritate the stomach, cause vomiting, and always cause water to flow into the digestive tract from the tissues at first, thereby temporarily worsening dehydration and impairing performance. As for potassium, avoid potassium supplements unless prescribed by a physician because, while they better some conditions, they worsen others.

Diets for Physically Active People

No one diet best supports physical performance. However, food choices and diet plans must be made within the framework of rules for diet adequacy presented in Chapter 7.

Choosing a Performance Diet

First, remember that water is the most important nutrient. Be sure to drink plenty of water. You will feel better, and your workout will seem easier if you consistently tend to your body's fluid needs. Table 6–2 in Chapter 6 offered a schedule of hydration for exercise and it is repeated here in the margin.

People need to eat both for adequacy and for energy. A person who plans to compete in athletic events may want full glycogen stores as well (see the Box, "Glycogen Loading"). Also, even athletes are not immune to heart disease or cancer and so must limit fats while still trying to eat enough food to provide all the needed energy. Simply stated, a diet that is high in carbohydrate works best to ensure full glycogen and other nutrient stores. Experts recommend that you derive 65 percent or more of your calories from carbohydrate, meaning that you need ample fruits, grains, and vegetables in your meals. Even for noncompetitors, such a diet helps to control weight (thus reducing risks of diabetes and other diseases) and provides adequate fiber while supplying abundant nutrients.

Adding more carbohydrate-rich foods to the diet is a sound and reasonable option for increasing energy intake, up to a point, but suppose people need more calories than they can obtain this way. A person can eat only so many slices of bread, apples, and heads of cauliflower. It becomes unreasonable to keep adding bulky carbohydrate foods when the energy needed exceeds the energy in the foods the person has the capacity to eat. At that point, the person must add more concentrated carbohydrate sources, such as dried fruits, sweet potatoes, nectars, and

Hydration Schedule:

2 hours before exercise
- About 3 cups water

10 to 15 minutes before exercise
- About 2 cups water

Every 10 to 20 minutes during exercise
- About ½ cup water

After exercise
- Replace each pound of body weight lost with 2 cups fluid

7. Candy has no place in the diet of a healthy person.

False.

Candy can help add needed calories to the diets of physically active people when they cannot eat bulkier foods.

To make glycogen, muscles need carbohydrate, but they also need rest, so vary daily exercise routines to work different muscles on different days.

Glycogen Loading

When the facts about glycogen stores and endurance performance became known, athletes naturally wanted to make sure they were storing abundant glycogen in their muscles. Various techniques, called **glycogen loading,** have been used in the past to trick muscles into storing extra glycogen. These techniques involved sudden, drastic changes in diet that caused nausea or cramping in some athletes. Other athletes experienced more dangerous effects such as abnormal heart and kidney function.

Exercise physiologists now recommend a moderate plan of glycogen loading that confers benefits without such side effects. First, about two or three weeks before competition, the athlete increases exercise intensity while eating a normal, high-carbohydrate diet. Then during the last week before competition, the athlete does two things. With respect to exercise, the athlete gradually cuts back on exercise, and on the day before, rests completely. Meanwhile, with respect to foods, the athlete eats carbohydrate as usual until three days before competition, and then eats a very high-carbohydrate diet.[22] Endurance athletes who follow this plan can keep going longer than their competitors without ill effects. In a hot climate, extra glycogen confers an additional advantage: As glycogen breaks down, it releases water, which helps to meet the athlete's fluid needs.

Extra glycogen benefits only those who exercise long (at least 90 minutes) and hard enough to deplete their stores; the regular, everyday exerciser will not benefit from having larger stores. What that person does need, though, is *adequate* glycogen from eating a diet high in complex carbohydrates.

How much protein do you need?

1. Express your weight in kilograms (divide your weight in pounds by 2.2).

   Examples: A 110-pound person weighs 50 kilograms. A 132-pound person weighs 60 kilograms. A 165-pound person weighs 75 kilograms. A 220-pound person weighs 100 kilograms.

even high-fat foods such as avocados, nuts, cookies, candies, and ice cream. Don't forget, though, that a nutrient-rich basic diet must be at the core of all this. Energy alone is not enough to support performance.

In addition to carbohydrate and some fat (and the calories from them) physically active people need protein. How much of what kinds of foods supply enough protein to meet their needs? (To figure out how much protein you need, do the quick calculation in the margin.)

Of course, meats and milk are traditional protein-rich foods. We might simply recommend, then, that exercisers eat plenty of meat, but this advice would be narrow for many reasons. For one thing, everyone must take steps against heart disease and even lean meats contain fat, much of it saturated fat. Fortunately, most of the foods recommended to supply carbohydrate also offer protein—the plant foods.

You may recall that the Four Food Group Plan presented earlier (Chapter 7) was recommended as the foundation for an adequate diet.

2. The RDA would say that 0.8 grams for each kilogram each day is an ample protein intake. If you are physically active, you might aim slightly higher—say, for 1 gram per kilogram per day.

Examples: A 110-pound person might aim for 40 grams or (if physically active) 50 grams. A 220-pound person might aim for 80 grams or (if physically active), 100 grams.

Turn back to the third set of color photos in the Food Feature (Figure I–3) and note that the plan calls for only two servings of meat and two of milk, but recommends a minimum of eight servings of foods from the plant food groups—grains, fruits, and vegetables. The basic plan, with only two teaspoons of fat added, delivers about 1,200 calories and derives close to half of its calories from carbohydrate, as shown in the first set of figures in Table 9–3. It also delivers about 70 grams of protein, an ample intake for anyone weighing up to 185 pounds.

Now, how would you add foods to such a foundation to obtain calorie intakes higher than this with the recommended balance of nutrients—mostly carbohydrate? Since meats contribute no carbohydrate, and milk contributes more protein than is necessary, you would do it mostly by

TABLE 9–3 • Examples of Food Patterns to Deliver Various Energy and Protein Amounts

		Calories Provided						
		1,200[a]	1,500[b]	2,000[b]	2,500[b]	3,000[b]	4,000[b]	5,000[b]
		Grams of Protein						
		70	80	90	100	150	180	200
Type of Food	**Serving Size**	**Number of Servings**						
Lowfat milk	1 cup	2	2	3	3	4	6	8
Vegetable	½ cup	2	5	6	7	10	12	14
Fruit	½ cup	2	5	7	10	11	14	20
Starchy vegetable or grain	½ cup or 1 slice	4	6	7	9	10	14	18
Meat[c] or meat alternate	2 ½ ounces	2	2	2	2	4	4	4
Fat	1 teaspoon	2	2	3	4	5	6	8

[a]The servings presented here represent only a core plan (the Basic Four Food Group Plan) to provide adequate protein and supply most of the vitamins and minerals people need daily. You should use this as a foundation for adequacy around which to plan each day's meals. Most people need more energy than this plan provides, and much of this energy should be obtained by adding nutrient-rich, complex carbohydrate foods, such as vegetables and fruits, and breads and whole-grain cereals. This basic plan provides about 50% of its energy as carbohydrate, 20% as protein, and 30% as fat.

[b]These plans provide 55 to 61% of total energy as carbohydrate, 17 to 22% as protein, and 21 to 25% as fat.

[c]These are approximate values for medium-fat meat, but try to choose mostly low-fat meats. One egg, or ½ to ¾ cup of dry beans or peas count as one ounce of meat, poultry, or fish.

adding plant foods. (In the process, you would be adding protein.) The next columns of the table show recommended patterns of food intake for energy intakes up to 5,000 calories a day. Note that the highest ones deliver amounts of protein greater than even the highest intakes recommended for active people weighing over 200 pounds. Clearly, if you eat plenty of nutritious foods, mostly plant foods, you need not worry about getting enough protein.

To show you what a meal plan constructed according to these guidelines might look like, Figure 9–2 depicts meals suitable for a physically active, 150-pound person. The plan delivers 3,000 calories and 135 grams of protein.

This demonstration shows that if foods are chosen wisely, the more food energy a person consumes, the more carbohydrate and protein that person receives. The relationship between high calorie intakes and high protein intakes breaks down only if people meet too much of their energy need with high-fat, high-sugar confections.

In summary, active people need a nutrient-dense diet composed mostly of unprocessed foods, the kind that supply maximum vitamins and minerals for the energy they provide. When people rely heavily on processed foods that have suffered nutrient losses and contain added-sugar and fat, nutrient status suffers. Even if these foods are fortified or enriched, manufacturers cannot replace the full array of nutrients lost in processing. This does not mean that you can *never* choose a white bread, bologna, and mayonnaise sandwich for lunch, but only that later, you should eat a large, fresh salad or big portions of vegetables and drink milk to compensate. That way, the nutrient-dense foods provide the needed nutrients; the bologna sandwich, high in fat and salt, was extra.

By this time, it should be clear that supplements are not necessary, even for high-performance athletes, so long as they eat well. Research confirms this statement: Studies indicate that those who take supplements gain no performance advantage.[23] What the studies consistently find, however, is that compromised nutrient status impedes performance. Not all, or even most, physically active people are well nourished, for they often choose nutrient-poor diets. A human body, even one in superb condition, cannot wring from high-fat, empty-calorie foods the nutrients it needs. For the most part, active people who choose foods with care can be sure of meeting their vitamin and mineral needs without supplements. After all, vitamins, minerals, and energy occur together in food, and people who are active need more food to maintain their weight. Many foods supply energy, including snack foods and sweets, but only one kind of food is nutritious enough to supply the nutrients needed by athletes, along with that energy—whole foods.

Caffeine and Alcohol

Beverages that contain caffeine or alcohol are well liked and widely used. What are their effects on physical performance? Do they offer any benefits? Are they harmful?

8. People who exercise vigorously on a regular basis need to take protein supplements.

False.

Active people can easily meet their protein needs by choosing nutritious foods.

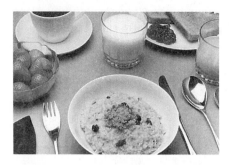

Breakfast
  1 cup coffee
  1 cup oatmeal with ¼ cup raisins
  1 cup 2% low-fat milk
  1¼ cup strawberries
  2 pieces whole-wheat toast
  4 teaspoons of jelly
  ½ cup orange juice
  2 teaspoons of brown sugar on the
    oatmeal

Total cal: **3,119**
61% cal from carbohydrate
24% cal from fat
15% cal from protein

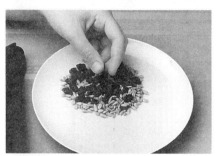

Morning Snack
  2 tablespoons of raisins
  2 tablespoons of sunflower seeds

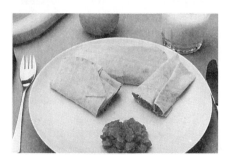

Lunch
  2 bean burritos
  1 banana
  1 orange
  1 cup 2% low-fat milk

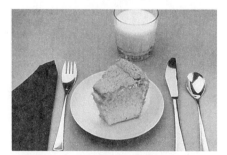

Afternoon snack:
  1 cup 2% low-fat milk
  1 piece angel food cake

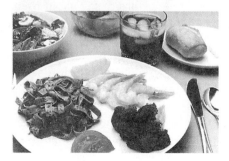

Dinner
  A salad made with:
    1 cup raw spinach leaves
    1 tablespoon sesame seeds
    ¼ cup fresh mushroom slices
    ¼ cup water chestnuts
    ⅓ cup garbonzo beans
    1 tablespoon vinaigrette dressing
  4 ounces of shrimp with ⅛ lemon
  1 cup of broccoli

  ¼ tomato
  1 glass iced tea with 1 teaspoon of
    sugar
  1 dinner roll
  2 teaspoons of butter
  ¾ cup noodles tossed with 2 teaspoons
    of butter and ¼ cup parsley
  1 cup sherbet

FIGURE 9-2 Meal Choices for Active People The meals shown here emphasize carbohydrate-rich plant foods and offer ample energy and protein.

Caffeine is a stimulant, and people sometimes use it to enhance performance. Taken in moderation before an event, caffeine offers one clear advantage: It mobilizes fat from stores, a process that normally does not become maximal until activity is under way. Of course, athletes and exercisers can accomplish the same thing by warming up with light activity before moving on to hard work. Caffeine cannot replace a warm-up activity because, as discussed in Chapters 3 and 4, activity warms the muscles and connective tissues, making them more flexible and less easily injured: Caffeine does not. If you are going to use caffeine for this purpose, though, stick with a cup or two of coffee or the equivalent because in college, national, and international competitions, it is a forbidden drug in amounts greater than the equivalent of about five cups of coffee.

In addition, caffeine is a diuretic. As such, it promotes the excretion of water, vitamins, and minerals. However, taken in moderation in the context of an adequate fluid intake and a nutritious diet, it does no significant harm.

Unlike caffeine, alcohol has no redeeming benefits in exercise metabolism and, in fact, impairs athletic performance. Alcohol is also a diuretic, and drinking it makes heat stroke likely (see Chapter 11). Furthermore, alcohol alters perceptions, slows reaction time, and deprives people of their judgment, all of which compromises performance and safety in sports. Many sports-related fatalities and injuries each year involve alcohol or other drugs.

Beer promoters have discovered that one of the most effective ways they can sell their product is to depict perspiring runners quaffing can after can of it to quench their thirst. Nothing could be more unwise. For each can of beer you drink, you'll excrete more than a can of water. Drink water. A beer at a party may be fine, but a beer at a marathon is a dumb thing to do.

The Pregame Meal

No single food improves speed, strength, or skill in athletic performance, although some kinds of foods do support performance better than others. An athlete may like a particular food, though, for psychological reasons. One eats steak the night before; another spoons up honey at the start of an event. These food rituals may be harmless, and if they are, why discourage them?

Still, athletes may want to know what science has to say about their pregame foods. The recommended pregame meal includes plenty of liquid and is light and easy to digest. The meal or snack should contain between 300 and 1,000 calories; and within this range, the lighter the better.[24] The competitor should finish it three to four hours before competition to allow time for the stomach to empty before exertion.

Breads, potatoes, pasta, and fruit juices—carbohydrate-rich foods that are low in fat, protein, and fiber—are the basis of the pregame meal. (Bulky, fiber-rich carbohydrate foods such as raw vegetables or high-bran

10. The best time to eat the pregame meal is just before your event.

False.

The recommended pregame meal should be finished three to four hours before competition.

cereals, while usually desirable, are best avoided at the pregame meal. Fiber in the digestive tract attracts water out of the blood and can cause stomach discomfort during performance.) Some athletes prefer liquid meals. These are easy to digest and many are commercially available. (You can make your own by mixing nonfat milk, a banana, and some flavorings in a blender.) Quick Tips for the pregame meal follow.

The person who wants to excel physically will apply the most accurate possible knowledge, along with dedication to rigorous training. A diet that provides ample fluid and consists of a variety of nutrient-dense, whole foods in quantities to meet energy needs will not only enhance athletic performance, but overall health as well. Training and genetics being equal, you can easily guess who would win a competition—the person who habitually consumes half or less of the needed nutrients, or the one who arrives at the event with a long history of full nutrient stores and well-met metabolic needs.

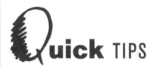

Quick TIPS

Suggestions for the Pregame Meal

- Good ideas: Apricot nectar, pineapple juice, grape juice, jello, sherbert, popsicles, jams, jellies, honey, toast, pancakes with syrup, baked white or sweet potatoes, pasta with steamed vegetables, raisins, figs, dates, frozen yogurt, graham crackers, sponge cake, angel-food cake.
- Not recommended: Stuffing, muffins, biscuits, croissants, french fries, onion rings, potato chips, meats, cheeses, pasta with meat and cheese, pies, ice cream, eggnog, creams, nuts, butter, gravy, mayonnaise, salad dressing, frosted cakes.

How to Calculate Your Carbohydrate Intake

For good health and to support athletic performance, you need a diet that provides adequate calories, of which about 60 percent or more come from carbohydrate. (Of course, there's a lot more to it than this—three chapters' worth in this book—but carbohydrate is worthy of emphasis for the active person.) To find out the percentage of carbohydrate calories you consume, follow the instructions given here and on Lab Report 9.

A. Begin by choosing a typical day and record on scratch paper all the foods you eat that day. Next, copy the foods onto the Lab Report form while consulting Appendix D, being careful to describe your food items in the same terms as they appear there, and to describe your portion sizes as multiples of those in the appendix. For example, suppose you ate a ham sandwich on whole wheat bread that contained two ounces of ham and a tablespoon of mayonnaise. Look up bread in Appendix D, choose the kind of bread you ate, and record the number of slices. For example:

Food description (Appendix D)	Portion size (Appendix D)	Portions I ate
Bread, whole-wheat	1 slice	2
Ham, canned	3 ounces	⅔
Mayonnaise, reg.	1 tablespoon	1

Now, copy the carbohydrate and calorie values *per portion* for these foods from Appendix D into columns 4 and 5 of the Lab Report form. So far you have done no calculating; now you have:

Food description (Appendix D)	Portion size (Appendix D)	Portions I ate	From Appendix D: Carb per portion (g)	From Appendix D: Energy per portion (cal)	My intake: Total carb (g)	My intake: Total energy (cal)
Bread, whole-wheat	1 slice	2	13	70		
Ham, canned	3 ounces	⅔	<1	140		
Mayonnaise, reg.	1 tablespoon	1	<1	100		

Next, on each line, multiply the number in column 3 (portions you ate) times the number in column 4 (carbohydrate per portion) to obtain the total carbohydrate you obtained from each food. Treat any number "<1" as a zero. Round off to a whole number. Enter the result in column 6. Total your carbohydrate intakes at the bottom of column 6.

Now do a similar thing for calories, only this time, on each line, multiply the number in column 3 times the number in column 5 (calories per portion) to obtain the total calories you obtained from each food. Enter the result in column 7. Total your calorie intakes at the bottom of column 7. Now, you have:

Food description (Appendix D)	Portion size (Appendix D)	Portions I ate	From Appendix D:		My intake:	
			Carb per portion (g)	Energy per portion (cal)	Total carb (g)	Total energy (cal)
Bread, whole-wheat	1 slice	2	13	70	26	140
Ham, canned	3 ounces	⅔	<1	140	0	93
Mayonnaise, reg.	1 tablespoon	1	<1	100	0	100
					26	333

Now you have your total carbohydrate intake in grams and your total energy intake in calories.

B. Convert the carbohydrate grams in your meals to carbohydrate calories and then calculate your carbohydrate-calorie intake as a percentage of your total energy intake.

1. Convert your carbohydrate intake into calories by multiplying it by 4 calories per gram:

   Example: 26 g carbohydrate × 4 cal/g = 104 cal carbohydrate.

2. Finally, express your carbohydrate-calorie intake as a percentage of your total energy intake:

   Example: (104 cal carb divided by 333 total cal) × 100 = 31% of calories from carbohydrate.

   In our example, this person needs a lot more carbohydrate or a lot less fat and protein to achieve a carbohydrate intake equal to 60 percent of total calories. It would have been a better choice nutritionally to eat two sandwiches with one slice of ham on each, and mustard instead of the mayonnaise.

Food description (Appendix D)	Portion size (Appendix D)	Portions I ate	From Appendix D:		My intake:	
			Carb per portion (g)	Energy per portion (cal)	Total carb (g)	Total energy (cal)
Bread, whole-wheat	1 slice	4	13	70	52	280
Ham, canned	3 ounces	⅔	<1	140	0	93
Mustard (no calories, no carbohydrate)					52	373

(4 × 52 = 108 cal, or 55% of calories from carbohydrate.)

C. Did you eat the kind of diet that best supports physical activity and overall health (60 percent of calories from carbohydrate and therefore 30 percent or less from fat)? If not, reconsider the earlier section that points

out carbohydrate sources and decide which you can include in your diet more often. Go over each meal and decide which high-fat foods you can replace with high-carbohydrate foods. Can you eat cereal with fruit and nonfat milk in place of biscuits and meat? At lunch, you might plan to replace a fast-food burger with fast-food chili and crackers (the beans in the chili provide abundant carbohydrate and equal the protein in the burger). For supper and snacks, how will you plan for more high-carbohydrate foods and fewer high-fat foods? Remember not to add much sugar to gain carbohydrate—add more starchy pasta, rice, potatoes, and don't neglect milk as a source of valuable nutrients, including carbohydrate.

You might want to write out a detailed plan for another day of meals and then analyze it as you did the first. If you do this, hand it, too, in to your instructor. Once you get into the habit of choosing high-carbohydrate foods, high-fat foods will seem less attractive, and your health and performance will benefit.

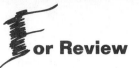

or Review

1. Describe how the body uses its energy fuels in the first few seconds of exercise (page 193).
2. Compare and contrast the exercising body's use of fat and carbohydrate during a long-duration, low-intensity session versus a short-duration, high-intensity session (page 195).
3. Describe a 35-year-old male athlete's needs for protein, vitamins, and minerals as compared to the RDA amounts listed for such a person in Appendix C (page 201).
4. Discuss some reasons why women athletes are especially prone to iron deficiency (page 202).
5. Describe briefly the kind of food and type of diet that best support athletic performance (page 203).

hapter Notes

1. J. P. Flatt, Dietary fat, carbohydrate balance, weight maintenance: Effects of exercise, *American Journal of Clinical Nutrition* 45 (1987): 296–306.
2. E. H. Christensen and O. Hansen, Arbeitsfahigkeit und ehrnahrung, *Skandinavisches Archiv fuer Physiologie* 8 (1939): 160–175, as cited in E. L. Fox, *Sports Physiology,* 2d ed. (New York: Saunders, 1984), pp. 40–57.
3. K. Keller and R. Schwartzkopf, Preexercise snacks may decrease exercise performance, *Physician and Sportsmedicine* 12 (1984): 89–91.
4. R. Bielinski, Y. Schutz, and E. Jequier, Energy metabolism during the postexercise recovery in man, *American Journal of Clinical Nutrition* 42 (1985): 69–82.
5. P. W. R. Lemon, K. E. Yarasheski, and D. Dolny, The importance of protein for athletes, *Sports Medicine* 1 (1984): 474–484.
6. P. Babij and F. W. Booth, Biochemistry of exercise: Advances in molecular biology relevant to adaptation of muscle to exercise, *Sports Medicine* 5 (1988): 137–143.
7. J. F. Hickson and coauthors, Failure of weight training to affect urinary indices of protein metabolism in men, *Medicine and Science in Sports and Exercise* 18 (1986): 563–567.
8. J. R. Brotherhood, Nutrition and sports performance, *Sports Medicine* 1 (1984): 350–389.
9. Lemon, Yarasheski, and Dolny, 1984.
10. Brotherhood, 1984.
11. P. W. R. Lemon, Protein and exercise: Update 1987, *Medicine and Science in Sports and Exercise* 19 (1987): S179–S188.
12. Lemon, 1987.
13. Position of the American Dietetic Association: Nutrition for physical fitness and athletic performance for adults, *Journal of the American Dietetic Association* 87 (1987): 933–939.

14. M. H. Williams, Use of nutritional supplements by athletes, in *Nutrition and Athletic Performance,* eds. W. Haskell, J. Scala, and J. Whitman (Palo Alto, Calif.: Bull Publishing, 1982), pp. 106–155.

15. A. Belko and coauthors, Effects of exercise on riboflavin requirements: Biological validation in weight reducing women, *American Journal of Clinical Nutrition* 41 (1985): 270–277.

16. M. H. Williams, The role of vitamins in physical activity, in *Nutritional Aspects of Human Physical and Athletic Performance,* 2d ed. (Springfield, Ill.: Charles C. Thomas, 1985), pp. 147–185.

17. V. Herbert, N. Colman, and E. Jacob, Folic acid and vitamin B$_{12}$, in R. S. Goodhart and M. E. Shils, eds. *Modern Nutrition in Health and Disease,* 6th ed. (Philadelphia, Pa.: Lea and Febiger, 1980), pp. 229–259.

18. W. W. Campbell and R. A. Anderson, Effects of aerobic exercise and training on the trace minerals chromium, zinc, and copper, *Sports Medicine* 4 (1987): 9–18.

19. Williams, 1985, p. 213.

20. P. A. Deuster and coauthors, Nutritional survey of highly trained women runners, *American Journal of Clinical Nutrition* 44 (1986): 954–962.

21. W. B. Strong and coauthors, The effect of iron therapy on the exercise capacity of nonanemic iron-deficient adolescent runners, *American Journal of Diseases of Children* 142 (1988): 165–169.

22. W. M. Sherman, Carbohydrate, muscle glycogen, and improved performance, *Physician and Sportsmedicine* 15 (1987). 157–161, 164.

23. M. H. Williams, Vitamin supplementation and physical performance, *Report of the Ross Symposium on Nutrient Utilization During Exercise* (Columbus, Ohio: Ross Laboratories, 1983), pp. 26–30.

24. Williams, 1983.

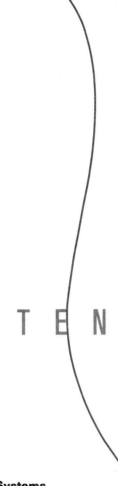

T E N

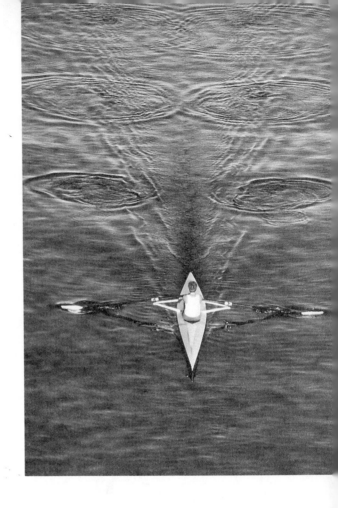

Contents

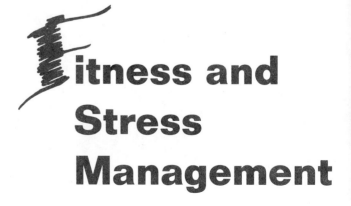

Fitness and Stress Management

JUST FOR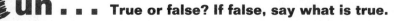

un . . . True or false? If false, say what is true.

1. Some stress is beneficial (page 216).

2. Buying a new car and taking a final exam are more similar than different as far as your body is concerned (page 217).

3. The fight-or-flight reaction is a tactical military maneuver designed to allow fighter jets to avoid enemy bullets (page 222).

4. Whether an event is stressful depends more on the person experiencing it than on the event itself (page 223).

5. Being able to talk to close friends about personal matters helps people manage stress (page 224).

6. You cannot change the way you react to stress (page 226).

7. You know you need to reduce your stress if you find that you are unable to make even the smallest decision (page 228).

8. Machines can help you to learn to relax (page 228).

stress: the effect of demands on the body that force it to adapt. Stress that provides a welcome challenge is *eustress;* stress that is perceived as negative is *distress.*

1. Some stress is beneficial.

   True.

Chapter 1 defined fitness as the characteristics of the body that enable it to engage in physical activity. A broader definition of fitness includes the body's ability to withstand **stress.** People normally think of stress as harmful and, indeed, it can be harmful when it occurs in excess of the body's ability to cope with it. However, stress can also be beneficial if it occurs in doses small enough to challenge, but not to overwhelm, that ability. Physical activity is itself a form of stress, and like all stresses, it can be harmful in excess, but it is usually beneficial because it is the one form of stress that leads to greater fitness. When the body practices meeting this stress, it becomes able to withstand other stresses as well. This relationship has many implications for your health and provides still another reason in addition to all the others you have already learned for engaging in regular physical activity.

Stress and the Body's Systems

Stress can be positive or negative, depending on your reaction to it. When one person claims to be under stress, he may mean that he is feeling an unwelcome strain. Perhaps he is ill, or his love life has gone awry, or he

adaptive: with respect to behavior, that which benefits the organism. Behavior that brings about results that are harmful to the organism is termed *maladaptive* behavior.

nervous system: the system of nerves, organized into the brain, spinal cord, and peripheral nerves, that send and receive messages and integrate the body's activities.

hormonal system: the system of glands—organs that send and receive bloodborne chemical messages—that integrate body functions in cooperation with the nervous system.

immune system: the cells, tissues, and organs that protect the body from disease; composed of the white blood cells, bone marrow, thymus gland, spleen, and other parts.

white blood cells: the blood cells responsible for the immune response (as opposed to the red blood cells, which carry oxygen).

antibodies: large protein molecules produced to fight infective or foreign tissue.

immunity: the body's capacity for identifying, destroying, and disposing of disease-causing agents.

homeostasis (HO-me-oh-STAY-sis): the maintenance of relatively constant internal conditions by corrective responses to forces that would otherwise cause life-threatening changes in those conditions. A homeostatic system is not static. It is constantly changing, but within tolerable limits.

is under financial pressure. In contrast, another person who says she is under stress may mean that she is excited and happy. She may have just started a new job or be about to buy the car she has always wanted. Stress is *any* change, and fitness derived from physical exertion helps enable you to cope with *any* kind of stress—desirable or undesirable. Therefore, your dedication to personal fitness can make a major contribution to your ability to manage all of the challenges your life presents.

First of all, though, what does a stress such as exercising, taking an exam, or buying a new car do to your body? You may say it is "scary" or "exciting" (as opposed to "relaxing"), but what does that mean physically? It means, among other things, that your heart beats faster and that you breathe faster than normal—in other words, that your body gets ready to exert itself physically. All external changes stimulate you this way to some extent, requiring your mind or body to change internally in some physical way—that is, to adapt. All environmental changes—changes in the temperature, the noise level around you, what is touching you, and countless others—require such adaptation. So do all psychological events, both desirable and undesirable (see Table 10–1). The greater the **adaptive** changes you must make internally, the greater the stress.

All of the body's systems are affected by stress, but of particular interest are the **nervous system,** the **hormonal system,** and the **immune system.** Figures 10–1 and 10–2 show the anatomy, and describe the workings of the nervous and hormonal systems. The immune system parts are so widespread in the body that to show them in a figure would require a picture of almost every organ and tissue. Many tissues characterize the system: **White blood cells** made in the bone marrow and incubated in other glands, **antibodies** made by white blood cells, and other tissues all work together to confer **immunity** on the body. These systems connect all the body's parts so that they act as a unit.

Whether a particular stressful event presents a mental challenge, such as an exam, or a physical one, such as a fistfight, the responses are always the same. The efficient functioning that results from the body's adjustment to changing conditions is **homeostasis.**

The stress of cold weather can serve as an example to show how the nervous system in particular works to maintain homeostasis. (Remember, all stresses have similar effects, so even if you never experience cold weather, this applies to you.) When you go outside in cold weather, your skin's temperature receptors send "cold" messages to the spinal cord and brain. Your nervous system reacts to these messages and signals your skin-surface capillaries to shut down so that your blood will circulate deeper in your tissues, where it will conserve heat. The system also signals involuntary contractions of the small muscles just under the skin surface: Goose bumps with their by-product heat. If these measures do not raise your body temperature enough, the nerves signal your large muscle groups to shiver. The contractions of these large muscles produce still more heat. All of this activity adds up to a set of adjustments that maintains your homeostasis (a constant temperature in this case) under conditions of external extremes (cold).

TABLE 10-1 • Physical and Psychological Challenges Experienced as Stressful

Physical Stresses[a]

Light and changes in light	Drugs/medicines/alcohol
Heat/cold and changes in temperature	Foodborne chemicals and contaminants
Sound and changes in sound level	Bacteria/viruses/other infective agents/allergens
Touch/pressure and changes in touch stimuli	Injury, including surgery
Airborne chemical stimuli (odors, smoke, smog, air pollution)	Exertion, work
Waterborne chemical stimuli	X rays/radioactive rays/other forms of radiation

Psychological Stresses[a]

Death of spouse or other loved one	Son or daughter leaving home
Divorce or marital separation (breakup with boyfriend/girlfriend)	Trouble with in-laws or parents
Jail term	Outstanding personal achievement
Marriage or marital reconciliation	Spouse beginning or stopping work
Being fired from a job or expelled from school	School beginning or ending (final exams)
Retirement	Change in living conditions
Change in health of a loved one	Revision of personal habits (self or family)
Pregnancy or sex difficulties	Trouble with boss or professor
Gain of new family member or change of roommate	Change in work or school hours or conditions
Business readjustment or change in financial state	Change in residence (moving to school, moving home)
Change to different line of work or change of major	Change in recreation, church activities, or social activities
Taking on a large mortgage or financial aid	Change in sleeping habits or eating habits
Foreclosure of mortgage or loan	Christmas or other vacation
Change in responsibilities at work or change in course demands	

[a]The items in this table are ranked in order of highest stress to lowest stress.

Source: Adapted from Lifescore: Holmes Scale. *Family Health*, January 1979, p. 32.

Now let's say you come in and sit by a fire and drink hot cocoa. You are warm, and you no longer need the body's heat-producing activity. At this point, the nervous system signals your skin-surface capillaries to open up again, your goose bumps to subside, and your muscles to relax. Your body is back in homeostasis. It has recovered.

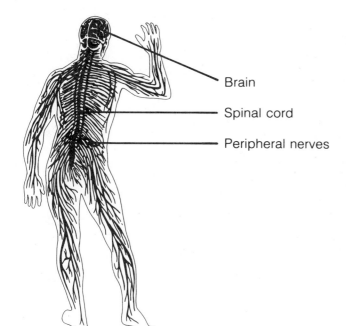

Brain

Spinal cord

Peripheral nerves

FIGURE 10-1 The Organization of the Nervous System The brain, spinal cord, and nerves make up a vast system of wiring that connects every body part. The nerves in the distant parts of the system gather information about the environment, both internal and external, and deliver it to the master control organ, the brain. The brain and spinal cord that make up the **central nervous system** act as a control unit for the body, and the nerves that make up the **peripheral nervous system** provide the wiring between the center and the parts.

A second distinction is between the part of the nervous system that controls the voluntary muscles (**somatic nervous system**) and the part that controls the internal organs (**autonomic nervous system**). Your conscious mind wills the movement of your legs, but your pancreas operates automatically with no conscious demand from you.

central nervous system: the central part of the nervous system, the brain and spinal cord.

peripheral nervous system: the outermost part of the nervous system, the vast complex of wiring that extends from the central nervous system to the body's outermost areas.

somatic nervous system: the division of the nervous system that controls the voluntary muscles, as distinguished from the autonomic nervous system, which controls involuntary functions.

autonomic nervous system: the division of the nervous system that controls the body's automatic responses. One set of nerves within this system helps the body respond to stressors from the outside environment. The other set regulates normal body activities between stressful times.

Now imagine that the system is constantly under stress—having to work to stay warm, to repair injuries, and to deal with fears and anxieties. You can see how, without periods of relaxation between times, this would be stressful.

The hormonal system, together with the nervous system, integrates the whole body's functioning so that all parts act smoothly together. And like the nervous system, the hormonal system is very busy during times of stress, frantically sending messages from one body part to another in an attempt to maintain order. Among the hormones important in stress, collectively called the **stress hormones,** are **epinephrine** and **norepinephrine,** which are secreted by the adrenal gland and mediate the stress response. A little practice (such as from the stress of physical activity) helps keep the hormonal system in good shape, but too much stress, unrelieved, is exhausting and debilitating.

The immune system is crucial in defenses against infectious disease agents, which are always present in all environments. It defends not only against colds, flu, measles, tuberculosis, pneumonia, and hundreds of other diseases, but even against some kinds of cancer. Cancerous tumors

stress hormones: epinephrine and norepinephrine, secreted as part of the reaction of the nervous system to stress.

epinephrine (EP-uh-NEFF-rin), **norepinephrine:** two hormones of the adrenal gland; sometimes called the stress hormones, although they are not the only hormones modulating the stress response. (The *adrenal gland* nestles in the surface of the kidney.)

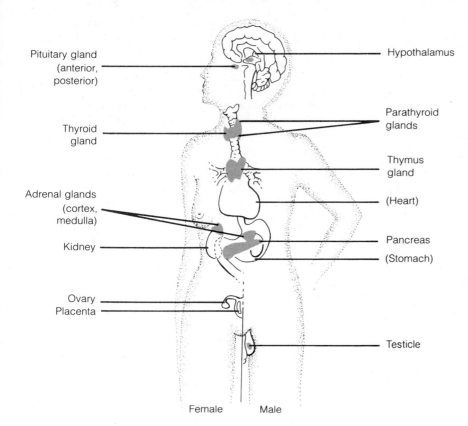

Pituitary gland
(anterior,
posterior)

Thyroid
gland

Adrenal glands
(cortex,
medulla)

Kidney

Ovary
Placenta

Hypothalamus

Parathyroid
glands

Thymus
gland

(Heart)

Pancreas

(Stomach)

Testicle

Female   Male

FIGURE 10-2 The Hormonal System These are the major glands that regulate the body's activities. The hormonal system coordinates body functions by transmitting and receiving messages. A hormonal system message originates in a **gland** and travels as a chemical compound (a **hormone**) in the bloodstream. The hormone flows everywhere in the body, but only its **target organs** respond to it because only they possess the equipment to receive it. Like the muscles at the ends of nerves, the target organs of the stress hormones respond by suppressing digestion, immunity, and circulation.

gland: an organ of the body that secretes one or more hormones.

hormone: a chemical messenger; it is secreted by a gland and travels to a *target organ,* where it brings about a response.

target organ: an organ of the body that responds to a hormone.

grow from the host's body tissues, but the immune system can often recognize them as abnormal tissue in their early stages and fight them off. Anything that impairs the immune system threatens life; anything that strengthens the system—such as improved fitness—supports health.

Like the other systems, the immune system is affected by stress. Small amounts of stress, alternating with times of relief from stress, are not harmful, but prolonged stress can impair immunity and make a person unusually vulnerable to disease.

The Experience of Stress

When students encounter stress, very often it is psychological and involves the pressure to achieve in school (see Figure 10–3). In addition to the demands of school are the need for parental approval and the need to meet students' own high standards. These are all psychological stressors that cause tension. Meeting these demands can lead to the satisfaction of achievement, but sometimes these demands cause stress that can lead to mental and physical harm. To avoid this harm, the student's physical systems must be able to mobilize their resources against stress. Fitness enhances the body's capacity to meet everyday challenges and can ease

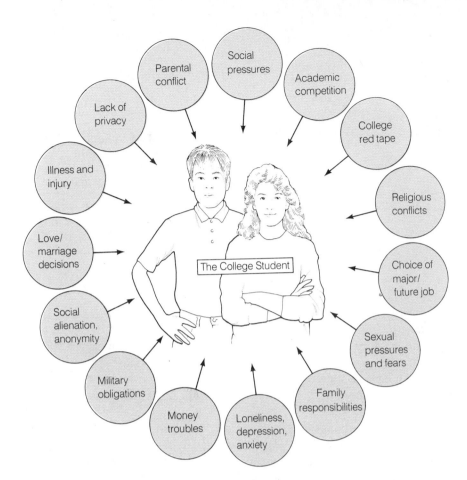

FIGURE 10-3 Psychological Challenges in the Lives of Students

the student's task of coping with both the physical and psychological effects of stress.

Consider what stress, whether it is physical, psychological, or both, does to the body. Whatever form of stress you encounter, the **stress response** has three phases—**alarm, resistance,** and **recovery** or **exhaustion** (see Figure 10–4). Alarm occurs when you perceive that you are facing a new challenge. Stress hormone secretion begins, activating all systems. Resistance is a state of speeded-up functioning in which stress hormone secretion continues, favoring muscular activity over other body functions (we'll describe this unbalanced state in more detail shortly). During the resistance phase, your resources are mobilized just as an army mobilizes its equipment and supplies to fight a battle. In the case of your body, the resources are your attention, strength, fuels, and others, but the principle is the same. You can use your resources until they run out or wear out; then you need to replace or repair them.

Hopefully, before your resources are exhausted, a recovery period is permitted. You relax and recuperate. Stress hormone secretion ceases, all systems slow down, normal functioning resumes, needed repairs take place, fuel stores are refilled, and you become ready for the next round of

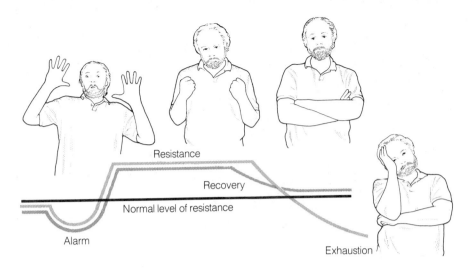

FIGURE 10-4 The Stress Response and Its Ending in Recovery or Exaustion Alarm briefly lowers resistance but is followed by a high level of resistance. Recovery restores the normal level. If resistance is required for too long, exhaustion sets in, and resistance temporarily falls below the level normally maintained.

excitement. It is because of the need for recovery between times of stress that the military provides "R and R" (rest and relaxation) times for its personnel.

If you have to stay in overdrive for too long, however, your resistance finally breaks down and recovery is delayed or becomes impossible. This is exhaustion.

The stress response evolved eons ago to permit our ancestors to react appropriately to immediate *physical* danger. It is often called the **fight-or-flight reaction** because fighting and fleeing are the two major alternatives when someone is faced with a physical threat. Every organ responds to an alarm and readies itself to take action. The heart rate and respiration rate speed up. The pupils of the eyes widen so that you can see better. The muscles tense up so that you can jump, run, or struggle with maximum strength. Circulation to the skin diminishes (to protect against blood loss from injury); circulation to the digestive system and internal organs (which can wait) also diminishes. Circulation to the muscles and brain (which are needed now) increases. The kidneys retain water (in case you should be injured and lose water by bleeding). The immune system temporarily shuts down, including the part of it that produces inflammation at a site of injury (the body can't afford to deal with irritation at a time when it needs to cope with external threats).

While the nerves bring about some of these effects, the hormones go to work, too. The brain initiates a hormone cascade that calls gland after gland into play and affects every organ in the body.

The nerves and hormones of the stress response produce not only the effects you feel—tense muscles, sharp eyesight, speeded-up heartbeat and respiration—but also other deep, internal responses that make you ready for fight-or-flight in other ways. They alter the metabolism—the chemical changes affecting energy—of every cell.

We called the state of stress resistance an *unbalanced state* earlier. The description just given shows how unbalanced it is. It is a state in which

fight-or-flight reaction: the response to immediate physical danger; the stress response.

3. The fight-or-flight reaction is a tactical military maneuver designed to allow fighter jets to avoid enemy bullets.

False.

The fight-or-flight reaction is the body's stress response that prepares it to cope with danger.

muscular activity is favored over other necessary body functions such as digestion and immune defenses. The state of stress resistance represents the body's effort to restore normal times when digestion and normal immune defenses can resume. Both states are important—normal functioning to keep you running smoothly during peaceful times, and stress resistance to get you through emergencies and back to normal functioning during times of change.

The stress response occurs each time you exercise vigorously, and especially when you compete. Think about it: What is the physical difference between running from a man-eating tiger or running a race in the Olympics? The emotion you feel may be fear or joy, but in either case, the hormones you secrete are the same; the reactions of the nerves, muscles, cardiovascular system, immune system, and all other body systems are the same. Afterward, the recovery process is the same: You relax. Either the running away or the athletic event can also progress to exhaustion.

It should be becoming clear that stress can either benefit you or harm you, depending on your response to it. Suppose, for example, that you experience alarm (anxiety, fear), but that you *don't* fight or flee—that is, your body takes no physical action. The body gets *ready* to exercise, mobilizes its resources, but doesn't use them. You have been drained, but you haven't improved your response capability. Alarm without a physical response is harmful. If you experience stress repeatedly and don't have sufficient recovery periods between times, that, too, is harmful, and explains the importance of rest, relaxation, and sleep, which are discussed next.

If a round of stress leads to recovery and to a greater ability to adapt to the next round, then it has benefited you. On the other hand, if it leaves you drained and *less* able to adapt the next time, it has harmed you.

How can you make sure to obtain benefit, rather than harm, from your stressful experiences? By practicing for them—that is, by exercising regularly in appropriate ways and amounts and permitting yourself to recover adequately between times. A round of exercise is a sort of controlled round of stress—you choose when to start it, how intensely to engage in it, and when to stop. During each round, you are practicing for the next one—getting better at it. The wonderful thing about exercise, though, is that it makes you better not only at exercising, but at resisting all other stresses, because (remember?) the stress response is the same, no matter what its trigger. Can you see, then, why fit people withstand all stresses better and recover from them faster than unfit people do?

Fitness contributes to all aspects of health, as Figure 1–2 in Chapter 1 showed. Beyond cultivating fitness, you can also learn specific stress management strategies that will stand you in good stead when stress is unavoidable.

Stress Management Strategies

Managing stress well involves two sets of skills. One set is for sailing along, when moment-to-moment adjustments can keep you on course; the other is for stormy times.

4. Whether an event is stressful depends more on the person experiencing it than on the event itself.

True.

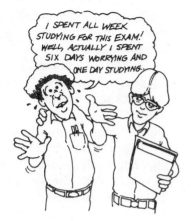

It only slows you down to worry about things you have to do.

Wise time management can help you to minimize stress. Time is similar to a regular income: You receive 24 hours of it each day. It is like money, too, in that you have three ways in which to spend it. You can save ahead (do tasks now so you won't have to do them later); you can spend as you go; or you can borrow from the future (have fun now and hope you will find the time later to do things you have to do). If you manage time wisely, you can gain the two advantages that wise money management also gives you—security for the future and enjoyment of the present. It takes skill to treat yourself to enough luxuries so that you enjoy your present life, while saving enough so that you will have time available when you need it. When your friends call on a Sunday to invite you out, you don't want to be caught with no money on hand, no clean clothes, and no studying done for the big exam on Monday. That is an avoidable stress, and planning ahead circumvents it. Make a time budget. Remember, you have to do it only once, and an hour of time spent organizing buys many hours of time doing what you choose.

Several planning techniques can help you get the most out of your day while keeping tabs on long-term time needs. One such technique is to make two records—one, a list of things to do, and the other, a weekly time schedule. Figure 10–5 shows how to use these tools for everyday tasks. Sometimes you will need to schedule special projects. To schedule a long-term assignment, such as a term paper, first identify every task you must do to complete the project. Then, working backward from the due date, schedule each task. For example, if it will take you six hours to type the paper, schedule those six hours on a grid that you have started for the due-date week. Back up and schedule time before that to write the final draft and time before that for the research. If you have been realistic about the time each step will take, you will not be caught short at the end.

In addition to effective time management, a person can take many other measures to maintain strong resistance to stress. Many of these have been described in earlier chapters. Obtain regular exercise, relaxation, and sleep. Eat nutritious, balanced meals that will maintain your appropriate body weight. Cultivate strong emotional and spiritual health, and stay drug-free. These strategies strengthen your resistance between stressful times. Now, consider the times of stress themselves. You have to cope.

The means of handling pain and stress are behaviors known as **coping devices,** and some are more adaptive than others (see the Box, "Coping Devices"). The less adaptive ones are ways of continuing to avoid the pain as much as possible, whereas the more adaptive ones are ways of dealing with it and working it through. The maladaptive coping behaviors are sometimes known as **defense mechanisms,** and they are listed in a box of their own.

An intermediate type of coping behavior is **displacement,** the application of energy to another area altogether. Displacement is suitable for a time. Healthy people have a hierarchy of displacement behaviors with which they handle life's ups and downs. A truly adaptive coping behavior is **ventilation.** Ventilating means letting off steam, by expressing feelings to another person.

coping devices: behaviors, both adaptive and maladaptive, used to deal with the reality of an unpleasant or painful situation. See the Box, "Coping Devices" (page 225).

defense mechanisms: automatic and often unconscious forms of emotional avoidance in reaction to emotional injury. See the Box, "Defense Mechanisms" (page 226).

5. Being able to talk to close friends about personal matters helps people manage stress.

True.

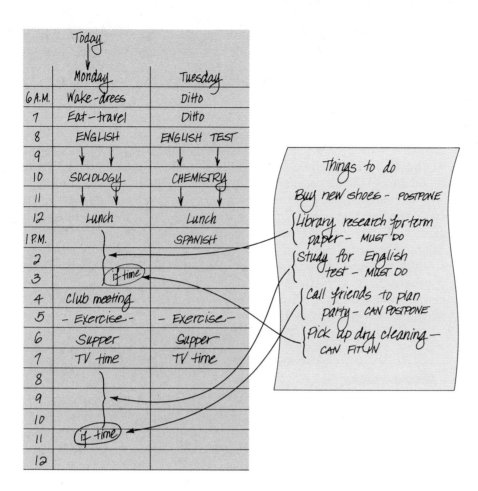

	Today ↓ Monday	Tuesday
6 A.M.	Wake-dress	Ditto
7	Eat-travel	Ditto
8	ENGLISH	ENGLISH TEST
9	↓	↓
10	SOCIOLOGY	CHEMISTRY
11	↓	↓
12	Lunch	Lunch
1 P.M.		SPANISH
2		
3	if time	
4	Club meeting	
5	- Exercise -	- Exercise -
6	Supper	Supper
7	TV time	TV time
8		
9		
10		
11	if time	
12		

Things to do

Buy new shoes - POSTPONE

Library research for term paper - MUST DO

Study for English test - MUST DO

Call friends to plan party - CAN POSTPONE

Pick up dry cleaning - CAN FIT IN

FIGURE 10–5 Time Management On a grid that lists the days of the week across the top and the hours of the day down the side, fill in your set obligations such as class meetings or work schedule. Allot a space for exercise each day. Prioritize other obligations such as bill paying or grocery shopping on a "things to do list," and find space throughout the week in which to do them. Check tasks off the schedule when you have completed them, and place any that you do not complete on next week's list of things to do. Be sure to plan time for nutrition, for sleep, and for play.

Too many people believe they must wait until the effects of stress are beginning to become severe before they take steps to relieve it. That's not true. At each step along the way, it's possible to intervene and obtain relief. The alarm step is the first step at which you can intervene. Recognize your own alarm reaction. You can then seek to identify the source of the stress and begin to deal with it immediately.

〰〰〰〰 Coping Devices

displacement: channeling the energy of suffering into something else—for example, using the emotional energy churned up by grief for work or recreation.

ventilation: the act of verbally venting one's feelings; letting off steam by talking, crying, swearing, or laughing.

---

6. You cannot change the way you react to stress.

False.

People can change the way they react to events so that the events aren't so stressful.

Stress management strategies:

1. Identify tensions when they first arise.
2. Recognize stress and identify its source.
3. Control responses. Identify inappropriate responses and change them.
4. Focus your attention and energy right on the task you are facing.

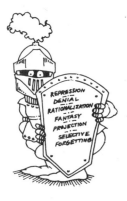

Defense mechanisms: Forms of mental avoidance.

We said earlier that the person's reaction, not the situation, determines the severity of stress. People can change the way they react to events so that the events aren't so stressful.

An example is public speaking. The stress response can help you get "up for it." Some excitement and anticipation ahead of the event, with the associated rapid heartbeat and breathing, will give you the physical energy to turn out a spectacular performance. You are at your most attractive when you are aroused and alert. But too much stress is debilitating. If you allow yourself to think about what a catastrophe it will be if you do less than a perfect job, you will be trembling visibly, your teeth will be chattering, and your knees will be knocking together. In such a state, you can hardly reach your audience at all, and you will be unduly exhausted afterward. It is to your advantage to learn to *perceive* the event as not so stressful.

This example illustrates another strategy: Use the stress response to your advantage. Direct and control the energy the stress response gives you. It is a magnificent, adaptive response to challenges, after all. It's only when the energy is scattered and wasted that it drains you without giving

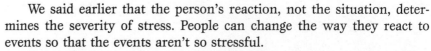

Defense Mechanisms

denial: the refusal to admit that something unpleasant or painful has occurred: "No, I don't believe it."

fantasy: delusion, in the face of a painful or unpleasant situation, that something positive has happened instead: "He hasn't really left me. He's gone to buy me a present."

oral behavior: ingesting substances such as drugs, alcohol, or unneeded food.

projection: the conviction, in the face of an unpleasant or painful situation you have caused, that it is the other person's fault: "The teacher asked the wrong questions on the exam."

rationalization: the justification of an unreasonable action or attitude by manufacturing reasons for it: "I couldn't prevent the accident because I had to pay attention to something else."

regression: the reversion to inappropriate childish ways of dealing with painful realities, such as chronic crying or whining.

repression: the refusal to acknowledge an unpleasant or painful event or piece of news: Not hearing it.

selective forgetting: memory lapse concerning an experience or piece of news too painful to bear: Not remembering it.

withdrawal: disengaging from people and activities to avoid pain. Examples: Engaging in extended periods of fantasy (daydreaming), refusing to talk with anyone, or sleeping excessively.

5. Recognize the warning signals of too much stress.

you anything in return. (In other words, it's OK to have butterflies in your stomach as long as they're all flying in formation.)

It is helpful to monitor your body for the many warning signals of too much stress. If you are alert to their appearance, you can initiate preventive action before exhaustion sets in and does damage. (See Table 10–2).

TABLE 10-2 • Signs of Stress

Physical Signs	Psychological Signs
Pounding of the heart, rapid heart rate.	Irritability, tension, or depression.
Rapid, shallow breathing.	Impulsive behavior and emotional instability; the overpowering urge to cry or to run and hide.
Dryness of the throat and mouth.	Lowered self-esteem; thoughts related to failure.
Raised body temperature.	Excessive worry; insecurity; concern about other people's opinions; self-deprecation in conversation.
Decreased sexual appetite or activity.	
Feelings of weakness, light-headedness, dizziness, or faintness.	Reduced ability to communicate with others.
Trembling; nervous tics; twitches; shaking hands and fingers.	Increased awkwardness in social situations.
Tendency to be easily startled (by small sounds and the like).	Excessive boredom; unexplained dissatisfaction with job or other normal conditions.
High-pitched, nervous laughter.	Increased procrastination.
Stuttering and other speech difficulties.	Feelings of isolation.
Insomnia—that is, difficulty in getting to sleep, or a tendency to wake up during the night.	Avoidance of specific situations or activities.
	Irrational fears (phobias) about specific things.
Grinding of the teeth during sleep.	Irrational thoughts; forgetting things more often than usual; mental "blocks"; missing of planned events.
Restlessness, an inability to keep still.	
Sweating (not necessarily noticeably); clammy hands; cold hands and feet; cold chills.	Guilt about neglecting family or friends; inner confusion about duties and roles.
Blushing; hot face.	Excessive work; omission of play.
The need to urinate frequently.	Unresponsiveness and preoccupation.
Diarrhea; indigestion; upset stomach nausea.	Inability to organize oneself; tendency to get distraught over minor matters.
Migraine or other headaches; frequent unexplained earaches or toothaches.	Inability to reach decisions; erratic; unpredictable judgment making.
Premenstrual tension or missed menstrual periods.	
More body aches and pains than usual, such as pain in the neck or lower back; or any localized muscle tension.	Decreased ability to perform difficult tasks.
	Inability to concentrate.
Loss of appetite; unintended weight loss; excessive appetite; sudden weight gain.	General ("floating") anxiety; feelings of unreality.
Sudden change in appearance.	A tendency to become fatigued; loss of energy; loss of spontaneous joy.
Increased use of substances (tobacco, legally prescribed drugs such as tranquilizers or amphetamines, alcohol, other drugs).	Nightmares.
	Feelings of powerlessness; mistrust of others.
Accident proneness.	Neurotic behavior; psychosis.
Frequent illnesses.	

Symptoms of stress indicate that you are exhausting your ability to cope if:

You know you are under severe stress.

The same symptoms, in the past, appeared just before your resistance failed.

7. You know you need to reduce your stress if you find that you are unable to make even the smallest decision.

True.

6. Identify which stressors you can control. Put the others out of your mind. List priorities and start taking action.

7. Learn to release tension whenever appropriate, by exercising, laughing, or willing yourself to relax.

relaxation response: the opposite of the stress response; the normal state of the body.

progressive muscle relaxation: a technique of achieving the relaxation response by systematically relaxing the body's muscle groups.

8. Machines can help you to learn to relax.

True.

The length of the lists of signs of stress is impressive. Some people have some of the symptoms all the time. Everyone has some of them some of the time. The presence of a few symptoms is not cause for alarm, but there is a time to take them seriously. You should be concerned about the appearance of these symptoms under conditions that you know are stressful for you and that have, in the past, proved to be the forerunners of serious illness or inability to cope.

The cumulative effects of stress create a situation in which even small details become overwhelming. The person under chronic stress may become unable to handle even small problems. Example: A student who is breaking up with his girlfriend, moving out of his home, and changing schools all at the same time is trying to get his personal effects packed. He picks up a paper clip and can't decide what packing box to put it in. He starts to sob; he can't cope.

At such a time, you need to reduce your stress. Ask yourself which elements of the situation you can control, and pay strict attention to only those. In the case of our friend, he needs to take a deep breath and calm down. Once the crying has relaxed him, he should ask himself what he can control right now and what he can't. The breakup, the move, and the change of schools are beyond his control right now. The packing is not. He can go on with it or stop. He may need to take a break—for food, sleep, or exercise. He may need to tap a friendship—get help moving boxes or just make plans for dinner. These are the tasks he has to handle right now. He can let go of the rest.

Finally, even in the midst of severe stress, you can learn to relax and indulge in moments of recovery.

Willed Relaxation

The exact opposite of the stress response is the **relaxation response** (see Table 10–3). Relaxation occurs naturally whenever stressors stop acting on you, and it permits your body to recover from the effects of stress. But you can also will it to happen, even in the midst of a stressful situation.

One way to relax is through **progressive muscle relaxation.** The technique involves lying flat and relaxing the muscles all over the body, beginning with the toes. The goal is to locate and erase tension wherever it is occurring in the body. People who have never tried this are astonished to discover the number of different muscles used in creating tension, especially in the abdomen, the upper back and neck, and the face.

A way to learn muscle relaxation is to use a machine (the electromyograph, or EMG) that can measure muscle tension. Harmless electronic sensors can be fastened to the forehead, neck, jaw, or anywhere muscles may be tense. A tone feeds back information to the person by changing pitch when the muscle tension changes. The pitch drops lower and lower as the person relaxes, and so the person learns what to do to become fully relaxed. Another biofeedback tool, the pulse monitor, can

TABLE 10-3 • **The Stress Response and the Relaxation Response**

Stress Response	Relaxation Response
Stress hormone activity	Normal hormonal activity
Rapid metabolism	Normal metabolism
Fast heart rate	Normal heart rate
Raised blood pressure	Normal blood pressure
Rapid respiration	Normal respiration
Tense muscles	Relaxed muscles
Blood supply to digestive organs and skin diverted to muscles	Normal blood circulation restored
Water retention	Normal water balance restored
Lowered immune resistance	Immune resistance restored

make the heartbeat audible, so that the subject can learn how to slow it down, thus achieving the same thing—relaxation.

You can practice muscle relaxation whenever you think of it—not only when you have time to lie down for 30 minutes. If your shoulders (for example) are tense while you are reading, what good does that do you? Relax them.

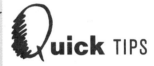

Quick TIPS

Steps to Relaxation

To relax at will:

1. Assume a comfortable sitting position.
2. Close your eyes.
3. Become aware of your breathing. Breathe in deeply, hold it, then breathe out. Each time you breathe out, say the word *one* silently to yourself.
4. Allow each of your muscles to relax deeply, one after another. Imagine that you are floating, drifting, or gliding.
5. Maintain a passive attitude and permit relaxation to occur at its own pace. (Any way that you are proceeding is correct.) Thoughts will pass through your mind; allow them to come and go without resistance.
6. Continue for 20 minutes. You may open your eyes to check the time, but do not use an alarm. When you finish, sit quietly for several minutes, and open your eyes when you are ready.

meditation, self-hypnosis: two methods of relaxing that involve closing the eyes, breathing deeply, and relaxing the muscles.

Two similar relaxation techniques are **meditation** and **self-hypnosis.** Both involve closing the eyes, breathing deeply, and relaxing the muscles. This chapter's Quick Tips section presents steps to relaxation. If you use them once or twice daily, after a while, the response will come with little effort. Practice the relaxation steps before meals; the digestive processes seem to interfere with the response.

To practice relaxation at intervals is to assume control of the body's responses, and it has a benefit beyond the simple pleasure it brings. Just as stress leads to disease, stress management helps to prevent it.

The joy of life is in meeting its challenges, developing new ways of dealing with them, and engaging in experiences that will facilitate new learning. The next chapter offers ways to prevent and deal with the physical stress of injuries and accidents that may occur when the challenges you take on prove to be greater than you anticipate.

PERSONAL FOCUS

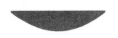

Your Need for Exercise and Relaxation

Fitness, derived from physical activity, permits you to deal with stress; relaxation enables you to recover from it. The more stress (other than physical activity) you experience in your life, the more you need physical activity and relaxation. To help you to discover your own needs for these parts of life, do the following two-part exercise.

First, consider how you, personally, respond to stress, for each person is different. Read carefully and answer each of the questions on Part A of this chapter's Lab Report: The Stress Mode Inventory. Check the boxes next to the symptoms that apply to you. Add up your points to determine your score as shown.

Compare your psychological and physical totals. Which is higher? These scores reflect whether you respond to stress with mostly physical symptoms or mostly psychological symptoms. Most people experience a mixture of both types, but often a trend is apparent.

Review the symptoms you checked. Watch for these symptoms to occur; they warn that stress is getting out of control.

An occasional bout of stress is easy to cope with, but when the stress is repeated, it may wear down resistance and threaten health. To discover which daily events are stressful for you, use Part B of the Lab Report, the Daily Stress Log, to keep an hourly log of the events of one day and your reactions to them. Try to pick a typical weekday; do not pick a day that you expect to be unusual in any way. You can also choose one weekend day to log; you may be stressed in some ways on weekdays and other ways on weekends. The example in Table PF-1 shows one way to record daily events and reactions; record your day the same way.

On Part B of the Lab Report, the Daily Stress Log, make a record of every hour of your day. In the first column, make note of the time of day when you begin to record events. In the next column, write down what you do during that time. Just a word or two to help you remember later is sufficient.

Under the heading *Environmental Conditions,* list anything you notice about the conditions around you. Are you too cold? Too hot? Is your chair too hard? Do your shoes pinch? Is the weather adverse? Notice your surroundings, both near and far, and make note of them. Next, note which social interactions or class activities you perceived as stressful or not stressful. Who was there? What was done or said that affected you? (Try to be specific.)

Even your own thoughts are important because your perceptions of events determine your reactions to them. In the column marked *Thoughts,* record how you react to each occurrence on your list. Write what occurs to you. Also list your emotions as they occur, without trying to change them.

Finally, list the physical and psychological signs of stress you experience. Be on the lookout for such subtle signs as frowning, jaw clenching, extra loud laughing, or reacting irritably with others, in addition to the symptoms you checked on Part A. Did you notice any symptoms that you didn't recognize before?

Now on Part C of your Lab Report, assess your stress log. Look over the first and last columns and write a paragraph or two answering the questions on the Lab Report.

Part D of the Lab Report asks you to list some ways you can change some things about your recurring stresses. Just writing down your recurring stresses may have made you aware that you can do something about them. For instance, in the sample form, the student recorded starting off the day with a stress reaction to traffic and fear of lateness. From now on, this student might be able to alter the morning routine to reduce stress. The student might, for example, leave the house at 7:45 instead of 8:00, change the route to school to avoid the traffic, or take public transportation to eliminate parking.

Part E of the Lab Report asks you how you might adjust you attitude to the stress-causing events that cannot be changed. For instance, the student in

TABLE PF-1 • Example Daily Stress Log

Time	Activity	Environmental Conditions	Social Interactions	Thoughts	Emotions/ Feelings	Stress Symptoms
8:00–9:00	Driving, parking	Loud traffic, parking lot full	—	"Traffic is making me late."	Fear of lateness; anger at traffic	Tight jaw, neck, shoulders
9:10–10:00	Spanish class	Quiet, comfortable	Greeted friends	"I made it on time."	Relief, paying attention	—
10:10–12:00	Study for exam	Chair is hard	Friends going to lunch	"It's too late to study. Go to lunch."	Worry, fear	Bored, can't concentrate
12:10–1:00	Lunch	Loud music, smoke in air	Discuss weight, then friend brags	"Don't order anything fattening."	Feel punished, jealous of others' food	Plan to eat cake later
1:10–2:00	Biology exam	Hot, I'm sweating	—	"Nothing I can do now will help."	Regret, confusion, guilt	Feel powerless, anxious
2:10–6:00	*Work on campus	Pleasant	Greeted boss, coworkers	"Now I can relax."	Competency	—
*At about 5:30	Patron came in to complain	—	Handled irate patron with diplomacy	"I will not get mad—I'll smile."	Pride, superiority satisfaction	Sweating, muscles tight
6:10–6:30	Driving to mall	Exciting, colorful	No one here I know	"I can't afford to buy the radio I want."	Unhappy	Bought and ate cake.

the example felt fearful and angry, and these feelings triggered the stress response. Next time, the student might choose to accept being late once in awhile and relax about it, as well as to plan not to be late as often in the future.

Still, you are bound to be left with some events and circumstances that are truly stressful for you. These signify a need for more physical activity and relaxation in your life. Part 6 of the Lab Report asks you how you might include these in your day. Better organization and more fun in all forms—activity, spiritual reflection, and socialization—can go a long way toward defusing the stress response.

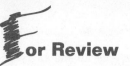

For Review

1. Define *stress* (page 216).
2. Describe the harmful side effects of prolonged stress on the body's systems (page 219).
3. Describe an effective time management strategy (page 224–225).
4. Describe some ways of dealing with emotional pain (defense mechanisms and coping devices), together with the limits of their utility (page 224–226).
5. Describe some of the physical and psychological signs of stress (page 227).
6. Describe the relaxation response and several different means of achieving it (page 228).

E L E V E N

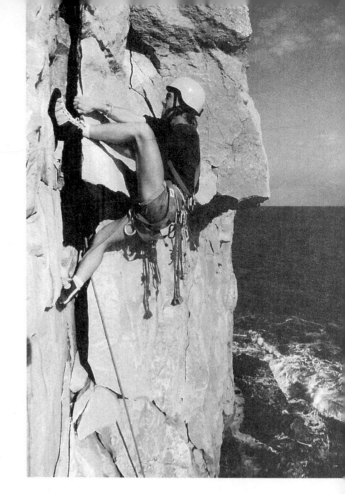

Contents

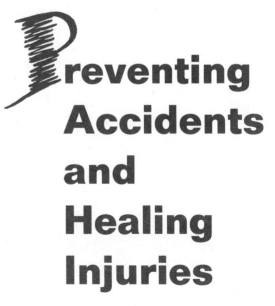

Preventing
Accidents
and
Healing
Injuries

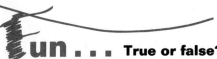
1. The person who learns how to prevent accidents can relax in the security of an accident-free future (page 237).

2. If you don't push yourself hard and fast in your fitness program, you won't progress satisfactorily (page 238).

3. Pain is your ally in safety (page 238).

4. If you are too busy during the week to exercise, a strenuous weekend session can help you to catch up (page 239).

5. Most runners' injuries are the result of falls (page 242).

6. People who exercise in rubber suits or heavy clothing to lose weight do not lose more fat than normal, but they do run the risk of heat stroke (page 246).

7. Coaches and trainers teach athletes to remember RICE in case of injury, because this wholesome grain best nourishes the injured part during recovery (page 250).

8. If you are injured, immediately apply heat (page 251).

injury: physical harm or damage to a person.

accident: an unexpected and undesirable event; an unintentional happening.

Is your response to **injury** prevention and treatment less than enthusiastic? Do you consider **accident** prevention to be unexciting? Does "boring" better describe what you think of these topics? Many people fail to realize the importance of injury and accident prevention in athletic training until they are actually injured. If you take a moment to think about the possible consequences of being injured, you may gain a new appreciation for the contents of this chapter.

Suppose you are a runner and you incur a minor injury such as an ankle sprain. You could be out of training for up to eight weeks. Not only would you suffer physical pain from the injury, but you would also spend valuable potential training time in recovery. Once you were able to resume training, you would then have to work extra hard to catch up to your pre-injury fitness level. Recovering from an injury and working to achieve your pre-injury fitness level can be tiresome and frustrating, especially if you watch your competition progress while you struggle to catch up. The more serious the injury, the longer the time away from training. If you have experienced this, or can imagine it, the value of injury prevention becomes clear.

1. The person who learns how to prevent accidents can relax in the security of an accident-free future.

False.

Even superior knowledge cannot stop some accidents—they just happen.

We should note right away that not all accidents are preventable, of course. Some just happen, and even superior knowledge of prevention techniques cannot stop them. But many accidents are preventable; this chapter is about those that never need to happen.

This chapter's mission is to help you maximize the benefits of your training within the limits of safety. It offers general guidelines for preventing injury both in the gym or pool and out-of-doors. In case you do suffer a sports injury, it offers basic guidelines for treatment and for seeking professional care. Its main points have appeared before (we could not have presented a whole book of activities without the safety precautions to go with them), but this chapter pulls those main points together and adds to them.

Preventing Exercise Injuries

The first step toward preventing exercise-related injuries and accidents is to ensure that you are physically healthy in the first place. It goes without saying that your judgment and coordination need to be at their best, unimpaired by the use of alcohol or any drugs. In addition, if you answered yes to any of the cautions provided in Table 3–1 in Chapter 3, consultation with a health care provider and possibly a physical examination are in order before you proceed with your exercise plan. Once you receive the OK to begin exercising, remember to progress slowly.

General Guidelines for Preventing Exercise Injuries

A few basic guidelines for preventing exercise-related injuries apply to any activity you pursue:

- Include a warm-up and cool-down in your program.
- Progress slowly and steadily (include at least one day a week of rest).
- Alternate heavy and light days.
- Pay attention to body signals.
- Be active all week (don't be a weekend athlete).
- Use proper equipment and attire.
- Perform approved exercises using proper form.

The following paragraphs expand on each of these.

Many people are tempted to skip the warm-up and cool-down segments of their workouts. Regardless of how fit you are, warming up and cooling down reduce muscle stiffness and cramping; minimize injury risk; help to prepare muscles, ligaments, and tendons for activity to come; and mobilize fuels to support strength and endurance activities. As you may recall from Chapters 3 and 4, warm muscles and connective tissues stretch more readily and are less vulnerable to pulls, **strains, sprains,** and muscle soreness.

strain: a muscle injury caused when the muscle is stretched beyond its limit.

sprain: a joint injury caused when the ligaments of the joint are torn.

2. If you don't push yourself hard and fast in your fitness program, you won't progress satisfactorily.

False.

If you push yourself hard and fast in your fitness program, you may injure yourself.

3. Pain is your ally in safety.

True.

The next guideline in injury prevention is to progress slowly. People who develop their fitness gradually are much less likely to incur injuries. For example, it is unrealistic (and dangerous) to expect to be able to run five miles on your first day of running. The reason marathon runners can run so far without joint damage is that they build slowly. Add small increments to your intensity or duration each session.

Another guideline is to alternate heavy and light days. To train hard every day is to invite overuse injuries. The body needs adequate time to repair or rebuild itself. By overtraining, people not only risk injury, they also impair the chances of reaping the full benefit of their training. People who overtrain are likely to become bored, fatigued, and sore. No wonder they often lose interest and quit their activity altogether.

It is tempting, sometimes, to ignore pain or other distress signals and keep on exercising. This is a mistake, and the consequences can be severe. Pain is your ally in safety—it warns you of danger or injury. An important guideline is to pay attention to your body signals. A persistent and sharp pain during exercise is a signal that something is wrong. Stop the activity and try to find out what is the matter. The pain may indicate improper form or technique. For example, if a runner feels leg pain, a change of posture may be indicated. But if the pain persists despite efforts to correct technique, discontinue the activity or get medical help. Once the pain is gone, gradually try performing the activity less strenuously. Symptoms such as abnormal heart action (pulse irregularity, fluttering, palpitations in the chest or throat, rapid heartbeats); pain or pressure in the middle of the chest, teeth, jaw, neck, or arm; dizziness; lightheadedness; cold sweat; or confusion demand immediate action: Stop the activity and seek medical advice.

Pay attention to pain *after* an injury, too, particularly the kind that "splints" parts of your body such as the shins or lower back, making it hard to move. That kind of pain arises when tears in an area need repair work: Adjacent muscle fibers cross-link to one another, making the area inflexible, much as a doctor's splint would do. If you do stretch or bend those muscles, the cross-linked fibers pinch nerves painfully, thus reminding you to keep the area still, much as a splint would do. The support and inhibited movement provide conditions that are optimal for healing: Rest and immobility. Go with the pain messages you receive from such areas; do not fight them by trying to move before they have healed. To respect pain is not being a sissy; it is being smart.

While we say you should be alert to symptoms, there are times when symptoms are not noticeable. This is because the body sometimes masks them. Physical activity elicits production of opium-like compounds that can mask pain exercisers would otherwise feel. These compounds are the body's natural painkilling drugs, endorphins (endogenous opiates), and they are produced in the brain whenever you exert yourself intensively. Endorphins suppress pain many times more effectively than the narcotic morphine, and they can mask the pain of the heart in trouble. They may also produce a dreamy, pleasant state that exercisers enjoy and learn to

exercise stress test: a record of the electrical activity of the heart (electrocardiograph) taken during exercise that may detect heart abnormalities.

4. If you are too busy during the week to exercise, a strenuous weekend session can help you to catch up.

False.

Those who exercise only on weekends increase their chances of injury.

seek. Runners have dubbed it the "runner's high," but it can occur in cross-country skiing, swimming, or any other aerobic sport.

It is prudent to seek an **exercise stress test** before proceeding with a new plan for exercise, particularly for those over 35 years of age and those who have been sedentary for several previous years. That way, you won't have to rely on symptoms (that could be masked by endorphins) to warn you of danger. If, during exercise, you notice any change in comfort or experience pain, stop exercising and consult a health care provider before continuing.

An inconsistent approach to physical activity (the so-called weekend athlete approach) invites injuries. The older weekend athlete is particularly susceptible to heart attack, and weekend athletes of all ages enhance their chances of injuries. Vigorous and sudden demands on out-of-condition muscles, ligaments, and tendons lead to sprains and strains. A regular program of activity helps to develop the fitness that safe weekend play demands.

No matter which activities you choose, make sure you use well-designed equipment to perform them. And, as mentioned in Chapter 6, both your performance and your safety benefit when you wear the appropriate shoes and clothing for your chosen activity. For example, if you want to bicycle, take the time and effort to find out which bike best meets your needs, and then invest in it. If you choose to run, wear shoes made especially for running; if you choose aerobic dance, wear aerobic dance shoes.

Another way you can prevent activity-related injuries is to learn to perform the activities correctly and avoid the methods that you know are harmful. For example, Chapters 4 and 5 offered detailed instructions on the correct positions for stretching and strength exercises and included cautions against improper form. The next sections revisit the main activities of Chapters 5 and 6 with an eye to injury prevention.

Weight Training

Injuries are common among weight trainers, especially among those who use free weights. Many people fail to warm up before exercising, lift with incorrect form, exercise too hard, and attempt to lift too much weight. General guidelines for injury prevention on page 237 are especially important in weight training. Increasing the workload gradually is crucial. Other helpful hints include:

- Use correct form and breathe properly.
- Raise and lower the weights with smooth motions.
- Use a spotter when necessary.
- Use a weight belt for lower back support when necessary.
- Use knee, ankle, and other wraps when appropriate.

When training with free weights, remember to practice guidelines for injury prevention not only during the exercise, but also while adding weights to the bars when setting up for an exercise and when returning weights or barbells to the racks when the exercise is completed. Cramps and lower back pain are especially likely to plague weight trainers who overwork, and Table 11–1 lists preventive strategies for these and other injuries.

TABLE 11–1 • Common Activity-Related Injuries and Their Prevention

Injury	Description	Prevention
Blisters	Swollen, liquid-filled areas of the skin	Wear socks and shoes that do not rub and slip on the feet.
Cramps	Painful cramping of muscles.	Drink plenty of fluids, eat balanced diet, increase workload gradually, stretch muscles.
Lower back pain	Pain in lower back area, sometimes running down the leg	Increase the back's workload gradually, stretch lower back, strengthen abdominal muscles.
Foot pain	Painful inflammation of the connective tissue along the sole	Perform calf stretches, and run, dance, or play on firm, springy surfaces. Wear proper shoes.
Runner's knee	Aching or soreness around or under the knee	Build up gradually. Use proper equipment and form. If untrained do not sprint. Slow your pace when cycling or running on hills. Stop at first sensation of pain.
Ankle or knee pain	Inflammation on the outer side of the ankle or knee joint	Practice on flat surface or alternate sides on sloping surface.
Shin splints	Pain in shin region	Progress more slowly and work out on proper surfaces.
Achilles tendon[a] pain	Stiffness or pain in Achilles tendon	Do gentle stretches of the heel and calf frequently. When running, avoid or go easy on steep hills. Wear running shoes with a slightly elevated heel.
Swimmer's shoulder	Painful inflammation of the soft tissues around the shoulder joint.	Build up gradually. Don't overdo overhand pulls.

[a]The Achilles tendon is shown in Figure 4–2.

Source: L. S. Weil, *Aches and Pains of Running* (Washington, D.C.: American Running and Fitness Association, 1989); Running Injuries You Can Avoid, *Executive Fitness,* March 1989, p. 3.

Walking

Walking can provide excellent fitness benefits with minimal risk of injury. Walking is less stressful to vulnerable joints than is running. In fact, walking-related injuries are relatively rare.

A good pair of walking shoes is the only necessary equipment. Well-cushioned, flexible walking shoes that have a low back tab to reduce pressure on the **Achilles tendon** are recommended. Shoes that have "breathable" upper materials keep the feet cool. The sides of a walking shoe should provide stability but need not be as strongly reinforced as running shoes. Loose-fitting, comfortable clothing that is appropriate for the climate is also advised.

Proper posture while walking minimizes back injury. Be sure to walk erect, look straight ahead, keep your shoulders back and your head up. Let your arms swing freely at your sides, and relax your hands and shoulders. Lean forward enough so that your weight is on the balls of your feet when they are under you. Push off for each step with your back foot rather than pulling yourself forward with your front foot. Keep your chest up, stomach in, and hips tucked under, not tilted back. Practice this posture in front of a mirror, then maintain that form outdoors.

Some people carry hand weights while walking to burn more energy. Carrying weights while walking increases the heart rate and energy expenditure slightly above that of walking without weights. However, some authorities caution against carrying weights while walking because it tends to elevates blood pressure.[1] Most authorities recommend against strapping weights to legs or ankles because they can alter the stride, impair balance, and strain joints, thus increasing the chances of leg injuries. (The knee and hip joints are not designed to lift weight while working.)

Aerobic Dancing

Aerobic dance often demands rapid turns and twists and intense jumping. Stress injuries from hopping, twisting, and jumping are common among aerobic dancers. Many of the complaints shown in Table 11–1, already referred to, trouble aerobic dancers who neglect safety precautions.

High-impact aerobics cause injuries because both feet are often off the ground simultaneously. Low-impact aerobics are less risky and therefore more popular because one foot is always firmly on the ground during exercise, reducing the risks of injury.

Aerobic dance or fitness programs should follow the recommended guidelines of the American College of Sports Medicine[2]:

- They should include warm-up, cardiovascular, and cool-down phases.
- They should occur at a frequency of two to three classes per week.
- They should occur at an intensity that maintains a heart rate between 75 percent and 80 percent of maximum

Achilles tendon: the tendon that connects the back of the heel to the muscles of the calf of the leg (see Figure 4–2).

- They should require preparticipation screening for medical problems and fitness.
- They should be taught by an instructor who is certified by one of the major aerobic dance certification groups (IDEA, AFFA, ACSM*) and trained in basic cardiac life support procedures.
- They should be conducted on wood floors. Concrete or carpet over concrete are not recommended for medium- or high-impact aerobic programs.
- Dancers should wear comfortable, well-fitting shoes designed specifically for aerobic dance. They are different from running shoes in that they support lateral movements. Many injuries occur from aerobic dancers' exercising barefoot or in running shoes.
- They should include proper warm-up and stretching exercises.
- They should discourage overly competitive aerobic programs.

The instructor should perform and demonstrate all exercises correctly. Form is of great importance in rapid dance movements, as in any fast-moving sport, because incorrect positions and movements lead to injuries.

Running

Running has been called the first exercise of the fitness era, and it is the workout of choice for millions of Americans. Unfortunately, more than half of the people who run are injured each year. The most common injuries (review Table 11–1, presented earlier) are to the feet, ankles, shins, knees, hips, and buttocks. Many runners complain of shin splints, "runner's knee," foot pain, calf muscle stress, and lower back pain. It is understandable that running injuries are so common: When you run, your feet strike the ground with a force of about two to three times your body weight. Most runners' injuries are the result of overuse or stress on the legs and feet. Some guidelines for preventing common running injuries include:

- Run on grass or dirt when possible. These surfaces are firm and supportive, yet softer than most other surfaces. (Beware of holes or uneven surfaces).
- When you run on paved roads, choose asphalt rather than concrete if possible. Asphalt has more yield and therefore stresses the feet and knees less.
- Run on a flat surface, if possible. If you run on the side of the road, the banked edge will turn your outside foot, stressing that ankle and leg. If you must run on such roadsides, alternate sides if traffic permits.
- Avoid running on an indoor track. It can increase the chance of injury because the continuous turns may strain the feet, ankles,

5. Most runners' injuries are the result of falls.

False.

Most runners' injuries are the result of overuse or stress on the legs and feet.

*International Dance Exercise Association: The Association for Fitness Professionals (IDEA), Aerobics and Fitness Foundation of America (AFFA), and American College of Sports Medicine (ACSM).

and knees. (It also is monotonous because of the repeated loops necessary to achieve distance).

- Do not run downhill too strenuously; this can injure your lower back.
- As mentioned previously, build endurance gradually. Do not push yourself too hard.

Most important:

- Wear a good pair of running shoes. The most important qualities in a running shoe are flexibility and heel support.
- Don't run barefoot, even on the beach.
- Replace shoes when necessary. When the shoes feel worn out, the heel support starts to collapse, the soles get thin, or new shoes feel significantly different, it's time for a new pair.
- Observe good running form. Hold your head up to help you maintain proper posture. Bend your elbows about 90 degrees, and move your arms forward and backward with the opposite leg. Your feet should land on an imaginary straight line each time they hit the ground, not on either side of a line. Avoid up-and-down motions. Develop a natural, fluid style and stay relaxed.

If you run on the beach, do so for relaxation and fun, not for serious training. The looseness of the sand stresses the arch of the foot, causing excessive foot rotation. The heel sinks too deeply in the sand straining the achilles tendon. Wear running shoes, warm up and stretch before running, and especially be sure to stretch the achilles tendon. Run as close to the water as possible, where the sand is flattest and firmest.

Swimming

Swimming is an excellent fitness activity for almost anyone. The injury rate among swimmers is low because swimming places no burden on the spine, hips, knees, or other joints. Still, form is important in swimming and, for most strokes, should be much the same as good walking posture—only horizontal, of course. Your chest should be out, stomach in, hips tucked, and back straight. Your shoulders should be relaxed, not hunched. Your legs should be parallel, with knees and feet straight, turned neither in nor out. An expert swimming coach has much to say about proper form for the sake of both performance and safety, and a skilled swimmer will comply.

Common complaints among swimmers include "swimmer's shoulder," "swimmer's itch," sunburn on shoulders and back, brittle hair, burning of the eyes, and ear infections. "Swimmer's shoulder" is a painful inflammation of the soft tissues around the shoulder joint. This is caused by pulling on the shoulder joint during overhand strokes and is common among swimmers who use hand paddles. A few days of rest will usually clear it up. The other complaints result from environmental influences and are discussed later in detail.

Cycling

Stress injuries from cycling are relatively rare because the bicycle absorbs the impact of the surface. Common injuries among bicyclists are tendinitis in the ankle, "runner's knee" (from too much hill work), sore shoulders, numb fingers, and saddle soreness. Many of these conditions can be avoided by practicing proper technique and wearing clothing that does not bind or restrict blood flow.

Proper cycling posture helps to prevent injury and promotes maximum comfort. The cyclist should lean forward, bend from the waist, and keep the back relatively straight. The knees should point forward, not splay out. The elbows should be bent so that the muscles, rather than the joints, absorb road shock.

Proper posture depends on a bicycle that fits the rider. To determine the appropriate frame size for you, measure your inseam and subtract 9 to 10 inches. This gives you the size bicycle you need. When you straddle the bicycle standing on the ground, the top tubular element of the frame should be about an inch lower than your crotch. It should be possible to adjust the seat so that the rider's leg is almost fully extended at the bottom of the stroke. The pedals should grip the feet, either with toe clips or cleats that fit in the tread of the shoes.

Proper cycling equipment can also help to prevent cycling injuries. Shoes designed specifically for cycling are advised because they stabilize the feet on the pedals and help to keep the feet from toeing out or toeing in. Cycling gloves with padded palms help to prevent soreness of the fingers. Clothes should be comfortable but not so loose as to get caught in the bicycle's moving parts.

Soreness from the bicycle seat (saddle) can occur when a person first takes up cycling or when the cyclist rides long distances. A beginner's soreness subsides as the tissues in the buttocks get tougher. However, here are some pointers to prevent or minimize soreness:[3]

- The saddle should be firm enough to absorb the person's body weight. One with gel or extra thick padding is recommended.
- The saddle should be wide enough in back to support weight, yet narrow enough in the front to keep out of the way. Seats that are too high or too wide cause chafing and rocking. Seats that are too narrow can cause numbness of the genital nerves.
- The saddle should be adjusted so that when the cyclist is seated, the knee is almost straight at the bottom of the pedal stroke. The front (nose) of the saddle should be parallel to the top tube of the frame, not pointing up or down.
- Set the handlebars high enough so that the cyclist doesn't have to sit with undue pressure on the nose of the saddle.
- If the saddle is uncomfortable, it can be cushioned with a saddle pad. If that doesn't work, a new saddle should be purchased.

Lined cycling shorts should be worn without underwear—underwear slides and causes chafing. If you take long rides, you should stand up on the pedals for 30 seconds at least once every 30 minutes. You should also stand up when riding over bumps, train tracks, and other rough surfaces.

General guidelines for preventing exercise injuries, as well as guidelines specific to individual sports, often require little more than common sense and attending to body signals. The discussion now turns to preventing environmental injuries and accidents.

Preventing Environmental Injuries and Accidents

The outside environment presents many injury risks to the athlete and can affect training.[4] This section discusses hyperthermia and heat stroke; hypothermia and frostbite; and pedestrian, cycling, and water safety.

Hyperthermia and Heat Stroke

Heat is a by-product of energy fuel breakdown, so muscles heat up during exertion and "burn" large amounts of fuel. To maintain a normal body temperature, blood penetrates the muscles, absorbs the heat, and transports it to the skin, where the surrounding air and the evaporation of sweat can carry it away. In hot, humid weather, sweat does not evaporate well because the surrounding air is already laden with water. Without the cooling effect of sweat evaporation, body heat builds up and triggers maximum sweating—the body's only defense against excess internal heat **(hyperthermia).** This excessive sweating can be extremely hazardous because fluid and electrolyte losses beyond a certain point compromise cellular functioning and can even be fatal.

The next step beyond excessive sweating is total failure of the body's heat-regulating mechanisms—**heat stroke.** The person stops sweating, the pulse and breathing rates grow rapid, dizziness and coma ensue, and the process can end in death.

The body sends signals of distress, such as cramps, nausea, chest pains, or diarrhea, which warn that heat stroke may be threatening during an activity. The most important preventive step is to stop the activity immediately, even if you must lose a competition. Other steps to prevent heat stroke include:

- Drink adequate fluid.
- Recognize dangerous environmental conditions—high humidity, high temperature, or both.
- Limit intentional exposure to heat.

In potential heat stroke weather:

- Wear lightweight, loose-fitting clothing.
- Drink several extra glasses of water in the hours before you exercise heavily (even if you are not thirsty).

hyperthermia: excess internal body temperature.

heat stroke: failure of the heat-regulating systems of the body that can lead to coma and death.

- Replace water lost during the activity with a dilute, cold beverage (about five ounces of cold, plain, or lightly flavored water, or one part fruit juice to four parts water) every 15 to 20 minutes.
- Recognize your body's distress signals, and heed the message to stop exercising—take a rest in the shade.

Because of the dangers of hyperthermia and heat stroke, it is unwise to exercise in a plastic or rubber suit as people sometimes do in hopes of losing pounds. The waterproof material prevents evaporation, causing the body to sweat excessively and bringing about a dangerous rise in body temperature. Similarly, too long a stay in a hot whirlpool bath, hot tub, or sauna can cause heat stroke.

Hypothermia and Frostbite

hypothermia: a dangerous drop in internal body temperature.

Another threat for athletes training outdoors is **hypothermia,** which is a dangerous loss of body heat. During winter weather, the body can lose heat, especially through the head, neck, and feet. The person may not even be aware of the drop in body temperature because the physical activity may have rendered the person insensitive. The warning signs of hypothermia are mental confusion, cold or pale skin, bloated face, trembling, slow pulse, shallow breathing, and stiff movements. An oral temperature below 95 degrees Fahrenheit warrants medical attention; recovery is rare when the oral temperature drops to about 80 degrees Fahrenheit.

frostbite: a destruction of tissue by freezing caused by exposure to intense cold. This is seen mainly on the nose, cheeks, ears, fingers, and toes.

A danger in extremely cold conditions, especially to exposed skin, is **frostbite.** It can occur without warning. The best preventive strategy is to cover as much body surface as possible. Creams and jellies help to prevent frostbite somewhat but not totally. For a man, it is important to protect the penis and testicles from frostbite by wearing sweatpants instead of nylon shorts.

Pedestrian Safety

Whenever you jog, bicycle, or walk along the roadside, traffic presents a hazard. Two-thirds of all pedestrian deaths and injuries occur when people are crossing or entering streets. Some drivers may not see you; some may be out of control. The Quick Tips offer some precautions.

When you breathe, you may also take in exhaust and dirt from passing cars, together with poisonous pollutants. To avoid inhaling them, stay at least 50 feet off major roads while jogging, running, or biking; at the least, avoid rush hour. If your city has no bike or jogging trails, you might be able to contact the elected public figures who represent you, such as city commissioners, and ask how to start such a project.

Another concern for the pedestrian is dogs. Some dogs may bite. The best action is to stop and face the dog and then slowly back away, trying not to antagonize it. It also may help to carry a stick or a can of mace.

Another environmental hazard is exposure to ultraviolet light. The declining level of ultraviolet-absorbing ozone in the earth's upper atmosphere is resulting in an increased risk of skin cancer for anyone who spends time in the sun, and especially for those who exercise outdoors because they expose more skin for longer times. A sunscreen with a sun protection factor (SPF) of at least 15 can minimize direct risks of ultraviolet exposure. Waterproof (not water resistant) sunscreen is recommended: It resists being washed off when you swim or sweat.

Unfortunately, the danger of rape is real. A woman who runs after dark should always run with a partner. Other precautions you can take are:[5]

- Leave word of where you plan to run (and when you will return) with family or friends.
- Stay alert to suspicious-looking people.
- Keep your arms free for defense.
- Stay on busy, well-lighted streets.
- Have your keys ready before you get to your front door.
- Carry a hatpin or stickpin in your hand. You will not have time to fumble for it.
- Carry a whistle.

If efforts fail and you are followed:

- Ring the nearest doorbell.
- Move away from shadowy areas into an open, well-lit area.

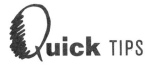

Roadside Precautions

Specific guidelines for pedestrians include:

- Run or walk against traffic.
- Use lights. Battery-operated flashing devices that clip to belts or strap onto legs are available.
- Carry a flashlight.
- Cross only at intersections or marked crosswalks; obey traffic signals.
- Whenever you bicycle alongside the street, always keep right, following the flow of traffic.
- Wear bright, easy-to-see clothing; wear flourescent or reflective materials made into vests, headbands, wrist and ankle bands, belts, or strips of tape at night.
- Don't look directly at approaching headlights; they'll blind you temporarily.
- Stay off high-speed roads.
- Don't wear headphones—they cut you off from the world, and you may not hear a car approaching.

If you are approached:

- Try to stall for time; someone may come along.
- Try to attract the attention of a passing motorist.

If you are attacked:

- Scream "fire" (not "police," since others are then likely to avoid becoming involved), and pull a fire alarm, if possible.
- Break a window; someone is likely to respond to the noise.
- Use your key or a stickpin to aim decisively for the attacker's eyes, temples, Adam's apple, or ears. Stab hard without warning.
- Try to disgust your attacker by urinating or by gagging yourself to induce vomiting. Tell him you have a sexually transmitted disease.

Cycling Safety

Head injuries account for 85 percent of the nation's 1,000 annual cycling deaths.[6] The American Academy of Pediatrics, the National Safety Council, and the Bicycle Federation of America unanimously favor the use of helmets. When you buy one, look for the seal of approval of an institution whose test standards are accepted nationwide.*

Besides using helmets, a series of safety measures are recommended to prevent accidents while cycling:[7]

- Wear bright clothing to make yourself more visible.
- Buy a new helmet; a secondhand one may be flawed.
- Use padded gloves to prevent forearm and hand injuries.
- Use a rearview mirror to check for passing cars.
- Ride with the traffic. Drivers expect you to follow the same rules they do.
- Be extra careful on wet and slippery roads. Rain or ice may pose visibility problems or make it difficult to stop abruptly.

Night cycling is much more dangerous than cycling during daylight hours because you can't see the road and cars can't see you. Some precautions for night cycling include:

- Use a headlight and taillight, preferably halogen (brighter than incandescent), powered by a generator or rechargeable battery. The headlight should be visible from 500 feet. The rear light should be visible from 600 feet.
- Wear reflective clothing and patches. Stick patches on your helmet, shirt, sleeves, seat, saddlebags, and the backs of your shoes.
- Use a spacer (a device to which you can attach a flag or disk high above the seat). It keeps traffic at bay during the daytime and, if the flag or disk is reflective, at night, too.
- Make sure your bike is equipped with front, side, rear, and pedal reflectors, which are now required by law on new bikes.

*The institutions are the American National Standards Institute (ANSI) or the Snell Memorial Foundation.

Often overlooked in bicycle injury reports are injuries to young children riding as passengers on adult bikes. The frequency of this type of injury is increasing. Child seats are not safe; the best protection is to use helmets approved for children by the American Academy of Pediatrics.

Water Safety

Drowning prevention stands out as the number one safety concern for water activities. Accidents can happen, even among experienced swimmers, so the most important guideline is **never swim alone.**

Other guidelines for swimming safety include:

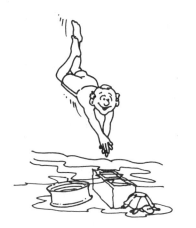

Don't dive where obstructions might lurk.

- Use good judgment when you choose a place to swim.
- When the water is cold, ease your way in.
- Swim only when you feel well, not when you are tired, sick, or overfull after eating.
- Do not dive where obstructions might lurk or where you don't know the water depth.
- Do not overestimate your ability.
- Do not dive too deep; come up promptly when you need to breathe.
- Have a boat accompany you on a distance swim.
- Never play rough in or near the water.
- Get out of the water when lightning threatens.
- Except in emergencies, rely on your own swimming ability, not on inner tubes or floats.

If you see someone in trouble in the water, help them by using the techniques described in Table 11–2. Only a trained lifeguard should attempt rescue by swimming out to the victim; a drowning person can easily overpower a novice and drown them both.

You may have heard that you should not swim until an hour after eating, to prevent stomach cramps. It is not necessarily dangerous to swim with a full stomach, especially if you exercise lightly. However, if you undertake an intense swimming workout after eating, you may indeed experience cramps, and they are just as likely to occur in your legs or arms as in your stomach. The reason may be that digestion requires energy and oxygen, robbing them from the hard-working muscles. You need not stay out of the lake altogether after a picnic—just take it easy while your stomach is full.

A minor complaint among swimmers is "swimmer's itch." This is an allergic reaction to the bite of a parasitic worm found in lakes and rivers. It often takes two weeks for the rash to heal. Alcohol or calamine help relieve the itching.

To prevent sunburn on the shoulders and back, use a waterproof sunscreen with an SPF of 15. Incidentally, though this is not a safety issue, wash your hair and condition it after each swim to combat the dryness. A swimcap is also helpful in taking care of the hair.

Burning of the eyes can result from the chlorine in a pool. Sand or microorganisms in open water can also irritate the eyes. In these circum-

TABLE 11-2 • Water Rescue Techniques

Even if you cannot swim, you can assist a swimmer who is nearby and in trouble. If the swimmer is near a dock or in a pool:

- Lie flat on the dock or pool ledge; extend an arm or leg, towel, shirt, fishing pole, oar, or other object, and pull the victim within reach of the edge. Most pools have long-handled cleaning tools around that work well. If there is a lifesaving cushion or float nearby, aim carefully and throw it to the victim.

If the troubled swimmer is farther away than you can reach:

- Wade into the water up to your waist, and extend an object or push a float or a board, or throw a rope where the victim can reach it.

If the victim fell from a boat, or you are in a boat:

- Allow the victim to hang onto the boat or to an object you hold out.

If the victim is too weak to hold on:

- Pull the victim into the boat carefully to avoid worsening any injuries.

If the victim fell through ice:

- Push a ladder or other long object, tied with a rope at the bottom rung and secured, out to the victim, or use ropes, poles, sticks, or a human chain to reach the person.
- If the victim is too weak to hold on, a rescuer can crawl along the ladder to help.

SOURCE: Adapted from American Red Cross, *Standard First Aid and Personal Safety* (New York: Doubleday, 1979) pp. 249–253.

stances, wear goggles. People prone to ear infections can use preswim eardrops to keep water out. Alternatively, after swimming, they can use eardrops containing alcohol to help dry the ear canals.

Treating Sports Injuries

If you have injured yourself, you have two options: To go to a health care provider, or to wait to see whether the injury clears up by itself. (If you are bleeding or badly hurt, of course, choose the former.) Pain is your guide. If the pain diminishes during the first few hours, chances are the injury is slight. If it increases or stays the same for several hours, you may have a more serious condition that requires attention. If, in two or three days, any injury fails to clear up, get medical help.

A set of guidelines applies to the treatment of many injuries to muscles, ligaments, and tendons. The guidelines apply to strains, sprains, suspected fractures, bruises, and joint inflammation. People who deal with sports injuries use the memory guide (RICE) to remember them:[8]

- Rest—to prevent additional damage to injured tissue, stop exercising immediately; if the lower extremities are affected, use crutches to move about.

7. Coaches and trainers teach athletes to remember RICE in case of injury, because this wholesome grain best nourishes the injured part during recovery.

False.

Coaches and trainers teach athletes to remember RICE for injury treatment because it stands for Rest, Ice, Compression, and Elevation, the four guidelines for injury treatment.

8. If you are injured, immediately apply heat.

False.

Never apply heat to an injured area at first. Apply ice.

- Ice—to limit blood flow to the injured part to prevent swelling, apply ice immediately for 15 to 30 minutes. Avoid direct ice contact with the skin, though; put the ice in a plastic bag, and wrap a towel around it.
- Compression—to limit swelling, firmly apply the ice to the injury using a towel or bandage to secure it.
- Elevation—to let gravity help drain excess fluid, raise the injured limb above heart level.

Rest continuously, and use the other treatments (ice, compression, and elevation) at intervals for at least 48 hours. On the fourth day, discontinue cold treatments and begin to apply moist heat or dry heat, or use a whirlpool twice daily for 15 to 30 minutes. Depending on the severity of the injury, mild exercise can resume in four or five days.

Never use heat at first. Use tape and bandages only to reduce swelling in conjunction with rest, ice, and elevation. Do not use them to enable you to keep playing despite an injury.

This chapter has offered guidelines for preventing and treating sports-related injuries and accidents. Chapter 12, the final chapter of the book, offers guidelines to help consumers recognize fraudulent practices and products.

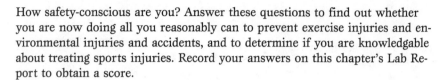

PERSONAL FOCUS

How Safety-Conscious Are You?

How safety-conscious are you? Answer these questions to find out whether you are now doing all you reasonably can to prevent exercise injuries and environmental injuries and accidents, and to determine if you are knowledgable about treating sports injuries. Record your answers on this chapter's Lab Report to obtain a score.

A. General Guidelines for Preventing Exercise Injuries

1. I consistently practice a warm-up before every workout and a cool-down at the end of each workout.
2. I increase my workload gradually.
3. I exercise consistently throughout the week, not only on weekends.
4. I wear appropriate clothing and use proper equipment for the activity I participate in.
5. I practice proper form when performing exercise activities.
6. I am knowledgable about exercises that cause injury and I avoid them.
7. I pay attention to the signals my body gives me and I act appropriately.

B. Preventing Environmental Injuries and Accidents

8. I take environmental precautions before exercising outdoors.
9. I never swim alone.
10. When I cycle, I always wear a helmet.

C. Treating Sports Injuries

11. When I suffer a minor injury, I discontinue the activity so that I can heal.
12. When I suffer an injury that does not clear up in a few days, I see a health care professional to obtain an accurate diagnosis and treatment.
13. When I suffer a minor injury, I apply the guidelines of RICE—Rest, Ice, Compression, and Elevation.

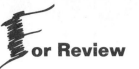

F or Review

1. List and describe general guidelines for preventing exercise injuries (page 237).
2. List and describe environmental injuries and strategies for preventing them (page 245).
3. List guidelines for treating sports injuries (page 250–251).

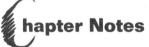

C hapter Notes

1. For walkers who carry weights, *Tufts University Diet and Nutrition Letter,* July 1989, p. 2.
2. Preventing injuries in aerobic dance, *Sports Medicine Digest,* May 1989, p. 3.
3. The cyclist's lament: Saddle soreness, *Sports Medicine Digest,* April 1989, p. 5.
4. C. C. Teitz, *Scientific Foundations of Sports Medicine* (Philadelphia, Pa.: B. C. Decker, Inc., 1989), pp.345–371.
5. Women running smart, *Sports Medicine Digest,* March 1990, p. 7.
6. Risks to the child as bicycle passenger, *Sports Medicine Digest,* April 1989, p. 5.
7. Accident among downtown cyclists, *Sports Medicine Digest,* May 1989, p. 5.
8. Teitz, 1989.

T W E L V E

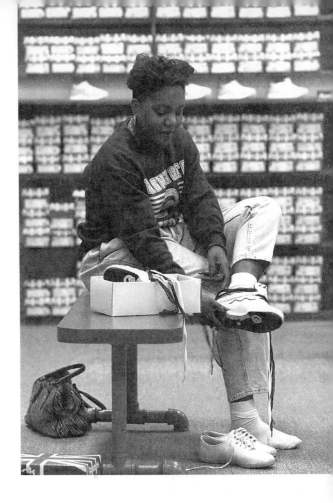

Contents

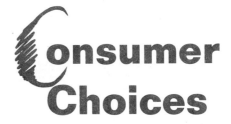

Consumer Choices

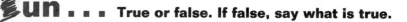

JUST FOR Fun . . . True or false. If false, say what is true.

1. An advertisement broadcast on nationwide television is likely to present the truth (page 258).

2. If a product label makes the claim ''organic'' or ''natural,'' this means the product has unusual powers to promote health (page 259).

3. Taking growth-promoting hormones is a safe way to develop your muscles (page 265).

4. The practice of injecting amphetamines into an athlete's blood to speed up performance is known as blood doping (page 265).

5. If a particular food or nutrient eaten just before a competition seems to benefit your performance, it's probably all in your head (page 266).

6. You can be sure you are getting a balanced workout if you follow one of the commercially available programs (page 274).

Overweight and out of shape? Want to lose pounds without dieting and eliminate inches without exerting any effort? If you do, you're not alone. Millions of Americans hope and believe that somehow, magically, they can be thin and firm.[1] Unwilling or unable to lose weight through diet and exercise, many people turn to weight-loss gimmicks. It is easy to be lured into the promise of losing inches without doing anything more strenuous than popping a pill or wrapping the flesh. It is difficult to resist ads that promise to burn away fat even during sleep.

The theme of this chapter is consumerism as it relates to health and fitness. Consumers face many problems in a free-enterprise market, where competition for their dollars encourages advertisers to push their products aggressively and not always honestly. Some promotions are so sophisticated that it is hard for even well-educated, mature adults to see through them.

This chapter gives pointers about sources of health and fitness information; strategies for evaluating health claims; ways to avoid gimmicks; and ways to evaluate fitness programs, facilities, and equipment. It concludes with guidelines for determining which programs and products are really necessary to achieve the fitness level desired.

Strategies for Evaluating Health and Fitness Claims

Many sources of information claim or imply that their statements are facts. Take television commercials, for example. Actors dressed as scientists or physicians make solemn pronouncements to the effect that "research has shown this product to be effective. . . ." But when you look closely, the evidence is nowhere to be found. Magazines do the same thing: Slick photographs of authority figures appear in them, but evidence to back their claims does not.

How, then, can the consumer of health and fitness information decide whether the claims made by the promoters of health products and services are legitimate? This section's main purpose is to enhance the consumer's skill in distinguishing between valid health information and health **fraud** or **quackery.**

fraud or **quackery:** conscious deceit practiced for profit.

When you see a claim for a product or service, you can use a set of basic strategies to evaluate it. The following paragraphs present these strategies with some example applications.

1. *Ask who is making the claim.* If the person or organization making the claim stands to profit by selling something, discount the claim. It is as simple as that. To get honest, unbiased information about any product or service, find an outside expert who can make an assessment. An example familiar to most people is buying a used car. The salesperson's word alone is not sufficient, nor is the word of someone who has another car to sell; an independent garage mechanic should be hired to assess the car. The mechanic is not personally involved in the sale and stands to gain most by telling the truth because the satisfied customer will give a favorable report to other customers. If the person making the claim does not appear to be motivated by personal gain, then go on to the next question.

2. *Ask about the person's education, training, skill, and reputation.* A person may be justly famed and admired for one specialty, but that does not indicate qualifications to speak in another specialty area. A noted poet is not as well qualified to speak on physical fitness as a trainer of Olympic athletes; a famed heart surgeon may not be knowledgeable about sex therapy; the governor of a state is not an authority on nutrition. When someone makes pronouncements on a given topic, ask whether the person is qualified to speak on that topic.

   The first of the four qualifications to look for is education. Education is indispensable; there is no substitute for the hundreds of hours of book learning that provide the foundation for a person's knowledge. Training is important, too, for all the book learning in the world is useless until the person has practiced using it in real-life situations. Skill is a third characteristic to evaluate; it normally develops as the result of education and training, but some people do not become skilled even with the best of both. Finally comes reputation: A person earns that by developing the first three assets.

3. *Ask where the claim is published: Newspaper, magazine, book written for the public, textbook, journal.* Health information purveyed by the mass communication media—newspapers, magazines, radio, television—is notoriously unreliable (see the Box, "The Truth of the Matter"). Books on health written for the public are also unreliable; most professional organizations maintain committees to combat the misinformation in them. Textbooks and the journals true scientists use to communicate their findings are not perfectly infallible, but they are more reliable than most other sources.

~~~~~~~~~ The Truth of the Matter

People who are interested in fitness and read about it in popular magazines come across advertisements such as these: "SWINDLE amino acids deposit slabs of muscle bulk," "Ram the body into turbo charge with HOODWINK enzymes," "Ultrapotent TECHNO-HYPE vitamins and minerals blast carbs through your system." Fortunately, ads like these are easy to see through—they are transparent in their purpose of extracting readers' money.

However, some advertising, though just as false, is more sophisticated and can fool all but the most tenacious quack-busters. It succeeds by creating the illusion of credibility. It convinces readers that amino acids or other products are needed and, further, that this or that company's products are superior to others on the market. You might open a magazine and find a professional-looking "review of the literature" that appears to lend support to the efficacy of the SCIEN-TIFIC Company's supplements in improving physical performance. The graphs and figures seem meaningful—all data point to the wisdom of using SCIENTIFIC Company's pills and potions. The references at the bottom of the page cite such credible sources as *The American Journal of Clinical Nutrition* and *The Journal of the American Medical Association.*

This looks scientific and it may be, but don't forget that you are reading an advertisement. The solidity of the claims may begin to crack when you probe into the listed references. A careful reading of the cited research will probably reveal that the company has taken the facts out of context. In one case, for example, the writers of such an ad reported a finding that supplements were useful in treating a disease—which was true—but then jumped to an invalid conclusion: They said that healthy athletes should use the supplements. The research they cited provided solid documentation for facts, but *not* for the facts stated in the advertisement. The original research was sound and reliable, and the authors clearly articulated their findings. The advertisers, on the other hand, selectively reported only facts that could be twisted to support sales of their products.

4. *Check with the professional society concerned with the subject of the claim.* Then decide whether to believe the speaker.*

   Many professional organizations have banded together to form the National Council Against Health Fraud (NCAHF), which has branches in many states. The NCAHF monitors radio, television, and other advertising; investigates complaints; and maintains a bimonthly newsletter to keep consumers informed on the latest health misinformation. If you do not know whom else to ask, write to the NCAHF.

5. *Be alert to the language in which claims are made.* Many buzzwords and phrases indicate false or misleading information — among them, the following:

   - "Organic, health, herbal, natural." These terms have no legal meaning on labels, and although they imply unusual power to promote health, they do not.
   - "Scientific breakthrough, medical miracle." Seldom do such popular reports prove true.
   - "Doctors agree, authorities agree." When the identity of the doctors is not revealed or when no reference to an authoritative publication is provided, these statements may mean only that the advertiser persuaded three doctors to agree.

   Some false claims are recognizable if you can spot the confused thinking that underlies them. Here are some examples:

   - "Tiredness is a symptom of iron-poor blood." This is true. "Therefore, if you are tired, you have iron-poor blood, and you need iron supplements." This is not true because tiredness is also a symptom of other conditions. You need a diagnosis by a health care professional.
   - "People need the essential nutrients or else they will get sick." This is true. "Therefore, they need food X, which contains nutrients." This is not true because no food is the unique possessor of any nutrient. Other foods can supply essential nutrients in the amounts needed.

6. *Recognize the child in yourself who frightens easily and delights in magic.* Some claims are outright tricks that work because every consumer has such a child inside. Even though the adult in you can see through these tricks, they still attract the child in you.

*If you have questions about a fitness book, product, or service, write to the American College of Sports Medicine, P.O. Box 1440, Indianapolis, Indiana, 46204; about a medical book, product, or service, to the American Medical Association, 535 North Dearborn Street, Chicago, Illinois, 60616; about an anticancer book, product, or service, to the American Cancer Society, 803 West Broad Street, Falls Church, Virginia, 22046; about a heart disease preventive, to the American Heart Association, 7320 Greenville Avenue, Dallas, Texas, 75231; about a diet or nutrient supplement, to the American Dietetic Association, 208 South LaSalle Street, Suite 1100, Chicago, Illinois, 60604. You can write to the National Council Against Health Fraud (NCAHF) at P.O. Box 1276, Loma Linda, CA. 92354.

Who has not been tempted to buy a product or try a service because it sounds so easy ("no effort"), because it costs so little and produces such a big reward ("something for nothing"), because it will protect you from terrible things (scare tactics), or because it will restore your vitality or youth or beauty or all of these (magical thinking)?

7. *Learn to recognize when an image is being used to "push your button," and sell a product.* The box presented earlier already gave the example of science appeal; here are some other claims that make other kinds of appeals:

- Rich people use our product (snob appeal).
- Famous people use our product (fame appeal).
- Ordinary people use our product (just plain folks appeal).
- Funny, happy people use our product (smile appeal).
- Beautiful people use our product (vanity appeal).
- Everyone uses our product (bandwagon appeal).
- Our product is new and improved. You can tell because the packaging has changed (newness appeal).
- Our product is better than theirs (brand loyalty appeal).
- We will give you bonuses and free merchandise if you buy our product (bribery).
- Our product is environmentally sound (ecology appeal).

Promoters also offer special machines (technology appeal), secret formulas (chemistry appeal), and medical breakthroughs (miracle appeal). These appeals work; otherwise, advertisers would not use them.

A new appeal is appearing on products and services today—the green appeal: "Our product or service is environmentally sound." Be especially discriminating about these. It is true that nothing is more urgent today than choosing products with an awareness of their environmental impacts. It is true that any conscientious consumer will pay close attention to this. But unfortunately, advertisers are beginning to abuse people's good intentions by making false or exaggerated claims about the "ecological" virtues of their products and services. Don't give up your environmental idealism, but arm yourself with knowledge so that you can make the right choices without unnecessary expense. For example, it is important to buy soaps that do not pollute the water when they go down the drain. It is not important to buy expensive, green soaps that call themselves names like "Ecosoap."

8. *Recognize attacks on your self-esteem as manipulations designed to sell you things you don't need.* The people who try to sell you products to improve your outward appearance are motivated to benefit themselves, not you. To benefit themselves, they have to extract your money. If you are satisfied with yourself as you are, they lose; they have nothing you'll be willing to buy. So their marketing strategy promotes your self-dissatisfaction, to convince you that

your appearance is not OK. You have a problem, and they have the solution. A person with low self-estcem to begin with is practically defenseless against these tricks; in fact, low self-esteem is one of the marks of a person who is vulnerable to quackery. The higher your self-esteem, the better you can see through these tricks, the more confidently you develop your own image, and the less you will feel compelled to mold yourself to fit theirs. The Quick Tips sum up these pointers.

The following sections evaluate a selection of products, programs, and services that claim to promote fitness and health. Some of these are truly effective, some are negative, and others are dangerous. They are under three headings—"Aids to Athletic Performance," "Weight-Loss Strategies," and "Fitness Programs and Equipment."

Aids to Athletic Performance

In a world where body condition and skill are hard won, athletes gravitate to promises that they can easily attain performance gains by taking pills or potions. Athletes too often hear well-intended, but unsubstantiated, advice from their coaches and peers that they should use special nutrients, drugs, or procedures.

Nutrition Supports to Performance

Valid nutrition supports of fitness have already been the subject of Chapters 7, 8, and 9 and are reviewed here. Ineffective and unnecessary nutrition products are found in the Box, "Nutrition Supplements."

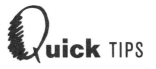

Strategies For Evaluating Health and Fitness Claims

1. Ask who is making the claim. Does that person stand to gain from your belief in it?
2. Ask about the person's education, training, skill, and reputation.
3. Ask where the claim is published: Newspaper, magazine, book written for the public, textbook, journal?
4. Consult the professional society concerned with the subject matter in question, or write to the National Council Against Health Fraud.*
5. Be alert to the language in which claims are made.
6. Recognize the child in yourself who frightens easily and delights in magic.
7. Recognize attacks on your self-esteem as manipulations designed to sell you things you don't need.

*See note on page 259 for addresses.

amino acids: isolated components of protein promoted to athletes on the mistaken notion that the body prefers single chemicals to those combined naturally in foods.

astragalus: see **herbal steroids.**

bee pollen: a product sold with the claim that it aids in weight loss and boosts athletic performance, but that in reality has no such effects.

branched-chain amino acids: amino acids that are burned for energy by muscle tissue; athletes do not need supplements of these because the liver liberates exactly the right amounts with exactly the right timing to support exercise; leucine, isoleucine, and valine.

brewer's yeast: a preparation of yeast cells promoted because it contains high concentrations of B vitamins; falsely promoted as an energy booster.

damiana: see **herbal steroids.**

DNA (deoxyribonucleic acid): a necessary chemical in protein synthesis; falsely promoted as an energy booster.

dong quai: see **herbal steroids.**

fo ti teng: see **herbal steroids.**

gelatin: protein used to thicken foods; sometimes falsely claimed to be a strength enhancer.

ginseng: a plant whose extract has been inappropriately promoted as an energy booster. See also **herbal steroids.**

ginseng root: see **herbal steroids.**

glandular products: extracts and concentrates of glands and tissues from cows, pigs, and sheep; falsely promoted to provide specific nutrition to the athlete's gland's and organs.

glycine: see amino acids.

growth hormone releasers: a product falsely promoted for enhancing athletic performance.

herbal steroids: curious mixture of "adaptogens" and "aphrodisiacs"; marketed with false claims that these herbs contain and enhance hormonal activity.[a]

isoleucine: see **branched-chain amino acids.**

leucine: see **branched-chain amino acids.**

licorice root: see **herbal steroids.**

octacosanol: an alcohol isolated from wheat germ; often falsely promoted to enhance athletic performance.

palmetto berries: see **herbal steroids.**

pangamic acid: also called vitamin B_{15} (but it is not a vitamin); falsely promoted as an energy booster.

continued

Balanced Diet.   A balanced diet is indispensable to health and fitness. The nutrients in food help to regulate energy-yielding processes in the body and promote growth, development, and repair of body tissues, including those involved in the generation of human energy. Sound nutrition is an important contributor to success in sports.

Glycogen Loading.   Some endurance athletes use glycogen loading (described in Chapter 9) to trick their muscles into storing extra glycogen. The technique recommended by exercise physiologists extends endurance with minimal side effects. The regular, everyday exerciser has no need of such extended endurance and so gains no benefit from this technique, but for all active people, a high-carbohydrate diet best supports physical activity.

Vitamin and Mineral Supplementation.   As described in Chapter 9, vitamins and minerals participate in many body processes that facilitate athletic performance. When athletes have experienced deficiencies of the B vitamins, supplementation has restored performance.[2] Athletes such as wrestlers consume low-calorie diets for prolonged periods, a practice that is not recommended by the American College of Sports Medicine. For those who persist in doing so, however, a one-a-day vitamin-mineral supplement may be recommended to prevent deficiencies. Even though vitamin-mineral supplementation has been and continues to be widely practiced by athletes, research indicates that it is not effective for enhancing performance in the well-nourished athlete.

As described in Chapter 9, some athletes have iron-deficiency anemia.[3] In those people, iron supplementation has been shown to improve aerobic performance. Although some research suggests that iron supplementation may also improve performance in people with iron deficiencies not severe enough to cause outright anemia, other research disputes this finding.[4] Iron supplementation does not, however, benefit individuals with normal iron status.

Drugs Athletes Use

Two drugs have been shown to enhance athletic performance: Anabolic steroids and caffeine. However, their use incurs risks.

Anabolic Steroids and Other Hormones. Men generally develop bulkier muscles than do women in response to exercise. This occurs because men produce larger amounts of certain **steroid hormones** in their bodies. (These hormones are called *anabolic,* signifying that they promote muscle growth.) These hormones are also available as drugs, developed to remedy deficiencies in people born without the ability to produce them, and like all drugs, they can be abused. Some athletes, both men and women, self-administer anabolic steroid drugs in the attempt to develop bulkier muscles. Studies of these practices show that anabolic steroid drugs can increase body weight (especially lean body weight) and, in combination with high-intensity weight training, can increase muscular strength in some highly conditioned athletes, but many users experience no such benefit.[5] No extra aerobic capacity is gained by steroid drug use.[6]

To athletes struggling to excel, the promise of bigger, stronger muscles beyond those that training alone can produce is tempting. Athletes who are not genetic superstar material, and who normally would not be able to break into the elite ranks, can suddenly compete with true champions. Such unfair competition compels other athletes to abuse the drugs. Especially in professional circles, where monetary rewards for excellence are enormous, steroid abuse is common, despite its illegality.

The medical community is concerned about the safety of steroid drugs. For one thing, all steroid users experience a sharp change in their blood lipid profiles reflecting an increased risk of heart disease.[7] In addition, steroids are known to impair liver function; cause cancerous liver tumors, liver rupture, and hemorrhage; promote permanent changes in the reproductive system; and alter facial appearance.[8]

Some of the side effects of hormone abuse occur in all users. Testicular shrinkage in men and masculinization of women are inevitable.[9] Psychological changes attributed to steroids include mood swings, aggressive behavior, and changes in sexual appetite.[10] A segment of users suffers the most deadly effects promptly; the symptoms that may result in other users after 20 years of abuse are unknown. For now, serious athletes are forced to make a hard choice—to use no steroids and face a field

steroid hormones: hormones of a certain chemical type that occur naturally in the body. Anabolic steroids that promote muscle growth are available as drugs and are misused by athletes seeking a shortcut to large muscles.

full of artificially endowed opponents, or to use the drugs and risk their side effects. Judging from athletes' extensive use of steroids, they must consider the drug risks less severe than the risk of facing disadvantages in competitive events.

Because steroids are detectable by urine testing, some athletes have resorted to the use of other hormones that are not detectable, with equally negative effects. Athletes who take human growth hormone (HGH) develop symptoms of the disease **acromegaly**—huge body size, widened jawline, widened nose, protruding brow and teeth, and an increased likelihood of death before age 50.[11]

The American Academy of Pediatrics and the American College of Sports Medicine condemn the use of hormones by athletes. They cite their known toxic side effects, state the belief that taking these drugs is another form of cheating, and say that competitors who use them put other athletes in the difficult position of either conceding an unfair advantage to the abusing competitors or "taking them and accepting the risk of untoward side effects."[12] Young athletes should not be placed in the situation of having to make such choices.

Caffeine.   Another drug often used to enhance athletic performance is caffeine. As described in Chapter 9, caffeine ingestion before exercise has been shown to extend endurance.[13] Caffeine is a stimulant that elicits a number of physiological and psychological effects in users. The possible benefits must be weighed against caffeine's adverse effects—stomach upset, nervousness, irritability, headache, and diarrhea. Caffeine induces fluid losses that can be potentially hazardous if caffeine-containing fluids are used in place of other fluids by athletes competing in hot environments.[14]

Blood Doping

Nutrient supplements and drugs are not the only substances athletes use in an effort to improve their performance. One of the most popular practices is to inject extra doses of their own blood—this is called **blood doping**.[15]

Blood doping may or may not improve athletic performance. Some studies say it does, some say it doesn't. World-class athletes—including members of the victorious U.S. bicycling team in the 1984 Olympics—have admitted to the practice, lending it credibility as a means of reducing race times. As a result, the issue is still alive and its ethics are often debated. Several studies confirm that blood doping increases the blood's oxygen-carrying capacity, but the practice also entails possible negative health consequences, such as effects on blood clotting and blood pressure. These effects remain to be studied.[16]

The search for a single food, nutrient, drug, or procedure that safely and effectively enhances athletic performance will no doubt continue for as long as people strive to achieve excellence in sports. So far, it seems that when athletic performance does appear to improve after use of a

---

acromegaly: a disease caused by above-normal levels of HGH, characterized in adults by thickening of the bones, hands, feet, cheeks, and jaw, thickening of the soft tissue of the eyelids, lips, tongue, and nose, and thickening and rumpling of the skin on the forehead and soles of the feet. Internally, the heart, liver, and other organs become distorted. A child with the condition is said to have *gigantism* because the bones grow abnormally long.

3. Taking growth-promoting hormones is a safe way to develop your muscles.

   False.

   Growth-promoting hormones have toxic side effects and may or may not be effective in developing muscle tissue.

4. The practice of injecting amphetamines into an athlete's blood to speed up performance is known as blood doping.

   False.

   Blood doping is the practice of injecting extra doses of the athlete's own red blood cells to increase the blood's oxygen-carrying capacity.

blood doping: an untested procedure that involves collecting and storing an athlete's own blood before competition, then adding it back to the person's blood supply in the attempt to overcome the limits on performance set by the oxygen-carrying capacity of the blood.

5. If a particular food or nutrient eaten just before competition seems to benefit your performance, it's probably all in your head.

True.

performance aid, the effect can probably be attributed to the psychological boost the aid provides.

Weight-Loss Strategies

It would be wonderful if people could lose body fat just by taking a pill, a powder, or a special food product; or if they could make their fat simply disappear by applying heat or rubbing their bulges. One survey of 29,000 weight-loss strategies found fewer than 6 percent of them effective—and 13 percent dangerous.[17] The consumer may react with the question, "What can the government do about that?" The government is active in pursuing and cracking down on health swindles, but most agencies have insufficient staff and resources to handle the massive number of reported cases. They can, at best, eliminate only the most dangerous schemes. The result is that promoters of less dangerous schemes can rake in billions of dollars. It is easy for a swindler to get a product on the market and hard for the government or other groups to get it off. That puts the burden of distinguishing weight-control frauds from reality on the consumer. To keep from being taken in, remember: If it sounds too good to be true, it probably is.

This section presents three kinds of weight-loss programs: Some are valid, some appear to work but are ineffective, and some are risky. Totally ineffective weight-loss gimmicks can be found in the Box "Weight-Control Gimmicks." The most valid criterion of a good weight-loss program's success is not the speed or the magnitude of weight loss, but maintenance of the goal weight, once achieved.

Effective weight-loss programs are characterized by a sensible approach based on:

- Selecting a diet that is realistic and that provides gradual weight loss.
- Incorporating a realistic, practical, and enjoyable exercise program into your schedule.
- Adopting new behavior patterns to achieve and maintain the desired body weight.

Few people are able to make these changes consistently on their own. Many people seek outside sources of guidance and support to help achieve weight loss in a healthy manner. Proven programs are Overeater's Anonymous, Weight Watchers, and individual diet counseling with a registered dietitian.

For some obese individuals, medically supervised very-low-calorie diets (such as Optifast) offer an alternative means of rapid weight loss that, for healthy people, sometimes proves effective. The very-low-calorie diet programs that teach behavior modification and train clients to change their eating behaviors are the better ones.

The preceding programs have been proven to be safe and effective when used appropriately. The remaining programs are either ineffective or unsafe. Table 12–1 offers guidelines for identifying weight-loss scams.

TABLE 12-1 • Guidelines for Identifying Weight-Loss Scams

Consider suspect any programs that:

- Promise or imply dramatic, rapid weight loss (that is, substantially more than one percent of total body weight per week).
- Include diets that are extremely low in calories (that is, below 800 calories per day; 1200 calories-per-day diets are preferred), unless under the supervision of competent medical experts.
- Attempt to make clients dependent upon special products rather than teaching how to make good choices from the conventional food supply (this does not condemn the marketing of low-calorie convenience foods, which may be chosen by consumers).
- Do not encourage permanent, realistic lifestyle changes including regular exercise and the behavioral aspects of eating wherein food may be used as a coping device (that is, programs should focus on changing the causes of overweight rather than simply the effect which is the overweight itself).
- Misrepresent salespeople as "counselors" supposedly qualified to give guidance in nutrition or general health. Even if adequately trained, such "counselors" would still be objectionable because of the obvious conflict of interest that exists when providers profit directly from products they recommend and sell.
- Require large sums of money at the start or require that clients sign contracts for expensive, long-term programs. Such practices too often have been abused as salespeople focus attention on signing up new people rather than on delivering continuing, satisfactory service to consumers. Programs should be on a pay-as-you-go basis.
- Fail to inform clients about the risks associated with weight loss in general or the specific program being promoted.
- Promote unproven or spurious weight-loss aids such as those described in the Box, "Weight-Control Gimmicks."
- Claim that "cellulite" exists in the body. (Cellulite is supposed to be a hard-to-lose form of fat, but in reality, there is no such thing as cellulite. All fat is hard to lose.)

Source: Adapted with permission from *National Council Against Health Fraud Newsletter*, March/April 1987.

Low-Carbohydrate Diets

As previously mentioned, the most valid criterion of a good weight-loss program is the maintenance of goal weight, once achieved. By this standard, low-carbohydrate diets are not effective ways to lose weight. Low-carbohydrate diets, by design, produce ketosis (defined in Chapter 8). The sales pitch is that "you will never feel hungry" and that "you will lose weight fast—faster than you would on any ordinary diet." Both claims are true, but both are misleading. Loss of appetite accompanies any low-calorie diet. Fast weight loss means lean tissue loss.

The body responds to a low-carbohydrate diet as it does to a fast. As described in Chapter 8, the body is receiving protein and fat (on a fast it draws on its own protein and fat), but it has used up its stored glycogen.

It therefore turns to its protein to make the needed glucose. When the body converts protein to glucose, it produces waste products, which it must excrete along with water in the urine. This produces a massive, rapid weight loss composed of lean tissue and water, which puts a burden on the kidneys. Other hazards of low-carbohydrate diets are high blood cholesterol, mineral imbalances, and other metabolic abnormalities.[18] Some low-carbohydrate diets, particularly protein-sparing fasts, have caused death due to heart failure.[19] These diets are never recommended by legitimate practitioners.

Low-carbohydrate diets have been around for many years under many names, and they are reintroduced with new names, too.* Watch out for them. Any diet that centers on meat, fat, or alcohol and limits carbohydrate is a member of this group. Bringing out new diet books and products is a profitable business and will continue to be successful as long as people are deceived by the initial rapid weight loss into thinking that the diets work.

One particularly objectionable focus of the low-carbohydrate diet is the liquid-protein diet based on a very-low-calorie liquid formula containing inadequate carbohydrate. Liquid-protein diets have caused abnormal heart rhythms in many users and deaths in quite a few. The Food and Drug Administration requires that all very-low-calorie (below 400 calories) protein diets carry warnings that their use as total diets without medical supervision "may cause serious illness or death."[20]

Water-Loss Inducers

Many products produce weight loss on the scale by temporarily depleting the body of water. The dieter sees the pounds disappear and concludes that this reflects fat loss. Water losses account for the weight losses seen when people take water pills or laxatives, or when they use steam baths, saunas, body wraps, or creams.

Water pills. Diuretics, or "water pills," have a legitimate medical use, but are of no use in controlling body fatness. The wishful thought behind their use by dieters is that excess weight is due to water accumulation. If *water* retention is a problem, a diuretic and possibly a mild degree of salt restriction can help, but the obese—that is, overfat—person has a *smaller* percentage of body water than the person of normal weight. Weight loss, accomplished this way, is accompanied by dehydration and electrolyte loss, and lasts less than a day.

Laxatives. Similar to diuretics, laxatives may be safe and effective for their intended purpose, but not for weight loss. Laxatives cause water loss, not fat loss.

*Names of low-carbohydrate diets popular in the past include the Air Force Diet, the Atkins Diet, the Calories Don't Count Diet, the Drinking Man's Diet, the Herbalife Diet, the Mayo Diet, the Protein-Sparing Diet, the Scarsdale Diet, the Simeons HCG Diet, the Ski Team Diet, and the Stillman Diet.

Steam baths and saunas.   A person who takes a steam bath or sits in a sauna sweats abundantly and can lose several pounds in less than an hour—all water. If the person drinks water after such a sweat session, the body returns to its previous weight. Similarly, people sweat in hot water, although they may not realize it. A whirlpool bath may feel wonderful and yield a noticeable weight change on the scale, but it does not "melt fat" or "burn calories," as some people claim.

Body wraps and creams.   Advertisements claim that body wraps will melt fat away in a short time and promise that people will lose 4 to 6 inches the first day. Body wraps are constricting or nonporous plastic or rubber garments. Some are worn around the waist; some cover the waist, hips, and thighs; still others cover nearly the entire body. Some are used after creams, gels, or lotions are applied. The Food and Drug Administration has investigated a number of these products and has taken action against their promoters for making unsubstantiated medical or therapeutic claims.[21]

The garments and wraps, with or without lotions and creams, reduce body dimensions by removing fluids. Most medical experts agree that such treatments cause loss of inches and perhaps pounds due to profuse perspiration, but the reductions are temporary. Rapid and excessive fluid losses are potentially dangerous, of course, because they bring on severe dehydration and upset the body's electrolyte balance.[22]

Some salons, gyms, or clubs advertise that wrapping the body in bandages soaked in a "magic solution" will cause a permanent reduction in body girth. This so-called treatment is pure quackery.[23] Tight, constricting bands can temporarily indent the skin and squeeze body fluids into other parts of the body, but the body regains its original shape within minutes or hours. Body-wrapping is potentially dangerous; at least one fatality has resulted.

Exercising in nonporous wraps is an especially dangerous practice because it prevents heat loss and sweat evaporation. The body's core temperature can rise to a dangerous level during exercise.

Wraps and creams have no chemical effect either. They do not dissolve fat, even temporarily. Nor does perspiration break down fat.[24] Fat breaks down only when less food energy is consumed than that needed to meet the body's requirements.

The person who goes to the gym and uses the steam bath, sauna, and whirlpool, and gets a massage and a body wrap may have a wonderful time socializing and relaxing. If the goal is to lose weight or to improve fitness, however, this person is in for a disappointment.

Diet Pills

A variety of diet pills are available by prescription or over the counter. Only one drug, a nervous system stimulant that suppresses the appetite, has been deemed safe and effective by the Food and Drug Administration for use in over-the-counter diet pills. It is **phenylpropanolamine.** Ap-

phenylpropanolamine (FEN-ill-prope-ah-NOLE-ah-meen): the active ingredient of over-the-counter diet pills; also an ingredient of many cold, cough, and allergy remedies.

proximately seventy diet products with different names line the shelves of drug stores, and they all contain this one active ingredient. (Even "Amazing Grapefruit Pills" labels list phenylpropanolamine.) On the label is a warning that the drug can induce strokes in those with a history of hypertension, and that it may harm people who suffer from any of a number of diseases. Even healthy people risk brain hemorrhages from the drug, especially if they exceed the suggested dose or combine it with other common drugs such as oral contraceptives, cold and cough remedies, or even caffeine.[25]

Another substance, **ephedrine,** may be approved for use as the active ingredient in some diet pills. Ephedrine is a common over-the-counter drug used in cold and asthma medicines. Ephedrine, administered with aspirin or caffeine, shows promise as a weight-control aid because it stimulates the body's heat output, thereby diminishing the amount of energy stored in fat.[26]

In contrast to these drugs, which are relatively safe, **amphetamines** are dangerous. They do reduce the appetite but are not appropriately used for this purpose except, perhaps, when obesity is life-threatening. Amphetamines are powerful, addictive, mind-altering drugs. Their milder side effects include nervousness, sleeplessness, and irritability; they also stress all body systems including the cardiovascular and nervous systems. A person who uses amphetamines for weight loss may indeed lose weight, but then is faced with the tough problem of how to kick the drug habit without regaining the weight. It can seldom be done. Short-term weight loss achieved by any means is not a permanent solution to a weight problem, and when it is achieved through drugs, it can leave a person with two problems—being overweight and being addicted as well.

Surgery

Surgery for obesity has dangerous side effects. *Bypass surgery,* which involves disconnecting or removing a portion of the small intestine to reduce nutrient absorption, is seldom performed anymore because results have been so disappointing. *Stapling* the stomach to reduce its capacity is preferred, but not perfect: Stomach tissue is damaged, scars are formed, and staples pull loose.

At intervals, medical researchers develop new approaches to limit the stomach's capacity. One approach is to slip a *balloon* into the stomach and inflate it; another is to confine the stomach within a web that keeps it from expanding. Risks of these procedures are unknown, but success, as measured by long-term weight maintenance, is seldom achieved.

Another surgery to reduce body fat is minor when compared with those just mentioned—**liposuction.** A competent plastic surgeon can suction the fatty deposits from beneath the skin to reduce the area's fatty appearance. Some obese people might wish they could get rid of their body fat this way but, unfortunately, excess body fat is usually distributed evenly all over the body, and no responsible surgeon would undertake to remove fat from such vast areas. Liposuction is not a valid weight-loss method; it is useful only for limited cosmetic purposes.

acupuncture: a system of medical treatment derived from ancient Chinese practice; it involves inserting slender needles into the skin at nerve junctions to influence the functioning of the nervous system. Possibly effective for some purposes (such as the treatment of pain), acupuncture has not been shown effective as a weight-control treatment.

amino acids: protein building blocks offered as nutrient supplements to quell the appetite and thus reduce food intake. (The amino acids most often used this way are arginine and ornithine.) At concentrations that make animals sick, they do reduce appetite, but such intakes are not safe. See also *human growth hormone.*

arginine: see *amino acids* and *human growth hormone.*

before-meal candies: candies promoted as "appetite spoilers." They contain a lot of sugar and a local anesthetic to "deaden" the taste buds; actually, they add calories before meals that can add to a weight problem. They are falsely promoted as having the ability to suppress appetite and thereby to control weight.

bulk producers, bulking agents: products that expand when they absorb water; they are taken about 10 to 30 minutes before meals. They are supposed to swell up in the stomach and quiet hunger contractions. Contrary to claims, bulk producers tend to pass fairly quickly into the small intestine. Even while they are in the stomach, no clear evidence indicates that their presence affects the stomach's hunger contractions.[a] These agents are ineffective for weight loss.

cholecystokinin (CCK): a hormone secreted into the blood by the intestine in response to the arrival of fat, which is known to signal the gallbladder to release bile; CCK reaches the brain and creates feelings of satiety. This hormone is widely available in health-food stores. It is sold in pill form; the pills contain ground-up animal intestines (CCK is produced there), supposedly to provide CCK and signal satiety. In reality, the amount of CCK in a pill's worth of animal intestine is almost too small to detect, let alone to suppress appetite. CCK is a protein; it is destroyed by digestion in the stomach, and none is absorbed from an oral dose.[b]

ear stapling: a special application of acupuncture that involves placing a staple permanently in the earlobe. The claim is that this reduces appetite and food intake; the reality is that it does not, except in believers prone to suggestibility.

electronic muscle stimulators (EMS): devices that can apply slight electric shocks through the skin to make muscles contract. In the hands of qualified medical personnel, muscle stimulators are valuable therapeutic devices. They can help to prevent atrophy in a patient who is unable to move, and they may decrease spasticity and contracture. However, when sold on the pretext that they "tone and firm," "spot reduce," and "improve body contours," as well as promote fat

continued

loss, these devices are fraudulent. Any effects are temporary (gone within hours); voluntary exercise directed by the brain is much more effective in developing fitness. The Food and Drug Administration has approved electronic muscle stimulators only for physical therapy. Electronic muscle stimulators should never be used by the layperson and have no place in a reducing or fitness program. One such device, the *Relax-A-Cizor* was issued a permanent injunction by a U.S. district court. The device was declared to be dangerous to health, having the potential effect of inducing abnormal rhythms of the heart, as well as causing miscarriages and aggravating such conditions as hernia, ulcers, varicose veins, and epilepsy.[c]

glucomannan (gloo-co-MAN-an): a preparation derived from a vegetable (konjac tuber) used in Japanese cooking; claims of weight-controlling properties are unsubstantiated.

human chorionic gonadotropin (HCG): a hormone from the placenta that supports early pregnancy, not useful in weight loss. Hormones are powerful body chemicals and many affect fat metabolism, but all have proved ineffective and often hazardous as weight-loss aids. Schemes that require injections of HCG are not only expensive and useless, but they also present risks of illness and shock from infected serum or amateur administration.

human growth hormone (HGH): a pituitary hormone that promotes growth and deposition of body protein and other lean tissue and breakdown of fat for energy; also called *somatotropin*. HGH releasers are really amino acids (arginine and ornithine) that supposedly correct a too-low level of HGH and promote weight loss during sleep. It is true that some obese people secrete less HGH in response to an arginine dose than thin people do, but this fact shows only that arginine is *not* effective precisely in those who need it the most.[d] As for the hormone itself, a true overdose causes acromegaly, a disfiguring disease.

massage: physical manipulation of the muscles, through the skin, by use of the hands, vibrator devices, or mechanical rollers. Massage has been used since ancient times to soothe tired painful joints and muscles and to induce relaxation. It causes a slight increase in surface blood flow and skin temperature. It can serve other therapeutic uses when it is administered in the clinical setting for medical reasons, but massage does not alter body shape or remove fat deposits under the skin. A six-week study of the effects of massage on body girth reported no significant decrease in girth when the unmassaged arm and leg were compared with the massaged arm and leg.[e]

metabolic accelerators: substances credited with speeding up the metabolic rate (see *thyroxine*).

motor-driven cycles and rowing machines: like all mechanical devices that "do the work" for the individual, these motor-driven machines are ineffective in a fitness program if the person merely re-

continued

laxes on the machine and lets it pull the limbs through the motions.[f] They may help to increase circulation, and some may even help maintain flexibility, but they do not replace active exercise. Nonmotorized cycles and rowing machines are appropriate equipment for developing fitness.

ornithine: see *amino acids* and *human growth hormone.*

Relax-a-Cizor: see *electronic muscle stimulators.*

rolling machines: types of equipment made of wood or metal, operated by an electric motor, that roll back and forth along the body parts to which they are applied. Contrary to claims, they do not remove, break up, or redistribute fat.

spirulina: a kind of algae ("blue-green manna") said to suppress appetite and to enhance athletic performance: It does neither.

starch blocker: a fraudulent product falsely promoted to impede starch digestion and therefore to help in weight control.

thyroxine: a hormone of the thyroid gland that regulates the body's metabolic rate; it promotes breakdown of glucose and protein, but not breakdown of fat. Thyroxine plays a role in remodeling of lean tissue during growth. Hormones top the list of potentially harmful diet aids, and *thyroxine* tops the list of such hormones. Thyroxine has long been promoted as a "metabolic accelerator," but it is dangerous in the amounts needed to overwhelm the human thyroid regulatory system. Its side effects include degradation of the body's lean tissue, including the heart muscle, and an irregular heart rate. At one point, a heart medicine and a diuretic were added to thyroxine to counter these effects, but they did not prevent the damage it caused; some people even died from the combined effects of the drugs.[g]

tummy trimmers and firmers: exercise machines and devices designed to firm and flatten the stomach; promoted by several television advertisements. They are sold under names such as *The Gut Buster, The Tummy Trimmer,* or *The Stomach Eliminator.* Testing of these gadgets by *Consumer Reports* showed that none of these exercisers deflates a "spare tire."[h] To do that, you need to burn fat. These gadgets do not burn fat and will not tone an overlarge abdomen. Most of the people testing the equipment felt the effects of the exercise in their fingers, arms, and shoulders but stated the springs had no effect on their abdominal muscles.

vibrating belts: wide canvas or leather belts designed to massage the chin, hips, thighs, or abdomen. These belts are driven by an electric motor and jerk back and forth, causing loose tissue of the body part to shake. Vibrating belts have no fitness or fat-loss-inducing benefits, and they are potentially harmful if used on the abdomen (especially if used by women during pregnancy or while an intrauterine device (IUD) is in place). They might also aggravate a back problem.

continued

vibrating devices: vibrating devices are common types of passive equipment. They come in the form of elaborate tables, couches, chairs, beds, cushions, belts, small hand-held appliances, and pillows. Contrary to advertisements, these passive devices do not improve posture, trim the body, reduce weight, or develop muscle tone. It is incorrect to assert, as has been done, that 45 minutes on a rocking table is equivalent to playing 36 holes of golf.[i] For some people, vibration can help induce relaxation, but it has no effect on body weight.

[a]Consumer Reports Books, *Health Quackery,* (Mount Vernon, N.Y.: Consumer's Union, 1980), pp. 123–155.

[b]Cholecystokinin (CCK): Weight-loss breakthrough or hoax?, *NCAHF Newsletter,* January/February 1985, p. 1.

[c]See note a above.

[d]J. Lowell, "Growth hormone releasers" don't cause weight loss, *Nutrition Forum,* December 1984, p. 24.

[e]See note a above.

[f]See note a above.

[g]L. Lasagna, Drugs in the treatment of obesity, in *Obesity,* ed. A. J. Stunkard (Philadelphia, Pa.: W. B. Saunders, 1980), p. 296.

[h]The wrong way to a trimmer tummy, *Consumer Reports,* May 1988, p. 285.

[i]See note a above.

Fitness Programs and Equipment

The consumer who chooses to invest money in fitness may ask any of the following questions:

- What programs shall I choose?
- What facilities shall I visit?
- What equipment shall I buy?

This section provides pointers to assist the consumer in exploring the variety of available answers.

Evaluating Fitness Programs

You have just learned that gimmicks promise results without effort or time. Contrary to these claims, a well-conditioned body costs effort and time. You know the importance of physical activity, and you are aware of your own fitness level. Perhaps you are considering using one of the many programs designed to help people develop fitness. If that is the case, Tables 12–2 and 12–3 can help you to rate the available programs according to the principles you have learned.

6. You can be sure you are getting a balanced workout if you follow one of the commercially available programs.

False.

Some commercially available programs are ineffective or unsafe.

TABLE 12-2 • Evaluating Fitness Programs

You can evaluate fitness programs objectively by using your knowledge of what fitness is and how it is gained and maintained. Ask the following questions, start with 100 points, and subtract points as indicated for shortcomings.

- Does the program include sufficient aerobic exercise for cardiovascular fitness (about 20 minutes, 3 days per week)? If not, **minus 10.**
- Does the program include exercises that promote muscle strength and endurance, such as sit-ups, push-ups, or weight training? If not, **minus 5.** Are strength exercises given for all large muscle groups? If some parts are left out, **minus 5.**
- Does the program include exercises for flexibility, such as gentle stretches? If not, **minus 10.**
- Does the program allow for varying initial fitness levels; that is, can you start out slowly and work your way up? If not, **minus 10.**
- Does the program take a reasonable time each day—say at least 20 minutes, but less than an hour—at least 3 days per week? If not, **minus 10.**
- Does the program include a warm-up and a cool-down period? If no to either, **minus 5**; if no to both, **minus 10.**
- Can the program be performed with only basic equipment, such as shoes, small weights, or a jump rope? Must you join an expensive club to participate? If specific or unusual products, perhaps sold by the promoters, must be used or if a large membership fee is required, **minus 10.**
- Is the program safe? If it suggests bouncy stretches, straight-leg sit-ups, or other exercises shown in this book to be unsafe, give it a **minus 10.** If it advocates clearly hazardous practices, such as running in heavy or rubber clothing, don't even consider using it: Its **total score is zero.**
- Does the promoter make claims backed up by legitimate research? If unorthodox claims are made, such as "no-work fitness," "redistribute your fat" (or cellulite), or "cures your heart disease" (or other diseases), **minus 10.**
- Does the program promote a lifetime fitness plan based on a variety of enjoyable activities? If the program is monotonous, it will soon become boring and hard to stay with, so give it a **minus 10.**

Evaluating Fitness Facilities

Many clues can assist you in distinguishing between a reputable fitness facility that promotes sound exercise practices and a facility that promotes ineffective or unsafe ones. To evaluate a fitness facility, ask yourself questions about all of the following:

- Its atmosphere
- Its location
- Its practices
- Its personnel qualifications
- Its approach
- Its reputation
- Your overall impression

TABLE 12-3 • Fitness Programs Compared

Fitness Program Name and Description	Question 1: Aerobic Exercise	Question 2: Muscle Strength	Question 3: Flexibility	Question 4: Initial Levels
The Aerobics Way (Dr. Kenneth Cooper). An aerobic system that favors cardiovascular over other fitness. It provides safety suggestions missing in previous versions. It is goal-oriented, and may lack fun for some, and it undervalues some enjoyable activities such as soccer.	Yes	No, insufficient strength exercises MINUS 10	No, insufficient flexibility exercises MINUS 10	Yes
Jogging (Bill Bowerman and Dr. W. E. Harris). A book that provides three jogging plans for various fitness levels. It presents no other types of exercise.	Yes	No, no strength exercises MINUS 10	No, insufficient flexibility exercises MINUS 10	Yes
Total Fitness (Dr. Lawrence Morehouse). A program that promises an excellent fitness level in just 12 hours, with many pounds of weight loss.	No, insufficient aerobic exercises MINUS 10	No, insufficient strength exercises MINUS 10	No, insufficient flexibility exercises MINUS 10	Yes
The Official YMCA Physical Fitness Handbook (Dr. Clayton R. Myers). A balanced program of aerobics, muscle strength, and flexibility exercises. YMCA membership may be required, but the cost is low. The emphasis is on health, not beauty.	Yes	Yes	Yes	Yes
The Fit Kit (Recreation Canada). The official fitness program of the National Health and Welfare Department of Canada.	Yes	Yes	Yes	Yes
The Royal Canadian Air Force Programs. Programs designed to develop fitness in 11 minutes of vigorous exercise each day. The programs are needlessly divided into sex groups and do not individualize advancement to higher levels.	No, only the advanced levels give sufficient aerobic work MINUS 10	Yes	Yes	Yes
Adult Physical Fitness (President's Council on Physical Fitness and Sports). A program intended to help men and women gain fitness at home. It needlessly separates men's and women's programs.	Yes, but only the advanced men's level provides meaningful aerobic work	Yes	Yes	Yes
Vigor Regained (Dr. Herbert de Vries). A home exercise program for the out-of-shape older individual; emphasizes good health by way of a fit body.	Yes	Yes	Yes	Yes

TABLE 12 – 3 • Continued

Question 5: Reasonable Time	Question 6: Warm-up/ Cool-down	Question 7: Equipment/ Membership	Question 8: Safety	Question 9: Accuracy of Claims	Question 10: Ability to Hold Interest	Total Score
Yes	Yes	Yes	No, the uniform advancement rate may not be safe for all MINUS 10	No, may overstate helpfulness for heart disease MINUS 10	Yes. Acknowledges that different sports can lead to fitness, but ratings are not accurate	60
Yes	Yes	Yes	Yes	Yes	No, monotonous MINUS 10	70
No, time required is insufficient MINUS 10	No, warm-up and cool-down periods are insufficient MINUS 10	Yes	Yes	No, makes unproved claims for fitness from minimal effort MINUS 10	No, doesn't include sports MINUS 10	30
Yes	Yes	Yes	No, includes some exercises of questionable safety MINUS 10	Yes	No, doesn't include sports MINUS 10	90
Yes	Yes	Yes	Yes	Yes	Yes	100
No, the 11 minutes per day is insufficient for aerobic work MINUS 10	No MINUS 10	Yes	Yes	Yes	No, a set routine is to be performed MINUS 10	60
No, too much of the 15 minutes per day is warm-up time MINUS 10	No, no cool-down period provided MINUS 5	Yes	No, includes some exercises of questionable safety MINUS 10	Yes	Yes, doesn't include sports, but does urge broadening of program	75
Yes	Yes	Yes	Yes	Yes	No, program repeats exercise routine MINUS 10	90

Table 12–3 continued on next page . . .

TABLE 12-3 • **Continued**

Fitness Program Name and Description	Question 1: Aerobic Exercise	Question 2: Muscle Strength	Question 3: Flexibility	Question 4: Initial Levels
Executive Fitness (Executive Health Examiners, Dr. Richard Winter, ed.). A program for male business executives but applicable to any healthy adults.	Yes	Yes	Yes	Yes
Jane Fonda's Workout Tape (1982). A tape recording of exercise to music with instruction booklet. A beginner's workout and an advanced workout are provided.	No, the segment of jogging is insufficiently aerobic MINUS 10	Strengthens the lower body only, not the upper body MINUS 5	Yes	Yes

Concerning the atmosphere, consider the surroundings and the immediate effect they have on your perception. (Some things to consider: Kinds of equipment—see next section for more information on equipment—equipment's condition, equipment's arrangement, amount of workout space available, the facility's appearance, staff members' appearance, members' appearance, and the like).

Regarding the location, ask yourself if the facility is conveniently located to meet your needs for time. This is important—the more conveniently located it is, the more likely you will attend your workout sessions. You may want to make a trial visit to the facility during the hours when you would normally expect to attend: Notice if it is overcrowded, if equipment is available, if the staff members are selling rather than assisting, and if you would enjoy the company of the other members.

To evaluate the facility's practices, ask a staff member to take you through a demonstration workout. What practices seem valid, according to the principles presented in this book? What practices seem unsound? Does the available equipment include mostly passive, "jiggle"-type machines, saunas, whirlpools, and the like, or equipment that requires real physical exertion? Is the facility's program designed to improve fitness in a balanced way, including exercise for flexibility, strength, and cardiovascular and muscular endurance? Do instructors or staff members emphasize the importance of exercise frequency, intensity, and duration? Does the program allow for varying fitness levels—can you start out slowly and work your way up? Does the program take a reasonable amount of time—say 20 minutes to 1 hour—at least 3 days per week? Does the program include a warm-up and cool-down period? Is the program safe?

It is important to determine the qualifications of the staff members and especially those of the individuals responsible for your program. Are

TABLE 12-3 • Continued

Question 5: Reasonable Time	Question 6: Warm-up/ Cool-down	Question 7: Equipment/ Membership	Question 8: Safety	Question 9: Accuracy of Claims	Question 10: Ability to Hold Interest	Total Score
Yes	Yes	Yes	No, includes body arching and unsafe yoga exercises MINUS 10	Yes	No, only the aerobics vary, so could be monotonous MINUS 10	80
Yes	Yes	Yes	No, recommends some questionable stretching and bouncing MINUS 10	Yes	No, the routine never varies MINUS 10	65

they exercise physiologists? Are the aerobic instructors certified by the IDEA, AFFA, or ACSM as described on p. 242? Or, are the personnel just attractive-looking salespeople dressed up in fancy exercise attire?

About the approach, determine what claims are made for the facility's practices. Do they seem sound, logical, and straightforward, or do they seem unrealistic, unhealthy, deceptive, or evasive? Why? Does the facility promise "miraculous" results? Do they offer drugs or food supplements? What do you get for how much money? Are you given a hard-sell approach to join? Do *NOT* join a spa during your visit for this experience. Take time to consider all your alternatives for exercise. Be prepared to haggle over prices—usually the membership prices are lowered if you start to walk out the door. Buying a spa membership is often similar to buying a car—the salespeople are prepared to sell for less than the "list" price.

It is also helpful to find out if the facility has a good reputation. Do the members seem pleased? Do you know anyone who is a member? How long has the facility been in operation? Consult with an independent expert if you have questions about the programs offered. Is the facility part of a national chain? Are there other associated facilities that you could use? Make certain that the club is well established and will not disappear overnight. You may want to check its reputation with the Better Business Bureau in your area.

To conclude your evaluation, make comparisons. Investigate all options. Programs offered by the YMCA or YWCA, local colleges or universities, and municipal park and recreation departments often have excellent fitness classes at lower prices than commercial establishments and usually employ qualified personnel. Finally, consider your overall impressions. Think about your answers to the preceding questions, and ask yourself which facilities look slick but lack substance, and which do the reverse. Do any fall somewhere between these extremes? Which would you join?

Evaluating Fitness Equipment

Health clubs may be too crowded, inconvenient, and time-consuming for some people. For these reasons, many people set up gyms in their own homes.

Some people's intentions to work out are delusions, so some money spent on exercise equipment is wasted. It is a mistake, however, to dismiss all such purchases as mere self-indulgence with new toys. According to a study commissioned by the National Sporting Goods Association, nearly 10 million people work out with their home equipment more than twice a week.[27] However, despite ads for exercise equipment that tout "high-efficiency methods" or "progressive resistance," not much exercise equipment is really indispensable for fitness. For aerobic training at home, all you really need are a pair of well-cushioned running shoes and perhaps a jump rope—total investment, $50 or so. To this you might add a mat and some dumbbells or ankle weights—perhaps another $20 to $30. Still, if you will use them, buy other items that will meet your exercise needs. This section discusses common pieces of exercise equipment, the components of fitness they develop, and some general purchasing guidelines.

Exercise bicycles.   Almost anyone can safely use a stationary exercise bicycle. Bicycling strengthens the legs, promotes lower body flexibility, and improves cardiovascular endurance. It is easy for those who are uncoordinated and kind to those who are out of shape.

Selecting a stationary bike is not so easy. More than 100 different brands and models of exercise bikes are available, ranging from $40 to $20,000 (for the kind used in laboratory testing). You may have to spend at least $150 or $200 for a bike that is sturdy and smooth enough for comfortable riding.[28] When selecting a bike, look for several features (see Table 12–4). *Consumer Reports* has rated exercise bikes for quality and comfort; consult their recommendations before you buy. Some bikes offer the advantage that you can work your arms and upper body as well as your legs, but they may be priced about twice as high as other top-rated bikes.

Exercise bikes can be adjusted to fit riders of all different sizes. Some designs may be better suited for one person than another, so try an exercise bike on for size before purchasing it. Adjust it as you would a regular bike before trying it out: The seat should be set so that when the pedal dips to its lowest position, the leg is almost fully extended. This lets the rider exercise the large leg muscles most efficiently, comfortably, and safely. Habitual use of a bike that has a seat at the wrong height can cause knee injuries.

Stair-climbing machines.   Stair-climbing machines are gaining popularity so fast that many fitness centers must set time limits for their use to

TABLE 12-4 • Features of a Good Exercise Bike

Seat	It should be wide, comfortable, and easy to adjust for height.
Handlebars	They should be adjustable to make long workouts more comfortable.
Resistance control	The resistance control should be calibrated — this makes it easy to reset.
Gauges	They should be clear and easy to read.
Resistance mechanism	Either of two ways to make pedaling harder is acceptable: A caliper brake or a belt around the flywheel.
Flywheel	Generally, the bigger and heavier it is, the smoother the ride. It should be made of cast iron or steel.
Frame	It should be rigid so that the rider's energy goes to spinning the flywheel, not to flexing the rest of the bike.
Pedals	Straps let you work on the upstroke and the downstroke. Weighted pedals keep the straps on top.

Source: Adapted from Exercise Bikes, *Consumer Reports,* August 1986, pp. 511–514.

keep people from fighting over them. Stair climbing, as many people are realizing, is one of the most effective activities they can do to burn energy and build cardiovascular endurance. Because stair-climbing machines provide low-impact workouts, the risks of injuries are minimal. As more and better machines are produced, home versions are now available for much less (about $400) than the expensive ($2,000 to $4,000) models found in health clubs. Some stair-climbing machines function by letting you push two paddles with your feet, and others are more like escalators that you climb on.

Rowing machines.   For those without back problems, a rowing machine may be a good exercise option to consider. Olympic rowers are among the fittest of athletes; their sport is one of the best for exercising the whole body. The sliding seat of the rowing scull allows the leg muscles to be used in a back-and-forth motion that is less punishing to the leg joints than running. Working the oars exercises the arms, shoulders, back, and abdominal muscles. Vigorous rowing burns as much energy as running at seven miles an hour; at a moderate pace, it is equivalent to walking. Rowing is an excellent aerobic exercise that develops overall muscular strength and endurance.

Rowing machines are rated mainly on their ability to provide a good aerobic workout. The most effective machine is one that lets you concentrate on the exercise instead of on the machine. Machines that produce a good stroke are usually designed so they do not force the body to work in potentially harmful positions. In general, the more expensive models are of better quality. The machine's arms have to be the right length and positioned correctly in relation to the footrests. If this position is incorrect, the rower has to lean too far forward at the beginning of a stroke, which can strain the back.

Another consideration is the angle of the footrests. A well-designed machine has rotating footrests that position the feet at a comfortable angle to the legs. Fixed footrests on several models force the ankles into a too-sharp angle, as do the freely rotating footrests on a few models. This kind of overextension can cause shin splints, foot strains, or overextension of the Achilles tendon. A comfortable seat that provides good back support is also important.

The foregoing equipment facilitates aerobic workouts. Some people also want to do strength work at home and need some kind of weights for this purpose.

Free weights. Free weights are recommended over home gyms for building muscle strength and muscle endurance. Free weights take up much less space than home gyms, and more and better equipment can be obtained for the money. A basic set of weights— 100 pounds or so, with one long and two short bars— costs as little as $30. Weight benches with a leg lift start at $60 or so.

Home gyms. The most basic home gym, as already described, might include a jump rope, a mat, and some dumbbells or ankle weights. Total cost: $50 to $80. A step up from that might include a stationary bike or rowing machine and a set of free weights or a "home gym" resistance machine. The cost of outfitting such a gym can range from $200 to $1,000.

The equipment sold as home gyms ranges from weight-stack machines that resemble *Universal* equipment to cable-strung racks. These devices are all designed to replace, and presumably improve upon, free weights. An advantage of this equipment is that you cannot drop a barbell on your chest or a dumbbell on your foot. A disadvantage is that bench-and-frame gyms require space.

In comparing home gyms, consider their ability to work different body parts. Weight-stack machines best duplicate a workout with free weights. Also inspect them to see if they are well or poorly made and how difficult they are to assemble.

Before purchasing a home gym, try it out. Tall or short people may have trouble fitting themselves to the preset machines of a gym. If the equipment forces your body into uncomfortable positions, do not buy it. It is also essential to get some instruction. A health club or a gym is a good place for this.

These pointers should help in the selection of exercise equipment. In addition, the following guidelines can be useful:

• Consult an expert if you want to know the effectiveness of a product. Individuals with degrees in physical education, physical therapy, corrective therapy, and exercise physiology should be able to give you good advice. Be sure to get an *outside* opinion; do not rely on salespeople's opinions alone—even if those people have impressive credentials, for after all, they stand to gain if you buy their wares.

• Buy from well-established, reputable companies that will not disappear overnight and that will back up warranties. Avoid mail order products. If a product is not available in a retail store where you can examine it, you probably should not buy it.

Finally, and most importantly, buy equipment only if you will use it. And remember: You already own the finest equipment ever made—the muscles, ligaments, tendons, and bones of your own wonderful body. Use and maintain that equipment with respect for its design and you will enjoy it in the best of health for years to come.

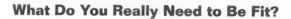

PERSONAL FOCUS

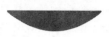

What Do You Really Need to Be Fit?

This chapter has presented information about fitness and the consumer. As previously mentioned, consumers face many problems in a free-enterprise market. Advertisers claim people need their products for fitness—products that are not only unnecessary but can even cause harm. This section offers help on recognizing the difference between a real need and a created one. By focusing only on what you truly need to develop fitness, you will be astonished at the number of items and the amount of expense you can eliminate from your life. The following steps can help you to decide what you need to be fit:

- Do not purchase any of the gimmick devices described in this chapter. Do not purchase any product that promises quick results with no effort.
- Determine which areas of fitness you want to develop: Flexibility, muscle strength, muscle endurance, or cardiovascular endurance.
- Now select physical activities that interest you and that will develop the fitness components you are seeking.
- Write down exactly what you *need* to participate in these activities on this chapter's Lab Report. For example:

Area of Fitness to Be Developed	Physical Activity	Items Needed
Cardiovascular endurance	Jogging	Running shoes, comfortable clothing

Record your conclusions on this chapter's Lab Report form.

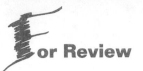

For Review

1. List elements a person should consider when evaluating health claims and explain why they are important (page 257).
2. Describe ways to recognize false or inflated health claims (page 259).
3. List several health and fitness gimmicks and describe why they are fraudulent (page 271).
4. Discuss the side effects of self-dosing with anabolic steroids (page 264).
5. List several valid ways to lose weight and describe why they are effective (page 266).

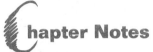

Chapter Notes

1. J. Willis, About body wraps, pills and other magic wands for losing weight, *FDA Consumer,* November, 1982, pp. 18–20.
2. M. H. Williams, Nutritional ergogenic aids and athletic performance, *Nutrition Today,* January/February 1989, pp. 7–14.
3. Williams, 1989.
4. E. R. Eichner, Nonanemic iron deficiency, *Sports Medicine Digest,* April 1989, p. 3.
5. P. G. Dyment and B. Goldberg, Anabolic steroids and the adolescent athlete, *Pediatrics* 83 (1989): 127–128.
6. H. Haupt and G. D. Rovere, Anabolic steroids: A review of the literature, *American Journal of Sports Medicine* 12 (1984): 469–484.
7. M. Alen and P. Rahkila, Reduced high-density lipoprotein-cholesterol in power athletes: Use of male sex hormone derivatives, an atherogenic factor, *International Journal of Sports Medicine* 5 (1984): 341–342; O. L. Webb, P. M. Laskarzewski, and C. J. Glueck, Severe depression of high-density lipoprotein cholesterol levels in weight lifters and body builders by self-administered exogenous testosterone and anabolic-androgenic steroids, *Metabolism* 33 (1984): 971–975.
8. Haupt and Rovere, 1984.
9. Haupt and Rovere, 1984.
10. Dyment and Goldberg, 1989.
11. D. R. Lamb, Anabolic steroids in athletics: How well do they work and how dangerous are they? *American Journal of Sports Medicine* 12 (1984): 31–38.
12. Dyment and Goldberg, 1989.
13. D. L. Costill, G. P. Dalsky, and W. J. Fink, Effects of caffeine ingestion on metabolism and exercise performance, *Medicine and Science in Sports* 10 (1978): 155–158.
14. F. T. O'Neil, M. T. Hynak-Hankinson, and J. Gorman, Research and application of current topics in sports nutrition, *Journal of the American Dietetic Association* 86 (1986): 1007–1015.
15. M. H. Williams, Introduction, in *Nutritional Aspects of Human Physical and Athletic Performance* (Springfield, Ill.: Charles C. Thomas, 1985), pp. 3–19.
16. Controversial blood doping revisited, *Science News,* May 1987, p. 344.

17. M. Simonton, An overview: Advances in research and treatment of obesity, *Food and Nutrition News,* March/April 1982.

18. F. Rickman, N. Michell, J. Dingman, and J. E. Dalen, Changes in serum cholesterol during the Stillman Diet, *Journal of the American Medical Association* 228 (1974): 54–58.

19. Very-low-calorie diets, *Berkeley Wellness Letter,* published in association with the School of Public Health, University of California, January 1989.

20. R. A. Lantigua and coauthors, Cardiac arrhythmias associated with a liquid protein diet for the treatment of obesity, *New England Journal of Medicine* 303 (1980): 735–738.

21. J. Willis, About body wraps, pills and other magic wands for losing weight, *FDA Consumer,* November 1982, pp. 18–20.

22. Willis, 1982.

23. *Health Quackery,* Consumer Reports Books (Mount Vernon, New York: Consumer's Union, 1980), pp. 123–155.

24. Willis, 1982.

25. Diet pills and stroke, *American Journal of Nursing* 87 (1987): 1970.

26. A. G. Dulloo and D. S. Miller, Aspirin as a promoter of ephedrine-induced thermogenesis: Potential use in the treatment of obesity, *American Journal of Clinical Nutrition* 45 (1987): 564–569; A. G. Dulloo and D. S. Miller, The thermogenic properties of ephedrine/methylxanthine mixtures: Animal studies, *American Journal of Clinical Nutrition* 43 (1986): 388–394.

27. Home exercise equipment, *Consumer Reports,* August 1985. p. 448–454.

28. Exercise bikes, *Consumer Reports,* August 1986, pp. 511–514.

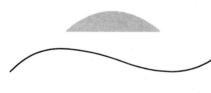

Appendix A
Lab Reports

The lab reports presented here correspond to the Personal Focus sections at the end of each chapter. The pages of this appendix are perforated so that as each lab report is completed, it can be turned in to the instructor.

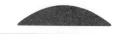

L A B   R E P O R T

## Chapter 1

How Physically Active Are You?

Name _____

Date _____

Instructor _____

Class _____

Record your point scores here for the questions on p. 17.

Category	*Score*	
A. Formal, Vigorous Exercise Routines	_____	(A high score would be 20)
B. Other Formal Exercise Routines	_____	(A high score would be 12)
C. Occupation and Daily Activities	_____	(A high score would be 12)
D. Leisure Activities	_____	(A high score would be 14)
Total:	_____	(A high score would be 50)

Evaluation of total score (circle one):

- Inactive (0 to 5 points)
- Moderately active (6 to 11 points)
- Active (12 to 20 points)
- Very active (21 points or over)

    If your score categorized you as inactive or only moderately active, return to the Personal Focus quiz, reread the questions, and choose some activities that you would like and could realistically undertake to raise your score to "Active" (12 points or more). List these activities below. You are not committing yourself to doing these things, just acknowledging that you could.

A. Formal, Vigorous Exercise Routines

I could: _____

_____

_____

_____

State for how long and how many times a week: _____

_____

B. Other Formal Exercise Routines

I could: _____

_____

_____

_____

State for how long and how many times a week: _____

_____

continued on next page

C. Occupation and Daily Activities

I could: _____

_____

_____

_____

State for how long and how many times a week: _____

_____

D. Leisure Activities

I could: _____

_____

_____

State for how long and how many times a week: _____

_____

LAB REPORT

Chapter 2

Name _____

Date _____

Instructor _____

Class _____

How's Your Fitness Motivation?

A. Discover Your Own Motivation

My chief motivators are:

1. _____
   _____
   _____

2. _____
   _____
   _____

B. Practice Setting Specific, Realistic Goals

Two fitness goals I have set:

1. _____
   _____
   _____

2. _____
   _____
   _____

C. Reward Yourself

I will reward myself as follows:

1. _____
   _____
   _____

2. _____
   _____
   _____

continued on next page

D. Anticipate Possible Barriers and Plan to Overcome Them

Barriers: *Strategies for Overcoming*

_____   _____

_____   _____

_____   _____

_____   _____

_____   _____

_____   _____

_____   _____

_____   _____

_____   _____

_____   _____

LAB REPORT

Chapter 3

Name _____

Date _____

Instructor _____

Class _____

How Fit Are You?

Record the results of your fitness tests here.

A. Body Composition: Fatfold Measures

Chest (Men) or Triceps (Women)

First measurement _____

Second measurement _____

Third measurement _____

Average of two closest measurements _____

Abdomen (Men) or Suprailium (Women)

First measurement _____

Second measurement _____

Third measurement _____

Average of two closest measurements _____

Thigh (Men and Women)

First measurement _____

Second measurement _____

Third measurement _____

Average of two closest measurements _____

Total of three averages _____

Percent of body fat from Table 3–3 (Women): _____

Percent of body fat from Table 3–4 (Men): _____

Body fat percentage classification from Table 3–5: _____

B. Flexibility:

1. Upper trunk flexibility: Body rotation

   Right side _____

   Rating (Table 3–6): _____

   Left side _____

   Rating (Table 3–6): _____

continued on next page

2. Lower back and hamstrings: Sit-and-reach test

_____ inches

   Rating (Table 3–6): _____

3. Shoulder flexibility: Shoulder rotation

Right shoulder _____ inches

Rating (Table 3–6): _____

Left shoulder _____ inches

Rating (Table 3–6): _____

C. Muscle Strength: Grip Strength

Grip score:

First trial: _____ kg.

Second trial: _____ kg.

Rating (Table 3–7)* _____

*Rating is based on the best of the two scores.

D. Muscle Endurance: Push-ups and Sit-ups

1. Number of push-ups or modified push-ups _____

   Rating (Table 3–8): _____

2. Sit-ups performed in 60 seconds: _____

   Rating (Table 3–8) _____

E. Cardiovascular Endurance: Cooper's Test

1. Distance covered in 12 minutes _____

   Rating (Table 3–9): _____

2. Resting pulse: _____

Have you identified any areas in which your fitness needs improvement?

Yes _____   No _____

If so, which ones?_____

_____

_____

LAB REPORT   How to Improve Your Flexibility

Chapter 4

Name _____

Date _____

Instructor _____

Class _____

1. Initial Flexibility Scores and Ratings

a. Upper trunk flexibility: Body rotation

Right side _____ inches

Rating (Table 3–6): _____

Left side _____ inches

Rating (Table 3–6): _____

b. Lower back and hamstrings: Sit and reach test

_____ inches

Rating (Table 3–6): _____

c. Shoulder flexibility: Shoulder rotation

Right shoulder _____ inches

Rating (Table 3–6): _____

Left shoulder _____ inches

Rating (Table 3–6): _____

2. Planned Flexibility Progress

	Day 1	2	3	4	5	6	7	8	9	10	11	12	13	14	15
# of seconds I will hold each stretch	—	—	—	—	—	—	—	—	—	—	—	—	—	—	—
# of times I will hold each stretch	—	—	—	—	—	—	—	—	—	—	—	—	—	—	—

continued on next page

3. Flexibility Log

Day/Date
performed
(example:
M 2/13,
Th 2/16)

— — — — — — — — — — — — — — —

Routine
Chosen
(long or short)

— — — — — — — — — — — — — — —

4. Flexibility Post-Test

a. Upper trunk flexibility: Body rotation

Right side _____ inches

Rating (Table 3–6): _____

Left side _____ inches

Rating (Table 3–6): _____

b. Lower back and hamstrings: Sit and reach test

_____ inches

Rating (Table 3–6): _____

c. Shoulder flexibility: Shoulder rotation

Right shoulder _____ inches

Rating (Table 3–6): _____

Left shoulder _____ inches

Rating (Table 3–6): _____

L A B   R E P O R T

Chapter 5

Name _____

Date _____

Class _____

Instructor _____

How to Improve Your Muscle Strength and Endurance

A. Initial Muscle Strength and Endurance Scores and Ratings

1. Muscle Strength: Grip strength

First trial: _____ kg

Second trial: _____ kg

Rating (Table 3–7):* _____

2. Muscle Endurance: Push-ups and Sit-ups

Number of push-ups or modified push-ups _____

Rating (Table 3–8): _____

Sit-ups performed in 60 seconds: _____

Rating (Table 3–8): _____

*Rating is based on the best of the two scores.

continued on next page

B. Weight Training and Calisthenic Logs

	Week 1					Week 2				
	Day	1	2	3	4	Day	1	2	3	4
Bench Press										
# Repeats										
# Sets										
Resistance										
Upright Rowing										
# Repeats										
# Sets										
Resistance										
Biceps Curl										
# Repeats										
# Sets										
Resistance										
Triceps Extension										
# Repeats										
# Sets										
Resistance										
Squat										
# Repeats										
# Sets										
Resistance										
Stomach Crunches										
# Repeats										
# Sets										
Diagonal Crunch										
# Repeats										
# Sets										
Push-ups										
# Repeats										
# Sets										

	Week 3					Week 4				
	Day	1	2	3	4	Day	1	2	3	4
Bench Press										
# Repeats										
# Sets										
Resistance										
Upright Rowing										
# Repeats										
# Sets										
Resistance										
Biceps Curl										
# Repeats										
# Sets										
Resistance										
Triceps Extension										
# Repeats										
# Sets										
Resistance										
Squat										
# Repeats										
# Sets										
Resistance										
Stomach Crunches										
# Repeats										
# Sets										
Diagonal Crunch										
# Repeats										
# Sets										
Push-ups										
# Repeats										
# Sets										

continued on next page

	Week 1					Week 2				
	Day	1	2	3	4	Day	1	2	3	4
Modified Push-ups										
# Repeats										
# Sets										
Pull-ups										
# Repeats										
# Sets										
Modified Pull-ups										
# Repeats										
# Sets										
Back Push-ups										
# Repeats										
# Sets										
Modified Back Push-ups										
# Repeats										
# Sets										
Pelvic Tilt										
# Repeats										
# Sets										
Bent-Leg Lift										
# Repeats										
# Sets										
Inner Thigh Lift										
# Repeats										
# Sets										
Hamstring Curl										
# Repeats										
# Sets										
Quadriceps Lift										
# Repeats										
# Sets										

	Week 3					Week 4				
	Day	1	2	3	4	Day	1	2	3	4
Modified Push-ups										
# Repeats										
# Sets										
Pull-ups										
# Repeats										
# Sets										
Modified Pull-ups										
# Repeats										
# Sets										
Back Push-ups										
# Repeats										
# Sets										
Modified Back Push-ups										
# Repeats										
# Sets										
Pelvic Tilt										
# Repeats										
# Sets										
Bent-Leg Lift										
# Repeats										
# Sets										
Inner Thigh Lift										
# Repeats										
# Sets										
Hamstring Curl										
# Repeats										
# Sets										
Quadriceps Lift										
# Repeats										
# Sets										

continued on next page

C. Muscle Strength and Endurance Post-test

1. Muscle Strength: Grip Strength

First trial: _____ kg.

Second trial: _____ kg.

Rating (Table 3–7): _____

2. Muscle Endurance: Push-ups and Sit-ups

a. Number of push-ups or modified push-ups _____

Rating (Table 3–8): _____

b. Sit-ups performed in 60 seconds: _____

Rating (Table 3–8): _____

*Rating is based on the best of the two scores.

L A B   R E P O R T   How to Improve Your Cardiovascular Endurance

Chapter 6

Name _____

Date _____

Class _____

Instructor _____

1. Activity

My chosen activity is: _____

_____

_____

Dates and durations I performed this activity were:

Date	Duration	Date	Duration
_____	_____	_____	_____
_____	_____	_____	_____
_____	_____	_____	_____
_____	_____	_____	_____
_____	_____	_____	_____
_____	_____	_____	_____
_____	_____	_____	_____
_____	_____	_____	_____
_____	_____	_____	_____
_____	_____	_____	_____
_____	_____	_____	_____
_____	_____	_____	_____
_____	_____	_____	_____

continued on next page

2. Cooper's Test
   a. My initial miles and rating (from Figure 3–5 and Table 3–9).

   Date: _____   Miles: _____   *Rating:* _____

   b. My miles and rating (from Figure 3–5 and Table 3–9) after beginning my cardiovascular program.

   Date: _____   *Miles:* _____   *Rating:* _____

   Date: _____   Miles: _____   *Rating:* _____

   Date: _____   Miles: _____   *Rating:* _____

3. Resting Pulse
   a. My initial resting pulse (from the Chapter 3 Lab Report).

   Date: _____   Pulse rate: _____ (beats per minute)

   b. My resting pulse rate after beginning my cardiovascular program.

   Date: _____   Pulse rate: _____ (beats per minute)

   Date: _____   Pulse rate: _____ (beats per minute)

   Date: _____   Pulse rate: _____ (beats per minute)

4. Personal comments

   _____

   _____

   _____

   _____

L A B   R E P O R T   How Is Your Nutrition?

Chapter 7

Name _____

Date _____

Instructor _____

Class _____

Record the total number of yes answers for each section of the Chapter 7 Personal Focus as indicated below. Each yes answer is worth one point.

Part	Score	
1. Milk and Milk Products	____	(A high score would be 4)
2. Meats and Meat Alternates	____	(A high score would be 6)
3. Vegetables and Fruits	____	(A high score would be 5)
4. Breads and Cereals	____	(A high score would be 5)
5. Extra Foods and Calories	____	(A high score would be 5)
Total:	____	(A high score would be 25)

Evaluation of total score (circle one):

Excellent diet (24 to 25 points)
Good diet (19 to 23 points)
Fair diet (14 to 18 points)
Poor diet (9 to 13 points)

If your diet is less than excellent, identify five ways you can improve it.

_____

_____

_____

_____

_____

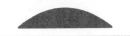

L A B   R E P O R T   What Is an Appropriate Weight for You?

Chapter 8

Name _____

Date _____

Class _____

Instructor _____

A. The safe range for a person of my height and sex:

    1. My height _____ feet _____ inches.

    2. My frame size is _____ .

    3. The appropriate weight range for a person my height, sex and frame size is _____ to _____ pounds.

    4. The extreme bottom end of the safe range of weights for a person my height, sex, and frame size is: _____ pounds.

    5. The extreme top end of the safe range of weights for a person my height, sex, and frame size is _____ pounds.

    6. My safe range: _____ to _____ pounds.

B. Record your current weight here: _____ pounds.
If your weight is above the top end of the safe range, record your Body Mass Index (BMI) here: _____ . Does your body mass index indicate the need for weight loss? If so, go on to question C. If not, go on to question D.

C. My family's health history.

    Do you or any close blood relative have a history of (circle one):

        Diabetes   yes   no

        Hypertension   yes   no

        High blood cholesterol   yes   no

D. Choosing my goal weight.

    1. My chosen occupation:

    _____ . Weight appropriate for this occupation: _____ pounds.

    2. My chosen sport: _____ .

    3. If female, planned pregnancy any time soon?   yes   no.

    4. My personal preference: _____ pounds.

E. My goal weight: _____ pounds.

Name _____

Date _____

Class _____

Instructor _____

A. Record all the foods you ate in a day in Table LR9–1 as instructed in the Personal Focus in Chapter 9. Day recorded: _____

B. Convert carbohydrate grams to carbohydrate calories and then calculate your carbohydrate-calorie intake as a percentage of your total energy intake:

1. Total carbohydrate (from column 6) = _____ grams × 4 calories/gram = _____ calories carbohydrate.

2. (Total carbohydrate calories: _____ divided by total calories: _____) × 100 = _____ % of calories from carbohydrate.

C. If your diet is not the kind of diet that best supports physical activity and health (60 percent of calories from carbohydrate and therefore 30 percent or less from fat), tell how might you improve it, based on the foods listed on this Lab Report.

_____

_____ .

TABLE LR9–1

Food description (Appendix D)	Portion size (Appendix D)	Portions I ate	From Appendix D: Carb per portion (g)	Energy per portion (cal)	My intake: Total carb (g)	Total energy (cal)

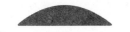

LAB REPORT Your Need for Exercise and Relaxation

Chapter 10

Name _____

Date _____

Class _____

Instructor _____

A. Stress Mode Inventory

When under stress, which of the following symptoms do you experience? Check each box next to responses appropriate to you.

☐   1. My heart pounds and beats faster.

☐   2. My breathing speeds up; I can't get a deep breath.

☐   3. My mouth and throat feel dry.

☐   4. I feel hot and feverish.

☐   5. I can't get in the mood for sex, or I can't reach orgasm.

☐   6. I feel nervous, touchy and irritable, or depressed.

☐   7. I feel an urge to run, cry, or behave impulsively.

☐   8. I have thoughts of how bad I am; I imagine I am a failure.

☐   9. I worry almost constantly; I fear other people think badly of me.

☐ 10. I can't think of what to say, or I run myself down.

☐ 11. I feel weak, dizzy, light-headed, or faint.

☐ 12. My hands shake; I get nervous tics or twitches.

☐ 13. I am easily startled; I am jumpy.

☐ 14. I laugh too much, too loudly, or at inappropriate times.

☐ 15. I stutter and stammer when I speak.

☐ 16. I don't know the right thing to do or say in company.

☐ 17. I get bored and dissatisfied with my life.

☐ 18. I postpone doing things.

☐ 19. I feel all alone.

☐ 20. I avoid seeing people or going places.

☐ 21. I have trouble sleeping.

☐ 22. My jaw is tired in the morning from jaw clenching or teeth grinding in the night.

☐ 23. I feel restless; I move about aimlessly.

☐ 24. My body sweats; my hands feel cold or clammy; I get cold chills.

continued on next page

- [ ] 25. I blush.
- [ ] 26. I fear certain things.
- [ ] 27. I become forgetful, misplace my possessions, or miss appointments.
- [ ] 28. I get confused about my duty to family or friends and I imagine I've let them down.
- [ ] 29. My work gives me comfort—I can't afford to play.
- [ ] 30. My thoughts are "somewhere else" and I fail to respond.
- [ ] 31. My bladder feels full more often.
- [ ] 32. My stomach gets upset; I get diarrhea, nausea, or abdominal pain.
- [ ] 33. I get toothaches, earaches, or headaches for no reason.
- [ ] 34. If I menstruate, I feel nervous beforehand or cease menstruating.
- [ ] 35. My body aches more, with pain in my neck, back, or shoulders.
- [ ] 36. I get disorganized, and small things upset me.
- [ ] 37. I just cannot decide, or I decide carelessly.
- [ ] 38. I can't work as well as I usually do.
- [ ] 39. I can't concentrate.
- [ ] 40. I can't pinpoint the cause of my ceaseless anxiety.
- [ ] 41. I lose my appetite, or eat excessively.
- [ ] 42. My appearance changes.
- [ ] 43. I rely more on chemicals, such as alcohol, tobacco, or other drugs.
- [ ] 44. I get clumsy or careless.
- [ ] 45. I get sick more often.
- [ ] 46. I feel so tired that I can't be happy.
- [ ] 47. I am awakened by nightmares; others report that I had nightmares.
- [ ] 48. I mistrust the motives of others.
- [ ] 49. I feel guilty.
- [ ] 50. I feel powerless.

Scoring

Give yourself 1 "physical" point for each item you checked that is numbered 1–5, 11–15, 21–25, 31–35, or 41–45.

Give yourself 1 "psychological" point for each item you checked that is numbered 6–10, 16–20, 26–30, 36–40, or 46–50.

Total points: physical _____ psychological _____

Note: Some of the symptoms listed here can also warn of serious conditions; if they persist, get them checked by a health care provider.

B. Daily Stress Log

Time	Activity	Environmental Conditions	Social Interactions	Thoughts	Emotions/ Feelings	Stress Symptoms

C. Stress Log Assessment

1. How often did you experience a stress symptom this day?

2. Is this amount of stress acceptable, beneficial, or excessive?

3. What time of day did stress symptoms occur?

4. If you repeated the log, would the stress occur again at the same time tomorrow?

continued on next page

D. Stress Management

How can you deal with the stresses that keep recurring in your life?

E. Attitude Adjustment

How can you adjust your attitudes toward stressful events that you cannot eliminate?

F. Activity Adjustment

How can you plan more physical activity and relaxation in your life?

L A B   R E P O R T How Safety Conscious Are You?

Chapter 11

Name _____

Date _____

Class _____

Instructor _____

A. General Guidelines for Preventing Exercise Injuries

1. I consistently practice a warm-up before every workout and a cool-down at the end of each workout. *Yes/No*

2. I increase my workload gradually. *Yes/No*

3. I exercise consistently throughout the week, not only on weekends. *Yes/No*

4. I wear appropriate clothing and use proper equipment for the activity I participate in. *Yes/No*

5. I practice proper form when performing exercise activities. *Yes/No*

6. I am knowledgable about exercises that cause injury and I avoid them. *Yes/No*

7. I pay attention to the signals my body gives me and I act appropriately. *Yes/No*

B. Preventing Environmental Injuries and Accidents

8. I take environmental precautions before exercising outdoors. *Yes/No*

9. I never swim alone. *Yes/No*

10. When I cycle, I always wear a helmet. *Yes/No*

C. Treating Sports Injuries

11. When I suffer a minor injury, I discontinue the activity so that I can heal. *Yes/No*

12. When I suffer an injury that does not clear up in a few days, I see a health care professional to obtain an accurate diagnosis and treatment. *Yes/No*

13. When I suffer a minor injury, I apply the guidelines of RICE—Rest, Ice, Compression and Elevation. *Yes/No*

D. Scoring: Give yourself 1 point for each yes answer.

12 to 13: You are a safety-conscious person.
10 to 11: You have a few more refinements to make on your choices.
8 to 9: You have some room for improvement.
7 or below: You need to attend to your safety awareness and behavior.

L A B R E P O R T What Do You Really Need to Be Fit?

Chapter 12

Name _____

Date _____

Class _____

Instructor _____

Area of Fitness to Be Developed	Physical Activity	Items Needed

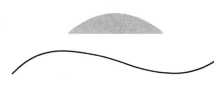

Appendix B

The Rockport Fitness Walking Test and Exercise Program*

The Rockport Fitness Walking Test estimates cardiovascular fitness based on age, gender, time it takes to walk one mile, and heart rate achieved at the end of the test. Based on these variables and standards from the American Heart Association, researchers devised the Relative Fitness Level chart and Exercise Program charts that are found in this appendix.

*No exercise test or program should be undertaken without the consent of your personal physician.

The Rockport Walking Test

1. Use a measured track, or measure out a mile on your own (make sure your measured course is flat).
2. Warm up for 5 to 10 minutes before you take the test. Your warm-up should include easy walking, jogging, or cycling, and a few minutes of leg stretches such as the quadriceps, hamstring, and calf stretches shown in Chapter 4.
3. Carry a stopwatch or a watch with a second hand and a pad and pencil to record your time and heart rate.
4. Walk one mile as fast as you can. Maintain a steady pace.
5. Record your time to the nearest second. Most people walk between 3.0 and 6.0 miles per hour, so an average time will be 10 to 20 minutes to walk the mile.
6. At the end of the mile, take your pulse immediately (your heart rate begins to slow as soon as you stop walking). Record your heart rate. (If you need a refresher course on taking your pulse, see Chapter 6.)
7. Find the appropriate Relative Fitness Level chart for your age and gender in Table B–1. The point at which your heart rate (vertical axis) and time (horizontal axis) intersect indicates your fitness level.

Evaluations

Once you have taken the test, you can determine your fitness level relative to people in your age and sex group by using Table B–1.

After evaluating your relative fitness level, progress to Table B–2. By using your heart rate and total walking time coordinates, you can find the appropriate exercise program category for your current fitness level. Note the background color of the section in which your coordinates intersect. Turn to Table B–3 and, using this color, find the corresponding exercise program.

The exercise programs outlined in Table B–3 are designed to help you maintain or improve your fitness level:

- If your test coordinates place you in the white or red exercise programs, you are in a program aimed at improvement, and, at the end of the 20-week program, you should retake the Walking Test to determine your new fitness level and exercise program.
- If your test coordinates place you in the charcoal exercise program, you may choose to retake the Walking Test at the end of the 20-week program to find your new fitness level and appropriate exercise program, or you may continue on the charcoal maintenance program, listed in Table B–3.
- If your test coordinate place you in the rose or grey exercise programs, you are in a program aimed at maintenance, and you should follow the maintenance guidelines given with those programs in Table B–3.

Note: For each program there are columns labeled *Pace* and *Heart Rate*. The pace listed is only an approximation. Rather than work for this mile-per-hour rate, you should concentrate on your heart rate. Your walking speed should be the speed that maintains your heart rate at the listed percentage of your maximum heart rate.

These charts are designed to tell you how fit you are compared to other individuals of your age and sex. For example, if your coordinates place you in the "above average" section of the chart, you're in better shape than the average person in your category.

The charts are based on weights of 170 lbs. for men and 125 lbs. for women. If you weigh substantially more, your relative cardiovascular fitness level will be slightly overestimated. If you weigh substantially less, your relative cardiovascular fitness level will be slightly underestimated.

Age	Males	Females

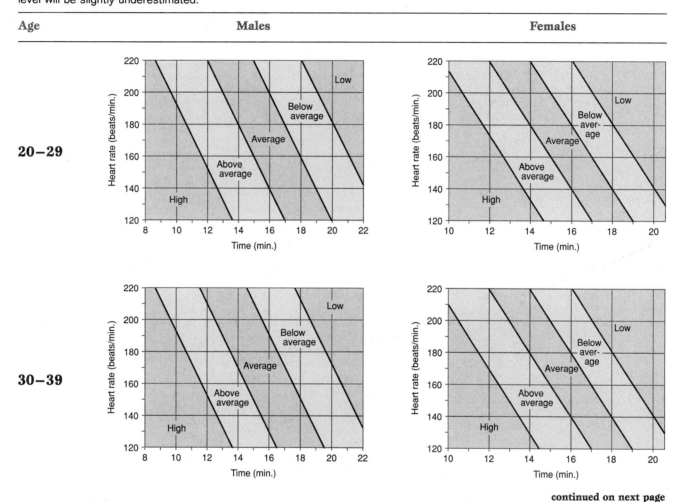

continued on next page

Age	Males	Females

40–49

50–59

60+

Age	Males	Females

20-29

30-39

40-49

continued on next page

THE ROCKPORT FITNESS WALKING TEST

Age	Males	Females

50–59

60+

TABLE B-3 • Exercise Programs

White Program*

Week	1–2	3–4	5	6	7–8	9	10	11	12–13	14	15–16	17–18	19–20
Warm-up (mins)	5–7	5–7	5–7	5–7	5–7	5–7	5–7	5–7	5–7	5–7	5–7	5–7	5–7
Mileage	1.0	1.25	1.5	1.5	1.75	2.0	2.0	2.0	2.25	2.5	2.5	2.75	3.0
Pace (mph)	3.0	3.0	3.0	3.5	3.5	3.5	3.75	3.75	3.75	3.75	4.0	4.0	4.0
Heart Rate (% of max)	60	60	60	60–70	60–70	60–70	60–70	70	70	70	70	70–80	70–80
Cooldown (mins)	5–7	5–7	5–7	5–7	5–7	5–7	5–7	5–7	5–7	5–7	5–7	5–7	5–7
Frequency (times per week)	5	5	5	5	5	5	5	5	5	5	5	5	5

*At the end of the twenty-week fitness walking protocol, retest yourself to establish your new program.

Red Program*

Week	1–2	3–4	5–6	7	8–9	10–12	13	14	15–16	17–18	19–20
Warm-up (mins)	5–7	5–7	5–7	5–7	5–7	5–7	5–7	5–7	5–7	5–7	5–7
Mileage	1.5	1.75	2.0	2.0	2.25	2.5	2.75	2.75	3.0	3.25	3.5
Pace (mph)	3.0	3.0	3.0	3.5	3.5	3.5	3.5	4.0	4.0	4.0	4.0
Heart Rate (% of max)	60–70	60–70	60–70	70	70	70	70	70–80	70–80	70–80	70–80
Cooldown (mins)	5–7	5–7	5–7	5–7	5–7	5–7	5–7	5–7	5–7	5–7	5–7
Frequency (times per week)	5	5	5	5	5	5	5	5	5	5	5

*At the end of the twenty-week fitness walking protocol, retest yourself to establish your new program.

continued on next page

TABLE B-3 • Continued

Charcoal Program*

Week	1	2	3–4	5	6–8	9–10	11–12	13–14	15	16–17	18–20
Warm-up (mins)	5–7	5–7	5–7	5–7	5–7	5–7	5–7	5–7	5–7	5–7	5–7
Mileage	2.0	2.25	2.5	2.75	2.75	3.0	3.0	3.25	3.5	3.5	4.0
Pace (mph)	3.0	3.0	3.0	3.0	3.5	3.5	4.0	4.0	4.0	4.5	4.5
Heart Rate (% of max)	70	70	70	70	70	70	70–80	70–80	70–80	70–80	70–80
Cooldown (mins)	5–7	5–7	5–7	5–7	5–7	5–7	5–7	5–7	5–7	5–7	5–7
Frequency (times per week)	5	5	5	5	5	5	5	5	5	5	5

*At the end of the twenty-week fitness protocol, you may either retest yourself and move to a new fitness walking category or follow the Charcoal Maintenance Program for a lifetime of fitness walking.

Rose Program

Week	1	2	3–4	5	6	7	8	9–10	11–14	15–20
Warm-Up (mins)	5–7	5–7	5–7	5–7	5–7	5–7	5–7	5–7	5–7	5–7
Mileage	2.5	2.75	3.0	3.25	3.25	3.5	3.75	4.0	4.0	4.0
Pace (mph)	3.5	3.5	3.5	3.5	4.0	4.0	4.0	4.0	4.5	4.5
Incline/Weight										−
Heart Rate (% of max)	70	70	70	70	70–80	70–80	70–80	70–80	70–80	70–80
Cooldown (mins)	5–7	5–7	5–7	5–7	5–7	5–7	5–7	5–7	5–7	5–7
Frequency (times per week)	5	5	5	5	5	5	5	5	5	3

*At the end of the twenty-week fitness protocol follow the Rose/Grey Maintenance Program for a lifetime of fitness walking.

Grey Program

Week	1	2	3	4	5	6	7–20
Warm-Up (mins)	5–7	5–7	5–7	5–7	5–7	5–7	5–7
Mileage	3.0	3.25	3.5	3.5	3.75	4.0	4.0
Pace (mph)	4.0	4.0	4.0	4.5	4.5	4.5	4.5
Incline/Weight							+
Heart Rate (% of max)	70	70	70	70–80	70–80	70–80	70–80
Cooldown (mins)	5–7	5–7	5–7	5–7	5–7	5–7	5–7
Frequency (times per week)	5	5	5	5	5	5	3

*At the end of the twenty-week fitness walking protocol turn to the Rose/Grey Maintenance Program for a lifetime of fitness walking.

Charcoal MAINTENANCE PROGRAM	Rose/Grey MAINTENANCE PROGRAM
Warm-Up: 5–7 minutes before walk stretches	Warm-Up: 5–7 minutes before walk stretches
Aerobic Work Out: mileage: 4.0 pace: 4.5 mph	Aerobic Work Out: mileage: 4.0 pace: 4.5 mph weight/incline: add weights to upper body or add hill walking as needed to keep heart rate in target zone (70–80% of predicted maximum).
Heart Rate: 70–80% of maximum	Heart Rate: 70–80% of maximum
Cooldown: 5–7 minutes after walk stretches	Cooldown: 5–7 minutes after walk stretches
Frequency: 3–5 times per week	Frequency: 3–5 times per week
Weekly Mileage: 12–20 miles	Weekly Mileage: 12–20 miles

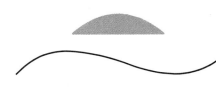

Appendix C
Recommended Dietary Allowances

Many countries have developed nutrient standards. Those of the United States (the Recommended Dietary Allowances, or RDA) are presented here. The main RDA table is presented in Table C–1. The energy RDA are presented in Table C–2. The estimated safe and adequate daily dietary intakes of selected vitamins and minerals appear in Table C–3, and Table C–4 presents the estimated minimum requirements of electrolytes.

TABLE C-1 • Recommended Dietary Alowances (RDA), 1989[a]

Age (years)	Weight (kg)	(lb)	Height (cm)	(inches)	Protein (g)	(µg RE) Vitamin A	(µg) Vitamin D	(mg α-Te) Vitamin E	(µg) Vitamin K	(mg) Vitamin C	(mg) Thiamin	(mg) Riboflavin	(mg NE) Niacin	(mg) Vitamin B$_6$	(µg) Folate	(µg) Vitamin B$_{12}$	(mg) Calcium	(mg) Phosphorus	(mg) Magnesium	(mg) Iron	(mg) Zinc	(µg) Iodine	(µg) Selenium
Infants																							
0.0–0.5	6	13	60	24	13	375	7.5	3	5	30	0.3	0.4	5	0.3	25	0.3	400	300	40	6	5	40	10
0.5–1.0	9	20	71	28	14	375	10	4	10	35	0.4	0.5	6	0.6	35	0.5	600	500	60	10	5	50	15
Children																							
1–3	13	29	90	35	16	400	10	6	15	40	0.7	0.8	9	1.0	50	0.7	800	800	80	10	10	70	20
4–6	20	44	112	44	24	500	10	7	20	45	0.9	1.1	12	1.1	75	1.0	800	800	120	10	10	90	20
7–10	28	62	132	52	28	700	10	7	30	45	1.0	1.2	13	1.4	100	1.4	800	800	170	10	10	120	30
Males																							
11–14	45	99	157	62	45	1,000	10	10	45	50	1.3	1.5	17	1.7	150	2.0	1,200	1,200	270	12	15	150	40
15–18	66	145	176	69	59	1,000	10	10	65	60	1.5	1.8	20	2.0	200	2.0	1,200	1,200	400	12	15	150	50
19–24	72	160	177	70	58	1,000	10	10	70	60	1.5	1.7	19	2.0	200	2.0	1,200	1,200	350	10	15	150	70
25–50	79	174	176	70	63	1,000	5	10	80	60	1.5	1.7	19	2.0	200	2.0	800	800	350	10	15	150	70
51+	77	170	173	68	63	1,000	5	10	80	60	1.2	1.4	15	2.0	200	2.0	800	800	350	10	15	150	70
Females																							
11–14	46	101	157	62	46	800	10	8	45	50	1.1	1.3	15	1.4	150	2.0	1,200	1,200	280	15	12	150	45
15–18	55	120	163	64	44	800	10	8	55	60	1.1	1.3	15	1.5	180	2.0	1,200	1,200	300	15	12	150	50
19–24	58	128	164	65	46	800	10	8	60	60	1	1.3	15	1.6	180	2.0	1,200	1,200	280	15	12	150	55
25–50	63	138	163	64	50	800	5	8	65	60	1.1	1.3	15	1.6	180	2.0	800	800	280	15	12	150	55
51+	65	143	160	63	50	800	5	8	65	60	1.0	1.2	13	1.6	180	2.0	800	800	280	10	12	150	55
Pregnant					60	800	10	10	65	70	1.5	1.6	17	2.2	400	2.2	1,200	1,200	320	30	15	175	65
Lactating																							
1st 6 mo					65	1,300	10	12	65	95	1.6	1.8	20	2.1	280	2.6	1,200	1,200	355	15	19	200	75
2nd 6 mo					62	1,200	10	11	65	90	1.6	1.7	20	2.1	260	2.6	1,200	1,200	340	15	16	200	75

[a]The allowances are intended to provide for individual variations among most normal, healthy people in the United States under usual environmental stresses. They were designed for the maintenance of good nutrition. Diets should be based on a variety of common foods in order to provide other nutrients for which human requirements have been less well defined.

Source: Reproduced from Food and Nutrition Board, *Recommended Dietary Allowances,* 10th ed. (Washington, D.C.: National Academy of Sciences, 1989), with permission.

TABLE C-2 • Median Heights and Weights and Recommended Energy Intakes (United States)

Age	Weight		Height		Average Energy Allowance			
(years)	(kg)	(lb)	(cm)	(inches)	REE[a] (kcal/day)	Multiples of REE[b]	kcal per kg	kcal per day[c]
Infants								
0.0–0.5	6	13	60	24	320		108	650
0.5–1.0	9	20	71	28	500		98	850
Children								
1–3	13	29	90	35	740		102	1,300
4–6	20	44	112	44	950		90	1,800
7–10	28	62	132	52	1,130		70	2,000
Males								
11–14	45	99	157	62	1,440	1.70	55	2,500
15–18	66	145	176	69	1,760	1.67	45	3,000
19–24	72	160	177	70	1,780	1.67	40	2,900
25–50	79	174	176	70	1,800	1.60	37	2,900
51+	77	170	173	68	1,530	1.50	30	2,300
Females								
11–14	46	101	157	62	1,310	1.67	47	2,200
15–18	55	120	163	64	1,370	1.60	40	2,200
19–24	58	128	164	65	1,350	1.60	38	2,200
25–50	63	138	163	64	1,380	1.55	36	2,200
51+	65	143	160	63	1,280	1.50	30	1,900
Pregnant (2nd and 3rd trimesters)								+300
Lactating								+500

[a]REE (resting energy expenditure) represents the energy expended by a person at rest under normal conditions.
[b]Recommended energy allowances assume light to moderate activity and were calculated by multiplying the REE by an activity factor.
[c]Average energy allowances have been rounded.
Source: *Recommended Dietary Allowances*, © 1989 by the National Academy of Sciences, National Academy Press, Washington, D.C.

TABLE C-3 • Estimated Safe and Adequate Daily Dietary Intakes of Selected Vitamins and Minerals[a]

Age (years)	Vitamins	
	Biotin (μg)	Pantothenic Acid (mg)
Infants		
0–0.5	10	2
0.5–1	15	3
Children		
1–3	20	3
4–6	25	3–4
7–10	30	4–5
11+	30–100	4–7
Adults	30–100	4–7

Age (years)	Trace Elements[b]				
	Chromium (μg)	Molybdenum (μg)	Copper (mg)	Manganese (mg)	Fluoride (mg)
Infants					
0–0.5	10–40	15–30	0.4–0.6	0.3–0.6	0.1–0.5
0.5–1	20–60	20–40	0.6–0.7	0.6–1.0	0.2–1.0
Children					
1–3	20–80	25–50	0.7–1.0	1.0–1.5	0.5–1.5
4–6	30–120	30–75	1.0–1.5	1.5–2.0	1.0–2.5
7–10	50–200	50–150	1.0–2.0	2.0–3.0	1.5–2.5
11+	50–200	75–250	1.5–2.5	2.0–5.0	1.5–2.5
Adults	50–200	75–250	1.5–3.0	2.0–5.0	1.5–4.0

[a]Because there is less information on which to base allowances, these figures are not given in the main table of the RDA and are provided here in the form of ranges of recommended intakes.

[b]Because the toxic levels for many trace elements may be only several times usual intakes, the upper levels for the trace elements given in this table should not be habitually exceeded.

Source: *Recommended Dietary Allowances,* 10th ed., © 1989 by the National Academy of Sciences, National Academy Press, Washington, D.C.

TABLE C-4 • Estimated Sodium, Chloride, and Potassium Minimum Requirements of Healthy Persons

Age (years)	Sodium[a] (mg)	Chloride (mg)	Potassium[b] (mg)
Infants			
0.0–0.5	120	180	500
0.5–1.0	200	300	700
Children			
1	225	350	1,000
2–5	300	500	1,400
6–9	400	600	1,600
Adolescents	500	750	2,000
Adults	500	750	2,000

[a]Sodium requirements are based on estimates of needs for growth and for replacement of obligatory losses. They cover a wide variation of physical activity patterns and climatic exposure but do not provide for large, prolonged losses from the skin through sweat.

[b]Dietary potassium may benefit the prevention and treatment of hypertension and recommendations to include many servings of fruits and vegetables would raise potassium intakes to about 3,500 mg/day.

Source: *Recommended Dietary Allowances,* 10th ed., © 1989 by the National Academy of Sciences, National Academy Press, Washington, D.C.

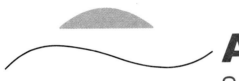

Appendix D
Selected Nutrients in Foods

This appendix offers information on most of the foods people commonly eat. The list of foods chosen is an expanded version of that presented in the 1986 edition of the USDA *Home and Garden Bulletin Number 72, Nutritive Value of Foods.* Many additional foods have been added (such as frozen yogurt, canola oil, and imitation seafood items) to reflect current food patterns.

To present all the available data would require hundreds of pages—space not available here. We have chosen to present calories (because everyone wants to know them) and grams of protein, carbohydrate, and fat in foods. This information facilitates the calculations needed to complete the Personal Focus and Lab Report for Chapter 9. The dietary fiber in foods is listed (current dietary guidelines encourage people to eat more high–fiber foods), and the sodium and cholesterol contents of foods are included as well (current dietary guidelines recommend limiting sodium and reducing cholesterol in diets).

Many factors influence the amounts of nutrients in foods, including the mineral content of the soil, the method of processing, the diet of the animal or the fertilizer of the plant, the season of the year, the method of analysis, the differences in the moisture content of the samples analyzed, the length and method of storage, and the methods of cooking the food. As a result, different nutrient values for the same food item are reported, even by reliable sources. Therefore, although each nutrient is presented as a single number, each number is actually an average of a range of data.

Considerable effort has been made to report the most accurate data available and to eliminate missing values. There will always be changes in the future, and the authors welcome any suggestions or comments.*

The items in this table have been organized into several food categories, which are listed at the head of each page. As the key shows, each group has a number and that number is indicated in the first column of the table. For ease in paging through this table, the category listed on the page you are on is highlighted with boldface type. Thus if 7–GRAIN is boldface and you are looking for dairy foods, turn back a few pages; if you are looking for sweets, turn forward.

---

*This table has been prepared for West Publishing Company and is copyrighted by ESHA Research in Salem, Oregon—the developer and publisher of *The Food Processor* computerized nutrition systems. The major sources for the data from the U. S. Department of Agriculture are supplemented by over 450 additional sources of information. Because the list of references is so extensive, it is not provided here, but it is available from the publisher.

Table D–1 Food Composition

Grp	Computer Code No.	Food Description	Measure	Wt (g)	H$_2$O (%)	Ener (cal)	Prot (g)	Carb (g)	Dietary Fiber (g)	Fat (g)	Chol (mg)	Sodi (mg)
BEVERAGES												
		Alcoholic:										
		Beer:										
1	1	Regular (12 fl oz)	1½ c	356	92	146	1	13	1	0	0	19
1	2	Light (12 fl oz)	1½ c	354	95	100[1]	1	5	1	0	0	10
		Gin, rum, vodka, whiskey:										
1	3	80 proof	1½ fl oz	42	67	97	0	<.1	0	0	0	<1
1	4	86 proof	1½ fl oz	42	64	105	0	<.1	0	0	0	<1
1	5	90 proof	1½ fl oz	42	62	110	0	<.1	0	0	0	<1
		Liqueur:										
1	1359	Coffee Liqueur, 53 proof	1½ fl oz	52	31	174	0	24	0	<1	0	4
1	1360	Coffee & cream liqueur, 34 proof	1½ fl oz	47	47	154	1	10	0	7	—	43
1	1361	Creme de menthe, 72 proof	1½ fl oz	50	28	186	0	21	0	<1	0	3
		Wine:										
1	6	Dessert (4 fl oz)	½ c	118	72	181[2]	<1	14[2]	0	0	0	11
1	7	Red	3½ fl oz	103	88	74	<1	2	0	0	0	6
1	8	Rosé	3½ fl oz	103	89	73	<1	2	0	0	0	5
1	9	White medium	3½ fl oz	103	90	70	<1	1	0	0	0	5
		Carbonated[3]:										
1	10	Club soda (12 fl oz)	1½ c	355	100	0	0	0	0	0	0	75
1	11	Cola beverage (12 fl oz)	1½ c	370	89	151	0	39	0	0	0	15
1	12	Diet cola (12 fl oz)	1½ c	355	100	2	0	<1	0	0	0	21[6]
1	13	Diet soda pop–average (12 fl oz)	1½ c	355	100	2	0	<1	0	0	0	21[6]
1	14	Ginger ale (12 fl oz)	1½ c	366	91	124	0	32	0	0	0	25
1	15	Grape soda (12 fl oz)	1½ c	372	89	161	0	42	0	0	0	57
1	16	Lemon-lime (12 fl oz)	1½ c	368	90	149	0	38	0	0	0	41
1	17	Orange (12 fl oz)	1½ c	372	88	177	0	46	0	0	0	46
1	18	Pepper-type soda (12 fl oz)	1½ c	368	89	151	0	38	0	0	0	38
1	19	Root beer (12 fl oz)	1½ c	370	89	152	<1	39	0	0	0	49
		Coffee[3]:										
1	20	Brewed	1 c	240	99	2[4]	<1	1	<1	0	0	5
1	21	Prepared from instant	1 c	240	99	2[4]	<1	1	0	0	0	8
		Fruit drinks, noncarbonated[5]:										
1	22	Fruit punch drink, canned	1 c	253	88	118	<1	30	0	<1	0	56
1	1358	Gatorade	1 c	230	99	39	0	11	0	0	0	123
1	23	Grape drink, canned	1 c	250	88	112	0	35	<1	<1	0	16
1	1304	Koolade, sweetened with sugar	1 c	240	100	100	0	25	0	0	0	0
1	1356	Koolade, sweetened with nutrasweet	1 c	240	100	4	0	0	0	0	0	0
		Lemonade, frozen:										
1	26	Concentrate (6-oz can)	¾ c	219	52	397	1	103	1	<1	0	8
1	27	Lemonade prepared from frozen concentrate	1 c	248	89	100	<1	26	<1	<1	0	8
		Limeade, frozen:										
1	28	Concentrate (6-oz can)	¾ c	218	50	408	<1	108	1	<1	0	<1
1	29	Limeade prepared from frozen concentrate	1 c	247	89	102	<1	27	<1	<1	0	<1
1	24	Pineapple grapefruit, canned	1 c	250	88	117	1	29	0	<1	0	34
1	25	Pineapple orange, canned	1 c	250	87	125	3	29	0	<1	0	9
		Fruit and vegetable juices: see Fruit and Vegetable sections										

[1] Calories can vary from 78 to 131 for 12 fl oz.

[2] Values are for sweet dessert wine. Dry dessert wines contain 149 cal and 5 g of carbohydrate.

[3] Mineral content varies depending on water source.

[4] Calorie values from USDA vary from 1 to 4 calories per cup.

[5] Usually less than 10% fruit juice.

[6] Value for product sweetened with aspartame only; sodium is 32 mg if a blend of aspartame and sodium saccharin is used; 75 mg if just sodium saccharin is used.

(For purposes of calculations, use "0" for t, <1, <.1, <.01, etc.)

Table D–1   Food Composition

Grp	Computer Code No.	Food Description	Measure	Wt (g)	H$_2$O (%)	Ener (cal)	Prot (g)	Carb (g)	Dietary Fiber (g)	Fat (g)	Chol (mg)	Sodi (mg)
BEVERAGES—Con.												
1	1357	Perrier® bottled water, 6.5 fl oz bottle	1 ea	192	100	0	0	0	0	0	0	3
1	30	Brewed Tea[8]:	1 c	240	100	2	<.01	1	0	0	0	7
1	31	From instant, unsweetened	1 c	237	100	2	0	<1	0	0	0	8
1	32	From instant, sweetened	1 c	262	91	86	0	22	0	0	0	1
DAIRY												
		Butter: see Fats and Oils, #158, 159, 160										
		Cheese, natural:										
2	33	Blue	1 oz	28	42	100	6	1	0	8	21	396
2	34	Brick	1 oz	28	41	105	6	1	0	8	27	159
2	35	Brie	1 oz	28	48	95	6	<1	0	8	28	178
2	36	Camembert	1 oz	28	52	85	6	<1	0	7	20	236
		Cheddar:										
2	37	Cut pieces	1 oz	28	37	114	7	<1	0	9	30	176
2	38	1″ cube	1 ea	17	37	69	4	<1	0	6	18	107
2	39	Shredded	1 c	113	37	455	28	1	0	37	119	701
		Cottage:										
2	40	Creamed, large curd	1 c	225	79	235	28	6	0	10	34	911
2	41	Creamed, small curd	1 c	210	79	215	26	6	0	9	31	850
2	42	With fruit	1 c	226	72	279	22	30	0	8	25	915
2	43	Low fat 2%	1 c	226	79	205	31	8	0	4	19	918
2	44	Low fat 1%	1 c	226	82	164	28	6	0	2	10	918
2	45	Dry curd	1 c	145	80	123	25	3	0	1	10	19
2	46	Cream	1 oz	28	54	99	2	1	0	10	31	84
2	47	Edam	1 oz	28	42	101	7	<1	0	8	25	274
2	48	Feta	1 oz	28	55	75	5	1	0	6	25	316
2	49	Gouda	1 oz	28	42	101	7	1	0	8	32	232
2	50	Gruyère	1 oz	28	33	117	8	<1	0	9	31	95
2	51	Gorgonzola	1 oz	28	39	111	7	0	0	9	25	513
2	52	Liederkranz	1 oz	28	53	87	5	0	0	8	21	390
2	53	Monterey jack	1 oz	28	41	106	7	<1	0	9	26	152
		Mozzarella, made with:										
2	54	Whole milk	1 oz	28	54	80	5	1	0	6	22	106
2	55	Part skim milk, low moisture	1 oz	28	49	80	8	1	0	5	15	150
2	56	Muenster	1 oz	28	42	104	6	<1	0	8	27	178
		Parmesan, grated:										
2	57	Cup, not pressed down	1 c	100	18	455	42	4	0	30	79	1862
2	58	Tablespoon	1 tbsp	5	18	23	2	<1	0	2	4	93
2	59	Ounce	1 oz	28	18	129	12	1	0	9	22	528
2	60	Provolone	1 oz	28	41	100	7	1	0	8	20	248
		Ricotta, made with:										
2	61	Whole milk	1 c	246	72	428	28	7	0	32	124	207
2	62	Part skim milk	1 c	246	74	340	28	13	0	19	76	307
2	63	Romano	1 oz	28	31	110	9	1	0	8	29	340
2	64	Swiss	1 oz	28	37	107	8	1	0	8	26	74
		Pasteurized processed cheese products:										
2	65	American	1 oz	28	39	106	6	<1	0	9	27	406
2	66	Swiss	1 oz	28	42	95	7	1	0	7	24	388
2	67	American cheese food	1 oz	28	44	93	6	2	0	7	18	337
2	68	American cheese spread	1 oz	28	48	82	5	2	0	6	16	381

[8]Mineral content varies depending on water source.

(Computer code number is for West Diet Analysis program)

GRP KEY: 1=BEV 2=DAIRY 3=EGGS 4=FAT/OIL 5=FRUIT 6=BAKERY 7=GRAIN 8=FISH 9=BEEF 10=POULTRY 11=SAUSAGE 12=MIXED/FAST 13=NUTS/SEEDS 14=SWEETS 15=VEG/LEG 16=MISC 22=SOUP/SAUCE

Grp	Computer Code No.	Food Description	Measure	Wt (g)	H₂O (%)	Ener (cal)	Prot (g)	Carb (g)	Dietary Fiber (g)	Fat (g)	Chol (mg)	Sodi (mg)
		DAIRY—Con.										
		Cream, sweet:										
		Half and half (cream and milk):										
2	69	Cup	1 c	242	81	315	7	10	0	28	89	98
2	70	Tablespoon	1 tbsp	15	81	20	<1	1	0	2	6	6
		Light, coffee or table:										
2	71	Cup	1 c	240	74	469	6	9	0	46	159	95
2	72	Tablespoon	1 tbsp	15	74	30	<1	1	0	3	10	6
		Light whipping cream, liquid:										
2	73	Cup	1 c	239	64	699	5	7	0	74	265	82
2	74	Tablespoon	1 tbsp	15	64	44	<1	<1	0	5	17	5
		Heavy whipping cream, liquid[9]:										
2	75	Cup	1 c	238	58	821	5	7	0	88	326	89
2	76	Tablespoon	1 tbsp	15	58	51	<1	<1	0	6	20	6
		Whipped cream, pressurized[9]:										
2	77	Cup	1 c	60	61	154	2	7	0	13	46	78
2	78	Tablespoon	1 tbsp	4	61	10	<1	<1	0	1	3	5
		Cream, sour, cultured:										
2	79	Cup	1 c	230	71	493	7	10	0	48	102	123
2	80	Tablespoon	1 tbsp	14	71	30	<1	1	0	3	6	7
		Cream products—imitation and part dairy:										
		Coffee whitener:										
2	81	Frozen or liquid	1 tbsp	15	77	20	<1	2	0	2	0	12
2	82	Powdered	1 tsp	2	2	11	<1	1	0	1	0	4
		Dessert topping, frozen:										
2	83	Cup	1 c	75	50	239	1	17	0	19	0	19
2	84	Tablespoon	1 tbsp	5	50	15	<1	1	0	1	0	1
		Dessert topping from mix:										
2	85	Cup	1 c	80	67	151	3	13	0	10	8	53
2	86	Tablespoon	1 tbsp	5	67	9	<1	1	0	1	<1	3
		Dessert topping, pressurized:										
2	87	Cup	1 c	70	60	185	1	11	0	16	0	43
2	88	Tablespoon	1 tbsp	4	60	11	<1	1	0	1	0	3
		Sour cream imitation:										
2	91	Cup	1 c	230	71	479	6	15	0	45	0	235
2	92	Tablespoon	1 tbsp	14	71	29	<1	1	0	3	0	14
		Sour dressing, part dairy:										
2	89	Cup	1 c	235	75	416	8	11	0	39	213	113
2	90	Tablespoon	1 tbsp	15	75	25	<1	1	0	2	1	7
		Milk, fluid:										
2	93	Whole milk	1 c	244	88	150	8	11	0	8	33	120
2	94	2% low-fat milk	1 c	244	89	121	8	12	0	5	22	122
2	95	2% milk solids added[10]	1 c	245	89	125	9	12	0	5	18	128
2	96	1% low-fat milk	1 c	244	90	102	8	12	0	3	10	123
2	97	1% milk solids added[10]	1 c	245	90	105	9	12	0	2	10	128
2	98	Skim milk	1 c	245	91	86	8	12	0	<1	4	126
2	99	Skim milk solids added[10]	1 c	245	90	91	9	12	0	1	5	130
2	100	Buttermilk	1 c	245	90	99	8	12	0	2	9	257

[9] For whipped cream, (non-pressurized), double the liquid cream volume of codes 75,76 or 73,74. One tablespoon liquid cream becomes 2 Tablespoons when "whipped".

[10] Milk solids added, label claims less than 10 g protein per cup.

(For purposes of calculations, use "0" for t, <1, <.1, <.01, etc.)

Table D–1 Food Composition

Grp	Computer Code No.	Food Description	Measure	Wt (g)	H₂O (%)	Ener (cal)	Prot (g)	Carb (g)	Dietary Fiber (g)	Fat (g)	Chol (mg)	Sodi (mg)

Grp	Code No.	Food Description	Measure	Wt (g)	H$_2$O (%)	Ener (cal)	Prot (g)	Carb (g)	Dietary Fiber (g)	Fat (g)	Chol (mg)	Sodi (mg)
DAIRY—Con.												
		Milk, canned:										
2	101	Sweetened condensed	1 c	306	27	982	24	166	0	27	104	389
2	102	Evaporated, whole	1 c	252	74	340	17	25	0	20	74	267
2	103	Evaporated, skim	1 c	255	79	200	19	29	0	1	10	293
		Milk, dried:										
2	104	Buttermilk	1 c	120	3	464	41	59	0	7	83	621
		Instant, nonfat:										
2	105	Envelope[12]	1 ea	91	4	326	32	48	0	1	16	500
2	106	Cup	1 c	68	4	244	24	36	0	1	12	373
2	107	Goat milk	1 c	244	87	168	9	11	0	10	28	122
2	108	Kefir[13]	1 c	233	82	122	9	9	0	5	10	50
		Milk beverages and powdered mixes:										
		Chocolate:										
2	109	Whole	1 c	250	82	210	8	26	4	8	31	149
2	110	2% fat	1 c	250	84	180	8	26	4	5	17	151
2	111	1% fat	1 c	250	84	160	8	26	4	3	7	152
		Chocolate-flavored beverages:										
2	112	Powder containing nonfat dry milk:	1 oz	28	1	100	4	23	<1	1	1	139
2	113	Drink prepared with water	¾ c	206	86	100	4	23	<1	1	1	139
2	114	Powder without nonfat dry milk:	¾ oz	22	<1	75	1	20	<1	1	0	45
2	115	Drink prepared with whole milk	1 c	266	81	226	9	31	<1	9	33	165
2	116	Eggnog, commercial	1 c	254	74	342	10	34	0	19	149	138
		Instant Breakfast:										
2	1027	Envelope, dry powder only	1 ea	37	3	130	7	23	0	0	0	166
2	1028	Prepared with whole milk	1 c	281	87	280	15	34	0	8	33	286
2	1029	Prepared with 2% milk	1 c	281	88	251	15	35	0	5	18	289
2	1283	Prepared with 1% milk	1 c	281	89	232	15	35	0	3	10	289
2	1284	Prepared with skim milk	1 c	282	89	216	15	35	0	<1	4	292
		Malted milk, chocolate flavor:										
2	117	Powder[14], 3 heaping tsp:	¾ oz	21	1	79	1	18	<1	1	1	53
2	118	Drink prepared with whole milk	1 c	265	81	229	9	30	<1	9	34	172
		Malted milk, natural flavor:										
2	119	Powder[14], 3 heaping tsp:	¾ oz	21	2	87	2	16	<1	2	4	103
2	120	Drink prepared with whole milk	1 c	265	81	237	10	27	<1	10	37	223
		Milk shakes:										
2	121	Chocolate (10 fl oz)	1¼ c	283	72	360	10	58	<1	11	37	273
2	122	Vanilla (10 fl oz)	1¼ c	283	75	314	10	51	<1	8	32	232
		Milk desserts:										
2	134	Custard, baked	1 c	265	77	305	14	29	0	15	13	209
		Ice cream, regular vanilla (about 11% fat):										
		Hardened:										
2	123	½ gallon	½ gal	1064	61	2153	38	254	0	115	478	926
2	124	Cup	1 c	133	61	269	5	32	0	14	59	116
2	125	Fluid ounces	3 oz	50	61	101	2	12	0	5	23	44
2	126	Soft serve	1 c	173	60	377	7	38	0	22	153	153
		Ice cream, rich vanilla (about 16% fat):										
		Hardened:										
2	127	½ gallon	½ gal	1188	59	2805	33	256	0	190	701	867
2	128	Cup	1 c	148	59	349	4	32	0	24	88	108

[12]Yields 1 qt fluid milk when reconstituted according to package directions.

[13]Most values provided by product labeling.

[14]The latest USDA data from *Handbook 8–14* on beverages updates previous USDA data.

(Computer code number is for West Diet Analysis program)

GRP KEY: 1 = BEV **2 = DAIRY** **3 = EGGS** **4 = FAT/OIL** 5 = FRUIT 6 = BAKERY 7 = GRAIN 8 = FISH 9 = BEEF 10 = POULTRY
11 = SAUSAGE 12 = MIXED/FAST 13 = NUTS/SEEDS 14 = SWEETS 15 = VEG/LEG 16 = MISC 22 = SOUP/SAUCE

Grp	Computer Code No.	Food Description	Measure	Wt (g)	H₂O (%)	Ener (cal)	Prot (g)	Carb (g)	Dietary Fiber (g)	Fat (g)	Chol (mg)	Sodi (mg)
		DAIRY—Con.										
		Milk Desserts—Con.										
		Ice milk, vanilla (about 4% fat):										
		Hardened:										
2	129	½ gallon	½ gal	1048	69	1467	41	232	0	45	146	838
2	130	Cup	1 c	131	69	184	5	29	0	6	18	105
2	131	Soft serve (about 3% fat)	1 c	175	70	223	8	38	0	5	13	163
		Pudding, canned, 5 oz can = .55 cup:										
2	135	Chocolate	1 ea	142	68	205	3	30	<1	11	1	285
2	136	Tapioca	1 ea	142	74	160	3	28	0	5	1	252
2	137	Vanilla	1 ea	142	69	220	2	33	0	10	1	305
		Puddings, prepared from dry mix with whole milk:										
2	138	Chocolate, instant	1 c	260	71	310	8	54	<1	8	28	880
2	139	Chocolate, regular, cooked	½ c	130	73	150	4	25	<1	4	15	167
2	140	Rice, cooked	½ c	132	73	155	4	27	<1	4	15	140
2	141	Tapioca, cooked	½ c	130	75	145	4	25	0	4	15	152
2	142	Vanilla, instant	½ c	130	73	150	4	27	0	4	15	375
2	143	Vanilla, regular, cooked	½ c	130	74	145	4	25	0	4	15	178
		Sherbet (2% fat):										
2	132	½ gallon	½ gal	1542	66	2158	17	469	0	31	113	709
2	133	Cup	1 c	193	66	270	2	59	0	4	14	88
2	144	Soy milk	1 c	240	93	79	7	4	0	5	0	30
2	1584	Yogurt, frozen, low fat[16]	½	87	70	110	4	17	0	2	7	45
		Yogurt, low fat:										
2	145	Fruit added[17]	1 c	227	74	231	10	43	<1	2	10	125
2	146	Plain	1 c	227	85	144	12	16	0	3	14	159
2	147	Vanilla or coffee flavor	1 c	227	79	193	11	31	0	3	11	150
2	148	Yogurt, made with nonfat milk (<.1% fat)	1 c	227	85	127	13	17	0	<1	4	173
2	149	Yogurt, made with whole milk (3.3% fat)	1 c	227	88	138	8	11	0	7	30	104
		EGGS[18]										
		Raw, large:										
3	150	Whole, without shell	1 ea	50	75	75	6	1	0	5	213	63
3	151	White	1 ea	33.4	88	17	4	<1	0	0	0	55
3	152	Yolk	1 ea	16.6	49	59	3	<1	0	5	213	7
		Cooked:										
3	153	Fried in margarine	1 ea	46	69	91	6	1	0	7	211	162
3	154	Hard-cooked, shell removed	1 ea	50	75	77	6	1	0	5	215	62
3	155	Hard-cooked, chopped	1 c	136	75	211	17	2	0	14	574	169
3	156	Poached, no added salt	1 ea	50	75	75	6	1	0	5	212	63
3	157	Scrambled with milk and margarine	1 ea	61	73	100	7	1	0	7	215	168
		FATS and OILS										
		Butter:										
4	158	Stick	½ c	113	16	813	1	<1	0	92	247	933[20]
4	159	Tablespoon	1 tbsp	14	16	100	<1	<1	0	12	31	116[20]
4	160	Pat (about 1 tsp)[19]	1 ea	5	16	34	<1	<1	0	4	11	41[20]

[16] Data is a composite of USDA information and several manufacturers.

[17] Carbohydrate and calories vary widely—consult label if more precise values are needed.

[18] This data is newest revised information from the USDA with 24% less cholesterol.

[19] Pat is 1″ square, ⅓″ thick; about 1 tsp; 90 per lb.

[20] For salted butter; unsalted butter contains 12 mg sodium per stick or ½ c, 1.5 mg/tbsp, or .5 mg/pat.

(For purposes of calculations, use "0" for t, <1, <.1, <.01, etc.)

Table D–1 Food Composition

Grp	Computer Code No.	Food Description	Measure	Wt (g)	H$_2$O (%)	Ener (cal)	Prot (g)	Carb (g)	Dietary Fiber (g)	Fat (g)	Chol (mg)	Sodi (mg)
		FATS and OILS—Con.										
		Fats, cooking:										
4	1363	Bacon fat	1 tbsp	14	<1	126	0	0	0	14	84	140
4	1362	Beef fat/tallow	1 c	205	0	1837	0	0	0	205	223	0
4	1364	Chicken fat	1 c	205	<1	1846	0	0	0	205	174	—
		Vegetable shortening:										
4	161	Cup	1 c	205	0	1812	0	0	0	205	0	0
4	162	Tablespoon	1 tbsp	13	0	15	0	0	0	13	0	0
		Lard:										
4	163	Cup	1 c	205	0	1849	0	0	0	205	195	<1
4	164	Tablespoon	1 tbsp	13	0	115	0	0	0	13	12	<1
		Margarine:										
		Imitation (about 40% fat), soft:										
4	165	8-oz container	8 oz	227	58	785	1	1	0	88	0	2178[22]
4	166	Tablespoon	1 tbsp	14	58	50	<.1	<.1	0	6	0	136[22]
		Regular, hard (about 80% fat):										
4	167	Cup	½ c	113	16	812	1	1	0	91	0	1066[22]
4	168	Tablespoon	1 tbsp	14	16	100	<1	<1	0	11	0	133[22]
4	169	Pat[19]	1 ea	5	16	36	<.1	<.1	0	4	0	47[22]
		Regular, soft (about 80% fat):										
4	170	8-oz container	8 oz	227	16	1626	2	1	0	183	0	2448[22]
4	171	Tablespoon	1 tbsp	14	16	100	1	<.1	0	11	0	153[22]
		Spread (about 60% fat), hard:										
4	172	Cup	½ c	113	37	610	1	0	0	69	0	1123[22]
4	173	Tablespoon	1 tbsp	14	37	75	<.1	0	0	9	0	139[22]
4	174	Pat[19]	1 ea	5	37	25	<.1	0	0	3	0	50[22]
		Spread (about 60% fat), soft:										
4	175	8 oz container	8 oz	227	37	1225	1	0	0	138	0	2256[22]
4	176	Tablespoon	1 tbsp	14	37	75	<.1	0	0	9	0	139[22]
		Oils:										
		Canola:										
4	1585	Cup	1 c	218	0	1927	0	0	0	218	0	0
4	1586	Tablespoon	1 tbsp	14	0	125	0	0	0	14	0	0
		Corn:										
4	177	Cup	1 c	218	0	1927	0	0	0	218	0	0
4	178	Tablespoon	1 tbsp	14	0	125	0	0	0	14	0	0
		Olive:										
4	179	Cup	1 c	216	0	1909	0	0	0	216	0	0
4	180	Tablespoon	1 tbsp	14	0	125	0	0	0	14	0	0
		Peanut:										
4	181	Cup	1 c	216	0	1909	0	0	0	216	0	0
4	182	Tablespoon	1 tbsp	14	0	125	0	0	0	14	0	0
		Safflower:										
4	183	Cup	1 c	218	0	1927	0	0	0	218	0	0
4	184	Tablespoon	1 tbsp	14	0	125	0	0	0	14	0	0
		Soybean:										
4	185	Cup	1 c	218	0	1927	0	0	0	218	0	0
4	186	Tablespoon	1 tbsp	14	0	125	0	0	0	14	0	0
		Soybean/cottonseed:										
4	187	Cup	1 c	218	0	1927	0	0	0	218	0	0
4	188	Tablespoon	1 tbsp	14	0	125	0	0	0	14	0	0

[19]Pat is 1″ square, ⅓″ thick; about 1 tsp; 90 per lb.
[22]For salted margarine.

(Computer code number is for West Diet Analysis program)

GRP KEY: 1 = BEV 2 = DAIRY 3 = EGGS **4 = FAT/OIL 5 = FRUIT** 6 = BAKERY 7 = GRAIN 8 = FISH 9 = BEEF 10 = POULTRY
11 = SAUSAGE 12 = MIXED/FAST 13 = NUTS/SEEDS 14 = SWEETS 15 = VEG/LEG 16 = MISC 22 = SOUP/SAUCE

Grp	Computer Code No.	Food Description	Measure	Wt (g)	H$_2$O (%)	Ener (cal)	Prot (g)	Carb (g)	Dietary Fiber (g)	Fat (g)	Chol (mg)	Sodi (mg)
		FATS and OILS—Con.										
		Oils—Con.										
		Sunflower:										
4	189	Cup	1 c	218	0	1927	0	0	0	218	0	0
4	190	Tablespoon	1 tbsp	14	0	125	0	0	0	14	0	0
		Salad dressings/ sandwich spreads:										
4	191	Blue cheese salad dressing	1 tbsp	15	32	75	1	1	<1	8	3	164
		French salad dressing										
4	192	Regular	1 tbsp	16	35	85	<.1	1	<1	9	0	188
4	193	Low calorie	1 tbsp	16	75	24	<.1	2	<1	2	0	306
		Italian salad dressing										
4	194	Regular	1 tbsp	14	34	80	<1	1	<1	9	0	162
4	195	Low calorie	1 tbsp	15	86	5	<.1	1	<1	1.5	0	136
		Mayonnaise:										
4	196	Regular	1 tbsp	14	15	100	<1	<1	0	11	8	80
4	197	Imitation, low calorie	1 tbsp	15	63	35	0	2	0	3	4	75
4	198	Ranch style salad dressing	½ c	119	35	435	4	6	0	45	47	522
		Mayo type salad dressing:										
4	199	Regular	1 tbsp	15	40	58	<1	4	0	5	4	105
4	1030	Low calorie	1 tbsp	15	63	35	<1	2	0	3	4	75
4	200	Tartar sauce	1 tbsp	14	34	74	<1	1	<1	8	4	182
		Thousand Island:										
4	201	Regular	1 tbsp	16	46	60	<1	2	<1	6	4	110
4	202	Low calorie	1 tbsp	15	69	25	<1	2	<1	2	2	153
		Salad dressings, prepared from home recipe:										
4	203	Cooked type[24]	1 tbsp	16	69	25	1	2	0	2	9	117
4	204	Vinegar and oil	1 tbsp	16	47	70	0	0	0	8	0	0
		FRUITS and FRUIT JUICES										
		Apples:										
		Fresh, raw, with peel:										
5	205	2¾" diam (about 3 per lb with cores)	1 ea	138	84	80	<1	21	3	<1	0	1
5	206	3¼" diam (about 2 per lb with cores)	1 ea	212	84	125	<1	32	5	1	0	1
5	207	Raw, peeled slices	1 c	110	84	65	<1	16	3	<1	0	1
5	208	Dried, sulfured	10 ea	64	32	155	1	42	8	<1	0	56[25]
5	209	Apple juice, bottled or canned	1 c	248	88	116	<1	29	<1	<1	0	7
		Applesauce:										
5	210	Sweetened	1 c	255	80	195	<1	51	4	<1	0	8
5	211	Unsweetened	1 c	244	88	106	<1	28	4	<1	0	5
		Apricots:										
5	212	Raw, without pits (about 12 per lb with pits)	3 ea	106	86	51	1	12	2	<1	0	1
		Canned (fruit and liquid):										
5	213	Heavy syrup	1 c	258	78	214	1	55	4	<1	0	10
5	214	Halves	3 ea	85	78	70	<1	18	1	<.1	0	3
5	215	Juice pack	1 c	248	87	119	2	31	4	<.1	0	9
5	216	Halves	3 ea	84	87	40	1	10	1	<.1	0	3
		Dried:										
5	217	Dried halves	10 ea	35	31	83	1	22	3	<1	0	4
5	218	Cooked, unsweetened, with liquid	1 c	250	75	210	3	55	7	<1	0	8
5	219	Apricot nectar, canned	1 c	251	85	141	1	36	2	<1	0	8

[24]Fatty acid values apply to product made with regular margarine.
[25]Sodium bisulfite used to preserve color; unsulfured product would contain lower levels of sodium.

(For purposes of calculations, use "0" for t, <1, <.1, <.01, etc.)

Table D–1 Food Composition

Grp	Computer Code No.	Food Description	Measure	Wt (g)	H$_2$O (%)	Ener (cal)	Prot (g)	Carb (g)	Dietary Fiber (g)	Fat (g)	Chol (mg)	Sodi (mg)
		FRUITS and JUICES—Con.										
		Avocados, raw, edible part only:										
5	220	California (½ lb with refuse)	1 ea	173	73	305	4	12	17	30	0	21
5	221	Florida (1 lb with refuse)	1 ea	304	80	340	5	27	29	27	0	14
5	222	Mashed, fresh, average	1 c	230	74	370	5	17	22	35	0	24
		Bananas, raw, without peel:										
5	223	Whole, 8¾″ long (weighs 175 g w/peel)	1 ea	114	74	105	1	27	2	1	0	1
5	224	Slices	1 c	150	74	138	2	35	3	1	0	1
5	1285	Bananas, dehydrated slices	1 c	100	3	346	4	88	8	2	0	3
5	225	Blackberries, raw	1 c	144	86	74	1	18	10	1	0	0
		Blueberries:										
5	226	Fresh	1 c	145	85	82	1	21	4	1	0	9
		Frozen, sweetened:										
5	227	10-oz container	10 oz	284	77	230	1	62	7	<1	0	4
5	228	Cup	1 c	230	77	185	1	51	5	<1	0	3
		Cherries:										
5	229	Sour, red pitted, canned water pack	1 c	244	90	90	2	22	3	<1	0	17
5	230	Sweet, raw, without pits	10 ea	68	81	49	1	11	1	1	0	0
5	231	Cranberry juice cocktail[28]	1 c	253	85	145	<1[29]	36	1	<1	0	5
5	232	Cranberry-apple juice	1 c	253	86	169	<1	43	1	1[30]	0	5
5	233	Cranberry sauce, canned, strained	1 c	277	61	419	1	108	6	<1	0	80
		Dates:										
5	234	Whole, without pits	10 ea	83	22	228	2	61	7	<1	0	2
5	235	Chopped	1 c	178	22	489	4	131	15	1	0	5
5	236	Figs, dried	10 ea	187	28	477	'6	122	21	2	0	21
		Fruit cocktail, canned, fruit and liquid:										
5	237	Heavy syrup pack	1 c	255	80	185	1	48	3	<1	0	15
5	238	Juice pack	1 c	248	87	115	1	29	3	<1	0	10
		Grapefruit:										
		Raw 3¾″ diam-weight with rind is 241g for one-half										
5	239	Pink/red, half fruit, edible part	1 half	123	91	37	1	9	2	<1	0	0
5	240	White, half fruit, edible part	1 half	118	90	39	1	10	2	<1	0	0
5	241	Canned sections with liquid	1 c	254	84	152	1	39	3	<1	0	4
		Grapefruit juice:										
5	242	Fresh, raw	1 c	247	90	96	1	23	1	<1	0	2
		Canned:										
5	243	Unsweetened	1 c	247	90	93	1	22	1	<1	0	2
5	244	Sweetened	1 c	250	87	115	1	28	1	<1	0	5
		Frozen concentrate, unsweetened:										
5	245	Undiluted, 6-fl-oz can	¾ c	207	62	300	4	72	3	1	0	6
5	246	Diluted with 3 cans water	1 c	247	89	102	1	24	1	<1	0	2
		Grapes, raw, European type (adherent skin):										
5	247	Thompson seedless	10 ea	50	81	35	<1	9	1	<1	0	1
5	248	Tokay/Emperor, seeded types	10 ea	57	81	40	<1	10	1	<1	0	1
		Grape juice:										
5	249	Bottled or canned	1 c	253	84	155	1	38	1	<1	0	8
		Frozen concentrate, sweetened:										
5	250	Undiluted, 6-fl-oz can	¾ c	216	54	385	1	96	4	1	0	15
5	251	Diluted with 3 cans water	1 c	250	87	128	<1	32	1	<1	0	5

[28] Data here are from the newest USDA *Handbook 8–14* on beverages. These data are somewhat different from that presented in *Handbook 8–9* on fruits and fruit juices.

[29] The newest USDA *Handbook 8–14* data on beverages indicates "0" for protein.

[30] The newest USDA *Handbook 8–14* data on beverages indicates "0" for fat.

(Computer code number is for West Diet Analysis program)

GRP KEY: 1 = BEV   2 = DAIRY   3 = EGGS   4 = FAT/OIL   **5 = FRUIT**   6 = BAKERY   7 = GRAIN   8 = FISH   9 = BEEF   10 = POULTRY
11 = SAUSAGE   12 = MIXED/FAST   13 = NUTS/SEEDS   14 = SWEETS   15 = VEG/LEG   16 = MISC   22 = SOUP/SAUCE

Grp	Computer Code No.	Food Description	Measure	Wt (g)	H₂O (%)	Ener (cal)	Prot (g)	Carb (g)	Dietary Fiber (g)	Fat (g)	Chol (mg)	Sodi (mg)
		FRUITS and FRUIT JUICES—Con.										
5	252	Kiwi fruit, raw, peeled (88g with peel)	1 ea	76	83	46	1	11	3	<1	0	4
5	253	Lemons, raw, without peel and seeds (about 4 per lb whole)	1 ea	58	89	17	1	5	1	<1	0	1
		Lemon juice:										
		Fresh:										
5	254	Cup	1 c	244	91	60	1	21	1	t	0	2
5	255	Tablespoon	1 tbsp	15	91	4	<.1	1	<1	t	0	<1
		Canned or bottled, unsweetened:										
5	256	Cup	1 c	244	92	52	1	16	1	<1	0	50[36]
5	257	Tablespoon	1 tbsp	15	92	3	<1	1	<1	<.1	0	3[36]
		Frozen, single strength, unsweetened:										
5	258	Cup	1 c	244	92	54	1	16	1	<1	0	4
5	259	Tablespoon	1 tbsp	15	92	3	<1	1	<1	<.1	0	<1
		Lime juice:										
		Fresh:										
5	260	Cup	1 c	246	90	65	1	22	1	<1	0	2
5	261	Tablespoon	1 tbsp	15	90	4	<1	1	<1	<.1	0	<1
5	262	Canned or bottled, unsweetened	1 c	246	92	50	1	16	1	1	0	39[36]
5	263	Mangos, raw, edible part (weighs 300 g with skin and seeds)	1 ea	207	82	135	1	35	7	1	0	4
		Melons, raw, without rind and cavity contents:										
5	264	Cantaloupe, 5″ diam (2⅓ lb whole (with refuse), orange flesh	½ ea	267	90	94	2	22	3	1	0	24
5	265	Honeydew, 6½″ diam (5¼ lb whole with refuse), slice = ⅒ melon	1 slice	129	90	45	1	12	1	<1	0	13
5	266	Nectarines, raw, without pits, 2½″ diam	1 ea	136	86	67	1	16	3	1	0	0
		Oranges, raw:										
5	267	Whole without peel and seeds, 2⅝″ dm. (weighs 180 g with peel and seeds)	1 ea	131	87	60	1	15	3	<1	0	<1
5	268	Sections, without membranes	1 c	180	87	85	2	21	4	<1	0	<1
		Orange juice:										
5	269	Fresh, all varieties	1 c	248	88	111	2	26	1	<1	0	2
5	270	Canned, unsweetened	1 c	249	89	105	1	25	<1	<1	0	5
5	271	Chilled	1 c	249	88	110	2	25	<1	1	0	2
		Frozen concentrate:										
5	272	Undiluted (6-oz can)	¾ c	213	58	339	5	81	2	<1	0	6
5	273	Diluted with 3 parts water by volume	1 c	249	88	110	2	27	<1	<1	0	2
5	1345	Orange juice, from dry crystals	1 c	248	89	114	2	27	0	<1	0	1
5	274	Orange and grapefruit juice, canned	1 c	247	89	105	1	25	<1	<1	0	7
		Papayas, raw:										
5	275	½″ slices	1 c	140	89	60	1	14	2	<1	0	9
5	276	Whole fruit, 3½″ diam by 5⅛″, without seeds and skin (1 lb with refuse)	1 ea	304	89	117	2	30	5	<1	0	8
5	1031	Papaya nectar, canned	1 c	250	85	142	<1	36	2	<1	0	14
		Peaches:										
5	277	Raw, whole, 2½″ diam, peeled, pitted (about 4 per lb whole)	1 ea	87	88	37	1	10	2	<1	0	0

[36] Sodium benzoate and sodium bisulfite added as preservatives.

(For purposes of calculations, use "0" for t, <1, <.1, <.01, etc.)

Table D–1 Food Composition

Grp	Computer Code No.	Food Description	Measure	Wt (g)	H$_2$O (%)	Ener (cal)	Prot (g)	Carb (g)	Dietary Fiber (g)	Fat (g)	Chol (mg)	Sodi (mg)
		FRUITS and FRUIT JUICES—Con.										
		Peaches—Con.										
5	278	Raw, sliced	1 c	170	88	73	1	19	3	<1	0	1
		Canned, fruit and liquid:										
		Heavy syrup pack:										
5	279	Cup	1 c	256	79	190	1	51	3	<1	0	16
5	280	Half	1 ea	81	79	60	<1	16	1	<1	0	5
		Juice pack:										
5	281	Cup	1 c	248	88	109	2	29	3	<1	0	11
5	282	Half	1 ea	77	88	34	<1	9	1	<1	0	3
		Dried:										
5	283	Uncooked	10 ea	130	32	311	5	80	11	1	0	9
5	284	Cooked, fruit and liquid	1 c	258	78	200	3	51	4	1	0	6
		Frozen, sliced, sweetened:										
5	285	10-oz package	1 ea	284	75	267	2	68	6	<1	0	17
5	286	Cup, thawed measure	1 c	250	75	235	2	60	4	<1	0	16
5	1032	Peach nectar, canned	1 c	249	86	134	1	35	1	<1	0	10
		Pears:										
		Fresh, with skin, cored:										
5	287	Bartlett, 2½″ diam (about 2½ per lb)	1 ea	166	84	98	1	25	5[38]	1	0	1
5	288	Bosc, 2½″ diam (about 3 per lb)	1 ea	141	84	85	1	21	4[38]	1	0	<1
5	289	D'Anjou, 3″ diam (about 2 per lb)	1 ea	200	84	120	1	30	6[38]	1	0	<1
		Canned, fruit and liquid:										
		Heavy syrup pack:										
5	290	Cup	1 c	255	80	188	1	49	4[38]	<1	0	13
5	291	Half	1 ea	79	80	59	<1	15	1[38]	<1	0	4
		Juice pack:										
5	292	Cup	1 c	248	86	123	1	32	4[38]	<1	0	10
5	293	Half	1 ea	77	86	38	<1	10	1[38]	<1	0	3
5	294	Dried halves	10 ea	175	27	459	3	122	19	1	0	10
5	1033	Pear nectar, canned	1 c	250	84	149	<1	39	2	<1	0	8
		Pineapple:										
5	295	Fresh chunks, diced	1 c	155	86	76	1	19	2	1	0	2
		Canned, fruit and liquid:										
		Heavy syrup pack:										
5	296	Crushed, chunks, tidbits	1 c	255	79	199	1	52	2	<1	0	3
5	297	Slices	1 ea	58	79	45	<1	12	1	<.1	0	1
		Juice Pack:										
5	298	Crushed, chunks, tidbits	1 c	250	84	150	1	39	2	<1	0	3
5	299	Slices	1 ea	58	84	35	<1	9	1	<.1	0	1
5	300	Pineapple juice, canned, unsweetened	1 c	250	86	140	1	34	1	<1	0	3
		Plantains, without peel:										
5	301	Raw slices (one whole plantain weighs 179 g without peel)	1 c	148	65	181	2	47	7[39]	1	0	6
5	302	Cooked, boiled, sliced	1 c	154	67	179	1	48	7	<1	0	8
		Plums, canned:										
		Fresh:										
5	303	Medium 2⅛″ diam	1 ea	66	85	36	1	9	1	<1	0	<1
5	304	Small, 1½″ diam	1 ea	28	85	15	<1	4	1	<1	0	<1

[38]Dietary fiber data vary 2.4 to 3.4 g/100 g for fresh pears; 1.6 to 2.6 g/100 g for canned pears.
[39]Dietary fiber value partially derived from data for bananas.

(Computer code number is for West Diet Analysis program)

GRP KEY: 1 = BEV   2 = DAIRY   3 = EGGS   4 = FAT/OIL   **5 = FRUIT**   **6 = BAKERY**   7 = GRAIN   8 = FISH   9 = BEEF   10 = POULTRY
11 = SAUSAGE   12 = MIXED/FAST   13 = NUTS/SEEDS   14 = SWEETS   15 = VEG/LEG   16 = MISC   22 = SOUP/SAUCE

Grp	Computer Code No.	Food Description	Measure	Wt (g)	H₂O (%)	Ener (cal)	Prot (g)	Carb (g)	Dietary Fiber (g)	Fat (g)	Chol (mg)	Sodi (mg)
		FRUITS—Con.										
		Plums—Con.										
		Canned, purple, with liquid:										
		Heavy Syrup pack:										
5	305	Cup	1 c	258	76	230	1	60	4	<1	0	49
5	306	Plums	3 ea	110	76	98	<1	25	2	<1	0	21
		Juice pack:										
5	307	Cup	1 c	252	84	146	1	38	4	<.1	0	3
5	308	Plums	3 ea	95	84	55	<1	14	2	<.1	0	1
		Prunes, dried, pitted:										
5	309	Uncooked (10 prunes weigh 97 g with pits 84 g without pits.):	10 ea	84	32	201	2	53	8[43]	<1	0	3
5	310	Cooked, unsweetened, fruit and liquid (250 g with pits)	1 c	212	70	227	2	60	9	<1	0	4
5	311	Prune juice, bottled or canned	1 c	256	81	181	2	45	3	<.1	0	10
		Raisins, seedless:										
5	312	Cup, not pressed down	1 c	145	15	435	5	115	9	1	0	17
5	313	One packet, ½ oz	½ oz	14	15	41	<1	11	1	<.1	0	2
		Raspberries:										
5	314	Fresh	1 c	123	87	60	1	14	8	1	0	0
		Frozen, sweetened:										
5	315	10-oz container	10 oz	284	73	293	2	74	15	<1	0	3
5	316	Cup, thawed measure	1 c	250	73	255	2	65	12	<1	0	3
5	317	Rhubarb, cooked, added sugar	1 c	240	68	279	1	75	5	<1	0	2
		Strawberries:										
5	318	Fresh, whole, capped	1 c	149	92	45	1	11	4	1	0	2
		Frozen, sliced, sweetened:										
5	319	10-oz container	10 oz	284	73	273	2	74	6	<1	0	9
5	320	Cup, thawed measure	1 c	255	73	245	1	66	8	<1	0	8
		Tangerines, without peel and seeds:										
5	321	Fresh (2⅜″ whole) 116g with refuse	1 ea	84	88	37	1	9	2	<1	0	1
5	322	Canned, light syrup, fruit and liquid	1 c	252	83	154	1	41	4	<1	0	15
5	323	Tangerine juice, canned, sweetened	1 c	249	87	125	1	30	1	<1	0	2
		Watermelon, raw, without rind and seeds:										
5	324	Piece, 1″ thick by 10″ diam (weighs 2 lb) with refuse (926g)	1 pce	482	92	152	3	35	2	2	0	10
5	325	Diced	1 c	160	92	50	1	12	1	1	0	3
		BAKED GOODS:										
		BREADS, CAKES, COOKIES, CRACKERS, PIES, PANCAKES, TORTILLAS										
6	326	Bagels, plain, enriched, 3½″ diam	1 ea	68	32	180	7	35	1	1	0	300
		Biscuits:										
6	327	From home recipe	1 ea	28	28	100	2	13	1	5	t	195
6	328	From mix	1 ea	28	29	94	2	14	1	3	t	265
6	329	From refrigerated dough	1 ea	20	30	65	1	10	<1	2	1	249
6	330	Bread crumbs, dry grated (see 364, 365 for soft crumbs)	1 c	100	7	390	13	73	4	5	5	736
		Breads:										
6	331	Boston brown bread, canned, 3¼″ slice	1 pce	45	45	95	2	21	2	1	3	113
		Cracked wheat bread (¼ cracked-wheat flour, ¾ enr wheat flour):										
6	332	1-lb loaf	1 ea	454	35	1190	42	227	23	16	0	1966
6	333	Slice (18 per loaf)	1 pce	25	35	65	2	13	1	1	0	106
6	334	Slice, toasted	1 pce	21	26	65	2	13	1	1	0	106

[43] Dietary fiber data can vary between 8 and 13 g for 10 prunes.

(For purposes of calculations, use "0" for t, <1, <.1, <.01, etc.)

Table D–1 Food Composition

Grp	Computer Code No.	Food Description	Measure	Wt (g)	H$_2$O (%)	Ener (cal)	Prot (g)	Carb (g)	Dietary Fiber (g)	Fat (g)	Chol (mg)	Sodi (mg)
		BAKED GOODS—Con.										
		Breads—Con.										
		French/Vienna bread, enriched:										
6	335	1-lb loaf	1 ea	454	34	1270	43	230	8	18	0	2633
6	336	French, slice, 5 × 2½ × 1″	1 pce	35	34	100	3	18	1	1	0	203
6	337	Vienna, slice 4¾ × 4 × ½″	1 pce	25	34	70	2	13	1	1	0	145
		French toast: see Mixed Dishes, and Fast Foods, code # 691										
		Italian bread, enriched:										
6	338	1-lb loaf	1 ea	454	32	1255	41	256	5	4	0	2656
6	339	Slice, 4½ × 3¼ × ¾″	1 pce	30	32	83	3	17	<1	<1	0	176
		Mixed grain bread, enriched:										
6	340	1-lb loaf	1 ea	454	37	1165	45	212	18	17	0	1870
6	341	Slice (18 per loaf)	1 pce	25	37	65	2	12	2	1	0	106
6	342	Slice, toasted	1 pce	23	27	65	2	12	2	1	0	106
		Oatmeal bread, enriched:										
6	343	1-lb loaf	1 ea	454	37	1145	38	212	16	20	0	2231
6	344	Slice (18 per loaf)	1 pce	25	37	65	2	12	1	1	0	124
6	345	Slice, toasted	1 pce	23	30	65	2	12	1	1	0	124
6	346	Pita pocket bread, enr, 6½″ round	1 ea	60	31	165	6	33	1	1	0	339
		Pumpernickel bread (⅔ rye flour, ⅓ enr. wheat flour):										
6	347	1-lb loaf	1 ea	454	37	1160	42	218	19	16	0	2461
6	348	Slice, 5 × 4 × ⅜″	1 pce	32	37	80	3	15	2	1	0	177
6	349	Slice, toasted	1 pce	29	28	80	3	15	1	1	0	177
		Raisin bread, enriched:										
6	350	1-lb loaf	1 ea	454	33	1260	37	239	12	18	0	1657
6	351	Slice (18 per loaf)	1 pce	25	33	68	2	13	1	1	0	92
6	352	Slice, toasted	1 pce	21	24	68	2	13	1	1	0	92
		Rye bread, light (⅓ rye flour, ⅔ enr. wheat flour):										
6	353	1-lb loaf	1 ea	454	37	1190	38	218	30	17	0	3164
6	354	Slice, 4¾ × 3¾ × ⁷⁄₁₆″	1 pce	25	37	65	2	12	2	1	0	175
6	355	Slice, toasted	1 pce	22	28	65	2	12	2	1	0	175
		Wheat bread (blend of enr. wheat flour and whole-wheat flour):[44]										
6	356	1-lb loaf	1 ea	454	37	1160	43	213	25	19	0	2447
6	357	Slice (18 per loaf)	1 pce	25	37	65	2	12	1	1	0	135
6	358	Slice, toasted	1 pce	23	28	65	2	12	1	1	0	135
		White bread, enriched:										
6	359	1-lb loaf	1 ea	454	37	1210	38	222	12	18	0	2334
6	360	Slice (18 per loaf)	1 pce	25	37	65	2	12	<1	1	0	129
6	361	Slice, toasted	1 pce	22	28	65	2	12	<1	1	0	129
6	362	Slice (22 per loaf)	1 pce	20	37	55	2	10	<1	1	0	103
6	363	Slice, toasted	1 pce	17	28	55	2	10	<1	1	0	103
		White bread cubes, crumbs:										
6	364	Cubes, soft	1 c	30	37	80	2	15	1	1	0	154
6	365	Crumbs, soft	1 c	45	37	120	4	22	1	2	0	231
		Whole-wheat bread:										
6	366	1-lb loaf	1 ea	454	38	1110	44	206	51	20	0	2887
6	367	Slice (16 per loaf)	1 pce	28	38	70	3	13	2	1	0	180
6	368	Slice, toasted	1 pce	25	29	70	3	13	2	1	0	180

[44]A blend of white and whole-wheat flour—no official ratio specified.

(Computer code number is for West Diet Analysis program)

GRP KEY: 1=BEV 2=DAIRY 3=EGGS 4=FAT/OIL 5=FRUIT **6=BAKERY** 7=GRAIN 8=FISH 9=BEEF 10=POULTRY
11=SAUSAGE 12=MIXED/FAST 13=NUTS/SEEDS 14=SWEETS 15=VEG/LEG 16=MISC 22=SOUP/SAUCE

Grp	Computer Code No.	Food Description	Measure	Wt (g)	H$_2$O (%)	Ener (cal)	Prot (g)	Carb (g)	Dietary Fiber (g)	Fat (g)	Chol (mg)	Sodi (mg)
		BAKED GOODS—Con.										
		Bread stuffing, prepared from mix:										
6	369	Dry type	1 c	140	33	500	9	50	4	31	0	1254
6	370	Moist type, with egg	1 c	203	61	420	9	40	4	26	67	1023
		Cakes, prepared from mixes:[45]										
		Angel food cake:										
6	371	Whole cake, 9 ¾″ diam tube	1 ea	635	38	1510	38	342	3	2	0	3226
6	372	Piece, 1/12 of cake	1 pce	53	38	125	3	29	<1	<1	0	269
6	373	Boston cream pie, 1/8 of cake	1 pce	120	35	260	3	44	1	8	20	225
		Coffee cake:										
6	374	Whole cake, 7¾ × 5⅛ × 1¼″	1 ea	430	30	1385	27	225	3	41	279	1853
6	375	Piece, 1/6 of cake	1 pce	72	30	230	5	38	2	7	47	310
		Devil's food with chocolate frosting:										
6	376	Whole cake, 2 layer, 8 or 9″ diam	1 ea	1107	24	3755	49	645	5	136	598	2900
6	377	Piece, 1/16 of cake	1 pce	69	24	235	3	40	1	8	37	181
6	378	Cupcake, 2½″ diam	1 ea	42	24	143	2	25	<1	5	23	110
		Gingerbread:										
6	379	Whole cake, 8″ square	1 ea	570	37	1575	18	291	3	39	6	1733
6	380	Piece, 1/9 of cake	1 pce	63	37	174	2	32	2	4	1	192
		Yellow, with chocolate frosting, 2 layer:										
6	381	Whole cake, 8 or 9″ diam	1 ea	1108	26	3735	45	638	5	125	576	2515
6	382	Piece, 1/16 of cake	1 pce	69	26	235	3	40	<1	8	36	157
		Cakes from home recipes with enriched flour:										
		Carrot cake, cream cheese frosting:[46]										
6	383	Whole, 9 × 13″ cake	1 ea	1792	23	6496	63	832	20	328	912	2336
6	384	Piece, 1/16 of 9 × 13″ cake 2¼ × 3¼″	1 pce	112	23	406	4	52	1	21	57	146
		Fruitcake, dark, 7½″ diam tube, 2¼″ high:[46]										
6	385	Whole cake	1 ea	1361	18	5185	74	783	38	228	640	2123
6	386	Piece, 1/32 of cake, ⅔″ arc	1 pce	43	18	165	2	25	2	7	20	67
		Sheet cake, plain, no frosting:[47]										
6	387	Whole cake, 9″ square	1 ea	777	25	2830	35	434	3	108	552	2331
6	388	Piece, 1/9 of cake	1 pce	86	25	315	4	48	<1	12	61	258
		Sheet cake, plain, uncooked white frosting:[48]										
6	389	Whole cake, 9″ square	1 ea	1096	21	4020	37	694	3	129	636	2488
6	390	Piece, 1/9 of cake	1 pce	121	21	445	4	77	<1	14	70	275
		Pound cake:[48]										
6	391	Loaf, 8½ × 3½ × 3¼″	1 ea	514	22	2025	33	265	4	94	555	1645
6	392	Piece, 1/17 of loaf, ½″ slice	1 pce	30	22	120	2	15	<1	5	32	98
		Cakes, commercial:										
		Pound cake:										
6	393	Loaf, 8½ × 3½ × 3″	1 ea	500	24	1935	26	257	4	94	1100	1857
6	394	Slice, 1/17 of loaf, ½″ slice	1 pce	29	24	110	2	15	<1	5	64	108
		Snack cakes:										
6	395	Chocolate w/creme filling, 2 small cakes per package	1 ea	28	20	105	1	17	<1	4	15	105
6	396	Sponge cake w/creme filling, 2 small cakes per package	1 ea	42	19	155	1	27	<1	5	7	155

[45] Excepting angel food cake, cakes were made from mixes containing vegetable shortening, and frostings were made with margarine. All mixes use enriched flour.
[46] Made with vegetable oil.
[47] Cake made with vegetable shortening.
[48] Made with margarine.

(For purposes of calculations, use "0" for t, <1, <.1, <.01, etc.)

Table D–1   Food Composition

Grp	Computer Code No.	Food Description	Measure	Wt (g)	H₂O (%)	Ener (cal)	Prot (g)	Carb (g)	Dietary Fiber (g)	Fat (g)	Chol (mg)	Sodi (mg)
		BAKED GOODS—Con.										
		Cakes—Con.										
		White cake with white frosting, 2-layer:										
6	397	Whole cake, 8 or 9″ diam	1 ea	1140	24	4170	43	670	5	148	46	2827
6	398	Piece, ¹⁄₁₆ of cake	1 pce	71	24	260	3	42	<1	9	3	176
		Yellow cake with chocolate frosting, 2-layer:										
6	399	Whole cake, 8 or 9″ diam	1 ea	1108	23	3895	40	620	5	175	609	3080
6	400	Piece, ¹⁄₁₆ of cake	1 pce	69	23	245	3	39	<1	11	38	192
		Cheesecake:										
6	401	Whole cake, 9″ diam	1 ea	1110	46	3350	60	317	5	213	2053	2464
6	402	Piece, ¹⁄₁₂ of cake	1 pce	92	46	278	5	26	1	18	170	204
6	1035	Cheese puffs/Cheetos®	1 oz	28.4	1	158	2	14	<1	10	5	344
		Cookies made with enriched flour:										
		Brownies with nuts:										
6	403	Commercial with frosting, 1½ × 1¾ × ⅞	1 ea	25	13	100	1	16	<1	4	14	59
6	404	Home recipe, 1¾ × 1¾ × ⅞″[49]	1 ea	20	10	95	1	11	<1	6	18	51
		Chocolate chip cookies:										
6	405	Commercial, 2¼″ diam	4 ea	42	4	180	2	28	<1	9	5	140
6	406	Home recipe, 2¼″ diam[50]	4 ea	40	3	185	2	26	1	11	18	82
6	407	From refrigerated dough, 2¼″ diam	4 ea	48	5	225	2	32	1	11	22	173
6	408	Fig bars	4 ea	56	12	210	2	42	3	4	27	180
6	409	Oatmeal raisin cookies, 2⅝″ diam	4 ea	52	4	245	3	36	1	10	2	148
6	410	Peanut butter cookies, home recipe, 2⅝″ diam[50]	4 ea	48	3	245	4	28	1	14	22	142
6	411	Sandwich-type cookies, all	4 ea	40	2	195	2	29	<1	8	0	189
		Shortbread cookies:										
6	412	Commercial, small	4 ea	32	6	155	2	20	1	8	27	123
6	413	From home recipe, large[51]	2 ea	28	3	145	2	17	1	8	0	125
6	414	Sugar cookies from refrigerated dough, 2½″ diam	4 ea	48	4	235	2	31	<1	12	29	261
6	415	Vanilla wafers	10 ea	40	4	185	2	29	<1	7	25	150
6	416	Corn chips	1 oz	28	1	155	2	16	1	9	0	233
		Crackers:[52]										
6	1034	Armenian cracker bread	4 pce	28.4	4	117	5	19	4	2	0	—
6	417	Cheese crackers	10 ea	10	4	50	1	5	<1	3	6	112
6	418	Cheese crackers with peanut butter	4 ea	30	3	150	4	19	<1	8	4	338
6	419	Graham crackers	2 ea	14	4	60	1	11	<1	1	0	86
6	420	Melba toast, plain	1 pce	5	4	20	1	4	<1	<1	0	44
6	421	Rye wafers, whole grain	2 ea	14	5	55	1	10	2	1	0	115
6	422	Saltine® crackers[53]	4 ea	12	4	50	1	9	<1	1	4	165
6	423	Snack-type crackers, round	3 ea	9	3	45	1	6	<1	3	0	90
6	424	Wheat crackers, thin	4 ea	8	3	35	1	5	1	1	0	69
6	425	Whole-wheat wafers	2 ea	8	4	35	1	5	1	2	0	59
6	426	Croissants, 4½ × 4 × 1¾″	1 ea	57	22	235	5	27	1	12	13	452
		Danish pastry:										
6	427	Packaged ring, plain, 12 oz	1 ea	340	27	1305	21	152	3	71	292	1302
6	428	Round piece, plain, 4¼″ diam 1″ high	1 ea	57	27	220	4	26	1	12	49	218

[49]Made with vegetable oil.
[50]Made with vegetable shortening.
[51]Made with margarine.
[52]Crackers made with enriched white (wheat) flour except for rye wafers and whole-wheat wafers.
[53]Made with lard.

(Computer code number is for West Diet Analysis program)

GRP KEY: 1 = BEV   2 = DAIRY   3 = EGGS   4 = FAT/OIL   5 = FRUIT   **6 = BAKERY**   7 = GRAIN   8 = FISH   9 = BEEF   10 = POULTRY
11 = SAUSAGE   12 = MIXED/FAST   13 = NUTS/SEEDS   14 = SWEETS   15 = VEG/LEG   16 = MISC   22 = SOUP/SAUCE

Grp	Computer Code No.	Food Description	Measure	Wt (g)	H₂O (%)	Ener (cal)	Prot (g)	Carb (g)	Dietary Fiber (g)	Fat (g)	Chol (mg)	Sodi (mg)
		BAKED GOODS—Con.										
		Danish Pastry—Con.										
6	429	Ounce, plain	1 oz	28	28	110	2	13	<1	6	24	109
6	430	Round piece with fruit	1 pce	65	30	235	4	28	1	13	56	233
		Desserts, 3 × 3 inch piece:										
6	1348	Apple crisp	1 pce	78	58	146	1	25	1	5	0	66
6	1353	Apple cobbler	1 pce	104	56	201	2	35	2	6	1	305
6	1349	Cherry crisp	1 pce	138	73	157	2	27	2	5	0	73
6	1352	Cherry cobbler	1 pce	129	65	199	2	34	1	6	1	311
6	1350	Peach crisp	1 pce	139	72	166	2	30	2	5	0	71
6	1351	Peach cobbler	1 pce	130	64	130	2	37	2	6	1	309
		Doughnuts:										
6	431	Cake type, plain, 3¼″ diam	1 ea	50	21	210	2	25	1	12	20	192
6	432	Yeast-leavened, glazed, 3¾″ diam	1 ea	60	27	235	4	26	1	13	21	222
		English muffins:										
6	433	Plain, enriched	1 ea	57	42	140	5	26	2	1	0	378
6	434	Toasted	1 ea	50	29	140	5	26	2	1	0	378
		Muffins, 2½″ diam, 1½″ high:										
		From home recipe:										
6	435	Blueberry[57]	1 ea	45	37	135	3	20	2	5	19	198
6	436	Bran, wheat[58]	1 ea	45	35	125	3	19	3	6	24	189
6	437	Cornmeal	1 ea	45	33	145	3	21	2	5	23	169
		From commercial mix:										
6	438	Blueberry	1 ea	45	33	140	3	22	2	5	45	225
6	439	Bran	1 ea	45	28	140	3	24	3	4	28	385
6	440	Cornmeal	1 ea	45	30	145	3	22	2	6	42	291
		Pancakes, 4″ diam:										
6	441	Buckwheat, from mix with egg and milk	1 ea	27	58	55	2	6	1	2	20	125
6	442	Plain, from home recipe	1 ea	27	50	60	2	9	1	2	16	115
6	443	Plain, from mix; egg, milk, oil added	1 ea	27	54	60	2	8	1	2	16	160
		Piecrust, with enriched flour, vegetable shortening, baked:										
6	444	Home recipe, 9″ shell	1 ea	180	15	900	11	79	4	60	0	1100
		From mix:										
6	445	Piecrust for 2-crust pie	1 ea	320	19	1485	21	141	6	93	0	2600
6	446	1 pie shell	1 ea	180	19	835	12	79	4	52	0	1462
		Pies, 9″ diam; pie crust made with vegetable shortening, enriched flour:										
		Apple pie:[59]										
6	447	Whole pie	1 ea	945	48	2420	22	360	19	105	0	2844
6	448	Piece, ⅙ of pie	1 pce	158	48	405	4	60	3	18	0	476
		Banana cream pie:[60]										
6	449	Whole pie	1 ea	1190	66	1915	38	282	10	77	90	2532
6	450	⅙ of pie	1 pce	198	66	319	6	47	2	13	15	422
		Blueberry pie:[59]										
6	451	Whole pie	1 ea	945	51	2285	23	330	22	102	0	2533
6	452	Piece, ⅙ of pie	1 pce	158	51	380	4	55	4	17	0	423

[57] Made with vegetable shortening.
[58] Made with vegetable oil.
[59] Recipes updated for latest USDA values for fruits/nuts/fruit juice.
[60] Recipe based on pie crust, cooked vanilla pudding, 2 bananas.

(For purposes of calculations, use "0" for t, <1, <.1, <.01, etc.)

Table D-1 Food Composition

Grp	Computer Code No.	Food Description	Measure	Wt (g)	H₂O (%)	Ener (cal)	Prot (g)	Carb (g)	Dietary Fiber (g)	Fat (g)	Chol (mg)	Sodi (mg)
		BAKED GOODS—Con.										
		Pies—Con.										
		Cherry pie:[59]										
6	453	Whole pie	1 ea	945	47	2465	26	363	15	107	0	2873
6	454	Piece, ⅙ of pie	1 pce	158	47	410	4	61	2	18	0	480
		Chocolate cream pie:[61]										
6	455	Whole pie	1 ea	1051	63	1863	45	255	4	76	90	2565
6	456	Piece, ⅙ of pie	1 pce	175	63	311	7	42	1	13	15	427
		Custard pie:										
6	457	Whole pie	1 ea	910	58	1760	46	204	4	84	705	2000
6	458	Piece, ⅙ of pie	1 pce	152	58	293	8	34	1	13	118	333
		Lemon meringue pie:[59]										
6	459	Whole Pie	1 ea	840	47	2140	31	317	5	84	822	2369
6	460	Piece, ⅙ of pie	1 pce	140	47	355	5	53	1	14	137	395
		Peach pie:[59]										
6	461	Whole pie	1 ea	945	48	2410	24	361	17	105	0	2533
6	462	Piece, ⅙ of pie	1 pce	158	48	405	4	61	3	17	0	423
		Pecan pie:[59]										
6	463	Whole pie	1 ea	825	20	3500	38	551	10	142	822	1823
6	464	Piece, ⅙ of pie	1 pce	138	20	583	6	92	5	24	137	304
		Pumpkin pie:[59]										
6	465	Whole Pie	1 ea	910	59	2200	54	308	15	94	655	2029
6	466	Piece, ⅙ of pie	1 pce	152	59	367	9	51	5	16	109	338
		Pies, fried, commercial:										
6	467	Apple	1 ea	85	43	255	2	32	2	14	14	326
6	468	Cherry	1 ea	85	43	250	2	32	1	14	13	371
		Pretzels, made with enriched flour:										
6	469	Thin sticks, 2¼″ long	10 ea	3	2	10	<1	2	<1	<1	0	48
6	470	Dutch twists, 2¾ × 2⅝″	1 ea	16	2	65	2	13	<1	1	0	258
6	471	Thin twists, 3¼ × 2¼ × ¼″	10 ea	60	3	240	6	48	2	2	0	966
		Rolls and buns, enriched:										
		Commercial:										
6	472	Cloverleaf rolls, 2½″ diam, 2″ high	1 ea	28	32	85	2	14	1	2	t	155
6	473	Hotdog buns	1 ea	40	34	115	3	20	1	2	0	241
6	474	Hamburger buns	1 ea	45	34	129	4	23	1	2	0	271
6	475	Hard rolls, white, 3¾″ diam, 2″ high	1 ea	50	25	155	5	30	1	2	0	313
6	476	Submarine rolls or hoagies, 11½ × 3 × 2½	1 ea	135	31	400	11	72	2	8	0	683
		From home recipe:										
6	477	Dinner rolls 2½″ diam, 2″ high	1 ea	35	26	120	3	20	1	3	12	98
6	478	Toaster pastries, fortified	1 ea	54	13	210	2	38	1	6	0	248
		Tortilla chips:										
6	1271	Plain	1 oz	28	4	139	2	17	1	8	0	140
6	1036	Nacho flavor	1 oz	28	1	139	2	18	1	7	0	107
6	1037	Taco flavor	1 oz	28	1	140	3	18	1	7	0	191
		Tortillas:										
6	479	Corn, enriched, 6″ diam	1 ea	30	45	65	2	13	2	1	0	1
6	480	Flour, 8″ diam	1 ea	35	27	105	3	19	1	3	0	134
6	1301	Flour tortilla, 10.5″ diam.	1 ea	57	27	168	4	31	2	4	0	215
6	481	Taco shells	1 ea	14	4	59	1	9	1	2	0	62

[59]Recipes updated for latest USDA values for fruits/nuts/fruit juice.
[61]Based on value for pie crust, cooked chocolate pudding with meringue.

(Computer code number is for West Diet Analysis program)

GRP KEY: 1 = BEV   2 = DAIRY   3 = EGGS   4 = FAT/OIL   5 = FRUIT   **6 = BAKERY**   **7 = GRAIN**   8 = FISH   9 = BEEF   10 = POULTRY
  11 = SAUSAGE   12 = MIXED/FAST   13 = NUTS/SEEDS   14 = SWEETS   15 = VEG/LEG   16 = MISC   22 = SOUP/SAUCE

Grp	Computer Code No.	Food Description	Measure	Wt (g)	H₂O (%)	Ener (cal)	Prot (g)	Carb (g)	Dietary Fiber (g)	Fat (g)	Chol (mg)	Sodi (mg)
		BAKED GOODS—Con.										
		Waffles, 7″ diam:										
6	482	From home recipe	1 ea	75	37	245	7	26	1	13	102	445
6	483	From mix, egg/milk added	1 ea	75	42	205	7	27	1	8	59	515
		GRAIN PRODUCTS: CEREAL, FLOUR, GRAIN, PASTA and NOODLES, POPCORN										
		Barley, pearled:										
7	484	Dry, uncooked	1 c	200	11	700	16	158	31	2	0	6
7	485	Cooked	1 c	157	69	193	4	44	4	1	0	5
		Breakfast cereals, hot, cooked:										
		Corn grits (hominy) enriched cooked:										
7	486	Regular and quick, prepared	1 c	242	85	146	4	31	5	<1	0	0[65]
7	487	Instant, prepared from packet, white	1 pkt	137	85	80	2	18	3	<1	0	343
		Cream of Wheat®, cooked:										
7	488	Regular, quick, instant	1 c	244	86	140	4	29	3	1	0	5[67,68]
7	489	Mix and eat, plain, packet	1 ea	142	82	100	3	21	2	<1	0	241
7	490	Malt-O-Meal® cereal, cooked	1 c	240	88	122	4	26	3	<1	0	2[68]
		Oatmeal or rolled oats, cooked:										
7	491	Regular, quick, instant, nonfortified	1 c	234	85	145	6	25	4	2	0	2[68]
		Instant, fortified:										
7	492	Plain, from packet	¾ c	177	86	104	4	18	3	2	0	285[64]
7	493	Flavored, from packet	¾ c	164	76	160	5	31	3	2	0	254[64]
7	494	Whole-wheat cereal, cooked	1 c	242	84	150	5	33	4	1	0	3
		Breakfast cereals, ready to eat:										
7	495	All-Bran®	⅓ c	28	3	70	4	22	9	<1	0	260
7	1306	Alpha Bits®	1 c	28	1	111	2	25	1	1	0	219
7	1307	Apple Jacks®	1 c	28	2	110	2	26	<1	<1	0	125
7	1308	Bran Buds®	1 c	84	3	217	12	64	23	2	0	516
7	1305	Bran Chex®	1 c	49	2	156	5	39	9	1	0	455
7	1309	Buc Wheats®	¾ c	28	3	110	2	24	2	1	0	235
7	1310	C.W. Post® plain	1 c	97	2	432	9	69	2	15	0	167
7	1311	C.W. Post® with raisins	1 c	103	4	446	9	74	2	15	0	160
7	496	Cap'n Crunch®	1 c	37	2	156	2	30	1	3	0	278
7	1312	Cap'n Crunchberries®	1 c	35	3	146	2	29	<1	3	0	243
7	1313	Cap'n Crunch®, peanut butter	1 c	35	2	154	3	27	<1	5	0	268
7	497	Cheerios®	1 c	23	5	89	3	16	2	1	0	246
7	1314	Cocoa Krispies®	1 c	36	3	139	2	32	<1	<1	0	275
7	1316	Cocoa Pebbles®	⅔ c	21	2	87	1	18	<1	1	0	102
7	1315	Corn Bran®	1 c	36	3	124	3	30	7	1	0	310
7	1317	Corn Chex®	1 c	28	2	111	2	25	<1	<1	0	271
7	498	Corn Flakes, Kellogg's®	1¼ c	28	3	110	2	24	1	<1	0	351
7	499	Corn Flakes, Post Toasties®	1¼ c	28	3	110	2	24	1	<1	0	297
7	1318	Cracklin' Oat Bran®	1 c	60	4	229	6	41	9	9	0	402
7	1038	Crispy Wheat 'N Raisins®	1 c	43	7	150	3	35	2	1	0	204
7	1319	Fortified oat flakes	1 c	48	3	177	9	35	1	1	0	429
7	500	40% Bran Flakes, Kellogg's®	1 c	39	3	125	5	35	5	1	0	363
7	501	40% Bran Flakes, Post®	1 c	47	3	152	5	37	6	1	0	431
7	502	Froot Loops®	1 c	28	2	111	2	25	<1	1	0	145

[64] Nutrient added (values sometimes based on label declaration).

[65] Cooked without salt. If salt is added according to label recommendation, sodium content is 540 mg.

[67] Values for regular and instant cereal. For quick cereal, phosphorus is 102 mg, and sodium is 142 mg.

[68] Cooked without salt. If added according to label recommendations, sodium content is 390 mg for Cream of Wheat; 324 mg for Malt-O-Meal; 374 mg for oatmeal.

(For purposes of calculations, use "0" for t, <1, <.1, <.01, etc.)

Table D–1 Food Composition

Grp	Computer Code No.	Food Description	Measure	Wt (g)	H$_2$O (%)	Ener (cal)	Prot (g)	Carb (g)	Dietary Fiber (g)	Fat (g)	Chol (mg)	Sodi (mg)
\multicolumn{13}{l}{GRAIN PRODUCTS—Con.}
		Cereals—Con.										
7	1320	Frosted Mini-Wheats®	4 ea	31	5	111	3	26	2	<1	0	9
7	1321	Frosted Rice Krispies®	1 c	28	3	109	1	26	1	<1	0	240
7	1323	Fruit & Fiber® w/apples	½ c	28	2	90	3	22	4	1	0	195
7	1324	Fruit & Fiber® w/dates	½ c	28	2	90	3	21	4	1	0	170
7	1325	Fruitful Bran® cereal	¾ c	34	3	110	3	27	5	0	0	240
7	1322	Fruity Pebbles® cereal	⅞ c	28	3	113	1	24	<1	2	0	157
7	503	Golden Grahams®	1 c	39	2	156	2	33	2	2	0	476
7	504	Granola, homemade	1 c	122	3	595	15	67	13	33	0	12
7	505	Grape Nuts®	½ c	57	3	210	6	46	5	<1	0	394
7	1326	Grape Nuts® flakes	⅞ c	28	3	102	3	23	2	<1	0	218
7	1327	Honey & Nut Corn flakes	¾ c	28	4	113	2	23	<1	2	0	225
7	506	Honey Nut Cheerios®	1 c	33	3	127	4	27	1	1	0	299
7	1328	Honey Bran	1 c	35	3	119	3	29	4	1	0	202
7	1329	Honeycomb®	1 c	22	1	86	1	20	<1	<1	0	166
7	1330	King Vitamin® cereal	1 c	21	2	85	1	18	<1	1	0	161
7	1039	Kix®	1 c	19	3	73	2	16	<1	<1	0	226
7	1331	Life®	1 c	44	5	162	8	32	1	1	0	229
7	507	Lucky Charms®	1 c	32	3	125	3	26	1	1	0	227
7	508	Nature Valley® Granola	1 c	113	4	503	12	76	12	20	0	232
7	1332	Nutri-Grain™—Barley	1 c	41	3	153	5	34	2	<1	0	277
7	1333	Nutri-Grain™—Corn	1 c	42	3	160	3	36	3	1	0	276
7	1334	Nutri-Grain™—Rye	1 c	40	3	144	4	34	3	<1	0	272
7	1335	Nutri-Grain™—Wheat	1 c	44	3	158	4	37	3	<1	0	299
7	1336	100% Bran	1 c	66	3	178	8	48	20	3	0	457
7	509	100% Natural® cereal, plain	¼ c	28	2	135	3	18	3	6	0	12
7	1337	100% Natural® with apples	1 c	104	2	478	11	70	5	20	0	52
7	1338	100% Natural® with raisins & dates	1 c	100	4	496	11	72	4	20	0	47
7	510	Product 19®	1 c	33	3	126	3	27	<1	<1	0	378
7	1339	Quisp®	1 c	30	2	124	2	25	<1	2	0	241
7	511	Raisin Bran, Kellogg's®	1 c	49	8	158	5	37	6	1	0	293
7	512	Raisin Bran, Post®	1 c	56	9	170	5	42	6	1	0	370
7	1040	Raisins, Rice & Rye™	1 c	46	9	155	3	39	<1	<1	0	350
7	1041	Rice Chex®	¾ c	19	3	75	1	17	1	1	0	158
7	513	Rice Krispies, Kellogg's®	1 c	29	2	112	2	25	<1	<1	0	340
7	514	Rice, puffed	1 c	14	3	55	1	13	<1	<1	0	<1
7	515	Shredded Wheat®	¾ c	32	5	115	3	25	4	1	0	3
7	516	Special K®	1½ c	32	2	125	6	24	<1	<1	0	298
7	1340	Sugar Corn Pops®	1 c	28	3	108	1	26	<1	<1	0	103
7	518	Sugar Frosted Flakes®	1 c	35	3	133	2	32	1	<1	0	284
7	517	Super Sugar Crisp®	1 c	33	2	123	2	30	<1	<1	0	29
7	519	Sugar Smacks®	¾ c	28	3	106	2	25	<1	<1	0	75
7	1341	Tasteeos®	1 c	24	2	94	3	19	1	1	0	183
7	1342	Team®	1 c	42	4	164	3	36	<1	1	0	259
7	520	Total®, wheat, with added calcium	1 c	33	4	122	3	26	2	1	0	330
7	521	Trix®	1 c	28	2	109	1	25	<1	1	0	179
7	1042	Wheat & Raisin Chex®	1 c	54	7	185	5	43	4	<1	0	306
7	1344	Wheat Chex®	1 c	46	3	169	5	38	3	1	0	308
7	1043	Wheat, puffed	1 c	12	3	44	2	10	2	<1	0	0
7	522	Wheaties®	1 c	29	5	101	3	23	3	1	0	363

(Computer code number is for West Diet Analysis program)

GRP KEY: 1 = BEV 2 = DAIRY 3 = EGGS 4 = FAT/OIL 5 = FRUIT 6 = BAKERY **7 = GRAIN** 8 = FISH 9 = BEEF 10 = POULTRY
11 = SAUSAGE 12 = MIXED/FAST 13 = NUTS/SEEDS 14 = SWEETS 15 = VEG/LEG 16 = MISC 22 = SOUP/SAUCE

Grp	Computer Code No.	Food Description	Measure	Wt (g)	H₂O (%)	Ener (cal)	Prot (g)	Carb (g)	Dietary Fiber (g)	Fat (g)	Chol (mg)	Sodi (mg)
		GRAIN PRODUCTS—Con.										
		Buckwheat:										
		Flour:										
7	523	Dark	1 c	98	12	338	12	71	8	3	0	1
7	524	Light	1 c	98	12	340	6	78	6	1	0	1
7	525	Whole grain, dry	1 c	175	11	586	23	128	16	4	0	3
		Bulgar:										
7	526	Dry, uncooked	1 c	140	9	479	17	106	31	2	0	24
7	527	Cooked	1 c	182	78	151	6	34	11	<1	0	9
		Cornmeal:										
7	528	Whole-ground, unbolted, dry	1 c	122	10	442	10	94	13	4	0	43
7	529	Bolted, nearly whole, dry	1 c	122	10	441	10	91	12	4	0	43
7	530	Degermed, enriched, dry	1 c	138	12	505	12	107	10	2	0	4
7	531	Degermed, enriched, cooked	1 c	240	88	120	3	26	3	<1	0	1
		Macaroni, cooked:										
7	532	Enriched	1 c	140	66	197	7	40	2	1	0	1
7	533	Vegetable, enriched	1 c	134	68	172	6	36	2	.1	0	8
7	534	Whole wheat	1 c	140	67	174	8	37	2	1	0	4
7	535	Millet, cooked	½ c	120	71	143	4	28	1	1	0	2
		Noodles:										
7	536	Egg noodles, cooked	1 c	160	69	213	8	40	4	2	50	11
7	537	Chow mein, dry	1 c	45	.73	237	4	26	2	14	0	197
7	538	Spinach noodles, dry	3½ oz	100	8	372	13	75	7	2	0	36
7	1343	Oat bran, dry	¼ c	25	6	61	4	17	4	2	0	1
		Popcorn:										
7	539	Air popped, plain	1 c	8	4	30	1	6	1	<1	0	<1
7	540	Popped in veg oil/salted	1 c	11	3	55	1	6	1	3	0	86
7	541	Sugar-syrup coated	1 c	35	4	135	2	30	1	1	0	<1
		Rice:										
7	542	Brown rice, cooked	1 c	195	73	217	5	45	3	2	0	10
		White, enriched, all types:										
7	543	Regular/long grain, dry	1 c	185	12	675	13	148	2	1	0	9
7	544	Regular/long grain, cooked	1 c	205	69	264	6	57	1	<1	0	4
7	545	Instant, prepared without salt	1 c	165	76	162	3	35	1	<1	0	5[69]
		Parboiled/converted rice:										
7	546	Raw, dry	1 c	185	10	686	13	151	4	1	0	9.3
7	547	Cooked	1 c	175	73	200	4	43	1	<1	0	5
7	548	Wild rice, cooked	1 c	164	74	166	4	35	3	<1	0	5
7	549	Rye flour, medium	1 c	102	10	361	10	79	15	2	0	3
7	1044	Soy flour, low fat	1 c	88	3	370	51	34	12	6	0	16
		Spaghetti, cooked:										
7	550	without salt, enriched	1 c	140	66	197	7	40	2	1	0	1
7	551	with salt, enriched	1 c	140	66	197	7	40	2	1	0	140
7	552	Whole-wheat spaghetti, cooked	1 c	140	94	174	7	37	5	1	0	4
7	1302	Tapioca, dry	1 c	152	11	518	.3	135	2	<.1	0	2
7	553	Wheat bran	½ c	30	10	65	5	19	8	1	0	.6
		Wheat germ:										
7	554	Raw	1 c	100	11	360	23	52	12	10	0	12
7	555	Toasted	1 c	113	6	432	33	56	16	12	0	5
7	556	Rolled wheat, cooked	1 c	240	80	142	4	32	5	1	0	2
7	557	Whole-grain wheat, cooked	⅓ c	50	86	28	1	7	1	<1	0	<1

[69] If prepared with salt according to label recommendation, sodium would be 608 mg.

(For purposes of calculations, use "0" for t, <1, <.1, <.01, etc.)

Table D–1 Food Composition

Grp	Computer Code No.	Food Description	Measure	Wt (g)	H₂O (%)	Ener (cal)	Prot (g)	Carb (g)	Dietary Fiber (g)	Fat (g)	Chol (mg)	Sodi (mg)

Grp	No.	Food Description	Measure	Wt (g)	H₂O (%)	Ener (cal)	Prot (g)	Carb (g)	Fiber (g)	Fat (g)	Chol (mg)	Sodi (mg)
GRAIN PRODUCTS—Con.												
		Wheat flour (unbleached):										
		All-purpose white flour, enriched:										
7	558	Sifted	1 c	115	12	419	12	88	3	1	0	2
7	559	Unsifted	1 c	125	12	455	13	95	3	1	0	3
7	560	Cake or pastry flour, enriched, sifted	1 c	96	12	348	8	75	3	1	0	2
7	561	Self-rising, enriched, unsifted	1 c	125	11	442	12	93	3	1	0	1587
7	562	Whole wheat, from hard wheats	1 c	120	10	407	16	87	15	2	0	6
MEATS: FISH and SHELLFISH												
8	1045	Bass, baked or broiled	3.5 oz.	100	70	125	24	0	0	4	80	75
		Bluefish:										
8	1046	Baked or broiled	3.5 oz.	100	68	159	26	0	0	5	63	77
8	1047	Fried in bread crumbs	3.5 oz.	100	61	205	23	5	0	10	60	67
		Clams:										
8	563	Raw meat only	3 oz	85	82	63	11	2	<1	1	29	47
8	564	Canned, drained	3 oz	85	64	126	22	4	t	2	57	95
8	1290	Steamed, meat only	20 ea	90	64	133	23	5	<1	2	60	100
		Cod:										
8	565	Baked with butter	3½ oz	100	75	132	23	0	0	3	60	224
8	566	Batter fried	3½ oz	100	61	199	20	8	0	10	55	100
8	567	Poached, no added fat	3½ oz	100	76	102	22	0	0	1	55	78
		Crab, meat only:										
8	1048	Blue crab, cooked	1 c	135	77	138	27	0	0	2	135	376
8	1049	Dungeness Crab, cooked	.75 c	101	74	85	18	<1	0	2	64	299
8	568	Canned	1 c	135	76	133	28	0	0	2	120	450
8	1587	Crab, imitation, from surimi	3 oz	85	74	87	10	9	0	1	17	715
8	569	Fish sticks, breaded pollock	2 ea	57	46	155	9	14	<1	7	64	332
		Flounder/sole, baked with lemon juice:										
8	570	With butter	3 oz	85	73	120	16	<1	0	6	68	145
8	571	With margarine	3 oz	85	73	120	16	<1	0	6	55	151
8	572	Without added fat	3 oz	85	78	99	21	0	0	1	58	89
		Haddock:										
8	573	Breaded, fried[70]	3 oz	85	61	175	17	7	<1	9	55	123
8	1050	Smoked	3.5 oz	100	72	116	25	0	0	1	77	763
8	574	Broiled with butter and lemon juice	3 oz	85	72	140	23	0	0	6	45	100
8	1051	Smoked	3.5 oz	100	49	224	21	0	0	15	100	480
8	1054	Raw	3.5 oz	100	78	110	21	0	0	2	32	54
8	575	Herring, pickled	3 oz	85	55	223	12	8	0	15	11	740
8	1052	Lobster meat, cooked w/ moist heat	1 c	145	77	142	30	2	0	1	104	551
8	576	Ocean perch, breaded/fried	3 oz	85	59	185	16	7	<1	11	46	138
8	1056	Octopus, raw	3.5 oz.	100	80	82	15	2	0	1	48	—
		Oysters:										
8	577	Raw, Eastern	1 c	248	85	170	18	10	0	6	136	277
8	578	Raw, Pacific	1 c	248	82	200	23	12	0	6	136	262
		Cooked										
8	579	Eastern, breaded, fried, medium	6 ea	88	65	173	8	10	<1	11	72	367
8	580	Western, simmered	3½ oz	100	71	135	19	7	0	2	48	210
		Pollock, cooked:										
8	581	Baked or broiled	3 oz	85	74	96	20	0	0	1	82	98
8	1055	Moist heat, poached	3.5 oz	100	72	128	23	0	0	1	70	98

[70] Dipped in egg, milk and bread crumbs; fried in vegetable shortening.

(Computer code number is for West Diet Analysis program)

GRP KEY: 1 = BEV   2 = DAIRY   3 = EGGS   4 = FAT/OIL   5 = FRUIT   6 = BAKERY   **7 = GRAIN**   **8 = FISH**   **9 = BEEF**   10 = POULTRY
11 = SAUSAGE   12 = MIXED/FAST   13 = NUTS/SEEDS   14 = SWEETS   15 = VEG/LEG   16 = MISC   22 = SOUP/SAUCE

Grp	Computer Code No.	Food Description	Measure	Wt (g)	H₂O (%)	Ener (cal)	Prot (g)	Carb (g)	Dietary Fiber (g)	Fat (g)	Chol (mg)	Sodi (mg)
		MEATS: FISH and SHELLFISH—Con.										
		Salmon:										
8	582	Canned pink, solids and liquid	3 oz	85	69	118	17	0	0	5	37	471
8	583	Broiled or baked	3 oz	85	62	183	23	0	0	9	74	56
8	584	Smoked	3 oz	85	72	99	16	0	0	4	20	666
8	585	Atlantic sardines, canned, drained, 2 = 24 g	3 oz	85	60	177	21	0	0	11	121	429
8	586	Scallops, breaded, cooked from frozen	6 ea	93	59	200	17	9	<1	10	57	431
8	1588	Scallops, imitation, from surimi	3 oz	85	74	84	11	9	0	<1	18	676
		Shrimp:										
8	587	Cooked, boiled, 18 large shrimp	3½ oz	100	77	99	21	0	0	1	195	224
8	588	Canned, drained	⅔ c	85	73	102	20	1	0	2	147	143
8	589	Fried, 4 large = 30g[70]	12 ea	90	53	218	19	10	<1	11	159	310
8	1057	Raw, large, about 7 g each	14 ea	100	76	106	20	1	0	2	152	148
8	1589	Shrimp, imitation, from surimi	3 oz	85	75	86	11	8	0	1	31	599
8	1053	Snapper, baked or broiled	3.5 oz	100	70	128	26	0	0	2	47	57
8	1060	Squid, fried in flour[72]	3 oz	85	65	149	15	7	<1	6	221	260
8	1590	Surimi[73]	3 oz	85	76	84	13	6	0	1	25	122
		Swordfish:										
8	1058	Baked or broiled	3.5 oz	100	76	121	20	0	0	4	39	90
8	1059	Raw	3.5 oz	100	69	155	25	0	0	5	50	115
8	590	Trout, baked or broiled	3 oz	85	63	129	22	<1	0	4	62	29
		Tuna, light, canned, drained solids:										
8	591	Oil pack	3 oz	85	60	163	25	0	0	7	27	301
8	592	Water pack	3 oz	85	71	111	25	0	0	1	28	303
8	1061	Tuna, raw, average	3.5 oz	100	68	144	23	0	0	5	38	39
		MEATS: BEEF, LAMB, PORK and others										
		BEEF, cooked:[74]										
		Braised, simmered, pot roasted:										
		Relatively fat, like chuck blade:										
9	593	Lean and fat, piece 2½ × 2½ × ¾″	3 oz	85	43	325	22	0	0	26	87	53
9	594	Lean only	3 oz	85	53	230	26	0	0	13	90	60
		Relatively lean, like round:										
9	595	Lean and fat, piece 4⅛ × 2¼ × ¾″	3 oz	85	54	222	25	0	0	13	81	43
9	596	Lean only	3 oz	85	57	189	27	0	0	8	81	44
		Ground beef, broiled, patty 3 × ⅝″:										
9	597	Extra lean, about 16% fat	3 oz	85	57	217	22	0	0	14	71	59
9	598	Regular, 21% fat	3 oz	85	54	246	21	0	0	18	76	70
		Roasts, oven cooked, no added liquid:										
		Relatively fat, rib:										
9	601	Lean and fat, piece 4⅛ × 2¼ × ½″	3 oz	85	46	324	19	0	0	27	72	54
9	602	Lean only	3 oz	61	58	204	23	0	0	12	68	63
		Relatively lean, round:										
9	603	Lean and fat, piece 2½ × 2½ × ¾″	3 oz	85	57	213	23	0	0	13	70	53
9	604	Lean only	3 oz	75	63	162	24	0	0	6	69	55
		Steak, broiled, relatively lean, sirloin:										
9	605	Lean and fat, piece 2½ × 2½ × ¾″	3 oz	85	54	238	22	0	0	16	67	54
9	606	Lean only	3 oz	72	60	172	24	0	0	8	65	57

[70]Dipped in egg, bread crumbs, and flour; fried in vegetable shortening.
[72]Recipe is 94.6% squid, 4.9% flour, and 0.6% salt.
[73]Surimi is processed from Walleye (Alaska) pollock. Also see Imitation crab, shrimp, scallops.
[74]Outer layer of fat removed to about 1/2″ of the lean. Deposits of fat within the cut remain.

(For purposes of calculations, use "0" for t, <1, <.1, <.01, etc.)

Table D–1 Food Composition

Grp	Computer Code No.	Food Description	Measure	Wt (g)	H₂O (%)	Ener (cal)	Prot (g)	Carb (g)	Dietary Fiber (g)	Fat (g)	Chol (mg)	Sodi (mg)
		MEATS: BEEF, LAMB, PORK and others—Con.										
		BEEF, Cooked—Con.										
		Steak, broiled, relatively fat, T-bone:										
9	1063	Lean and fat	3 oz	85	50	276	20	0	0	21	71	51
9	1064	Lean only	3 oz	85	60	182	24	0	0	9	68	56
		Variety meats:										
9	1086	Brains, pan fried	3 oz	85	71	167	11	0	0	14	1696	134
9	599	Heart, simmered	3 oz	85	64	140	25	<1	0	5	164	54
9	600	Liver, fried	3 oz	85	56	184	23	7	0	7	410	90
9	1062	Tongue, cooked	3 oz	85	56	241	19	<1	0	18	91	51
9	607	Beef, canned, corned	3 oz	85	58	213	23	0	0	13	73	855
9	608	Beef, dried, cured	1 oz	28	57	47	8	<1	0	1	18	984
		LAMB, domestic, cooked:										
		Chop, arm, braised (5.6 oz raw with bone):										
9	609	Lean and fat	2.5 oz	70	44	244	21	0	0	17	84	51
9	610	Lean part of #609	1.9 oz	55	49	152	19	0	0	8	66	41
		Chop, loin, broiled (4.2 oz raw with bone):										
9	611	Lean and fat	2.3 oz	64	52	201	16	0	0	15	64	49
9	612	Lean part of #611	1.6 oz	46	61	100	14	0	0	5	44	39
9	1067	Cutlet, avg of lean cuts, cooked	3 oz	85	62	175	24	0	0	8	78	64
		Leg, roasted, 3 oz piece = 4⅛ × 2¼ × ½″:										
9	613	Lean and fat	3 oz	85	57	219	22	0	0	14	79	56
9	614	Lean only	3 oz	85	64	162	24	0	0	7	76	58
		Rib, roasted, 3 oz piece = 2½ × 2½ × ¾″:										
9	615	Lean and fat	3 oz	85	48	305	18	0	0	25	82	62
9	616	Lean only	3 oz	85	60	197	22	0	0	11	74	69
		Shoulder, roasted:										
9	1065	Lean and fat	3 oz	85	56	235	19	0	0	17	78	55
9	1066	Lean only	3 oz	85	64	163	22	0	0	8	73	57
		Variety meats:										
9	1069	Brains, pan-fried	3 oz	85	61	232	14	0	0	19	2128	133
9	1068	Heart, braised	3 oz	85	64	158	22	2	0	7	212	54
9	1070	Sweetbreads, cooked	3 oz	85	62	196	16	0	0	13	347	179
9	1071	Tongue, cooked	3 oz	85	58	234	18	0	0	17	161	57
		PORK, CURED, cooked (see also #669–672):										
9	617	Bacon, medium slices	3 pce	19	13	109	6	<1	0	9	16	303
9	1087	Breakfast strips, cooked	3 pce	34	27	156	10	<1	0	13	36	714
9	618	Canadian-style bacon	2 pce	47	62	86	11	1	0	4	27	719
		Ham, roasted:										
9	619	Lean and fat, 2 pieces 4⅛ × 2¼ × ¼″	3 oz	85	58	207	18	0	0	14	53	1009
9	620	Lean only	3 oz	85	66	133	21	0	0	5	47	1128
9	621	Ham, canned, roasted	3 oz	85	66	140	18	<1	0	7	35	908
		PORK, fresh, cooked:										
		Chops, loin (cut 3 per lb with bone):										
		Braised:										
9	1291	Lean and fat	1 ea	71	44	261	19	0	0	20	73	46
9	1292	Lean only	1 ea	55	51	150	18	0	0	8	58	41
		Broiled:										
9	622	Lean and fat	3.1 oz	87	50	275	24	0	0	19	84	61
9	623	Lean only from #622	2.5 oz	72	57	166	23	0	0	8	71	56

(Computer code number is for West Diet Analysis program)

GRP KEY: 1 = BEV 2 = DAIRY 3 = EGGS 4 = FAT/OIL 5 = FRUIT 6 = BAKERY 7 = GRAIN 8 = FISH **9 = BEEF** **10 = POULTRY**
11 = SAUSAGE 12 = MIXED/FAST 13 = NUTS/SEEDS 14 = SWEETS 15 = VEG/LEG 16 = MISC 22 = SOUP/SAUCE

Grp	Computer Code No.	Food Description	Measure	Wt (g)	H₂O (%)	Ener (cal)	Prot (g)	Carb (g)	Dietary Fiber (g)	Fat (g)	Chol (mg)	Sodi (mg)
		MEATS: BEEF, LAMB, PORK and others—Con.										
		PORK, Fresh Cooked—Con.										
		Pan fried:										
9	624	Lean and fat	3.1 oz	89	45	334	21	0	0	27	92	64
9	625	Lean only from #624	2.4 oz	67	54	178	19	0	0	11	71	57
		Leg, roasted:										
9	626	Lean and fat, piece 2½ × 2½ × ¾″	3 oz	85	53	250	21	0	0	18	79	50
9	627	Lean only from #626	3 oz	85	60	187	24	0	0	9	80	54
		Rib, roasted:										
9	628	Lean and fat, piece 2½ × 2½ × ¾″	3 oz	85	51	270	21	0	0	20	69	37
9	629	Lean only	3 oz	85	57	210	24	0	0	12	67	40
		Shoulder, braised:										
9	630	Lean and fat, 3 pieces 2½ × 2½ × ¼″	3 oz	85	47	293	23	0	0	22	93	74
9	631	Lean only	3 oz	85	54	208	27	0	0	10	95	85
9	1088	Spareribs, cooked, yield from 1 lb raw with bone	6.25 oz	177	40	703	51	0	0	54	214	165
9	1095	Rabbit, roasted (1 cup meat = 140g)	3 oz	85	59	175	26	0	0	7	73	31
		VEAL, cooked:										
9	632	Veal cutlet, braised or broiled, 4⅛ × 2¼ × ½″	3 oz	85	60	166	27	0	0	6	100	76
9	633	Veal rib roasted, lean, 2 pieces 4⅛ × 2¼ × ¼″	3 oz	85	65	151	22	0	0	6	97	82
9	634	Veal liver, pan-fried	3 oz	85	53	208	25	3	0	10	280	112
9	1096	Venison (Deer meat) roasted	3.5 oz	100	65	158	30	0	0	3	112	54
		MEATS: POULTRY and POULTRY PRODUCTS										
		CHICKEN, cooked:										
		Fried, batter dipped:[78]										
10	635	Breast (5.6 oz with bones)	1 ea	140	52	364	35	13	<1	19	119	385
10	636	Drumstick (3.4 oz with bones)	1 ea	72	53	193	16	6	<1	11	62	194
10	637	Thigh	1 ea	86	52	238	19	8	<1	14	80	248
10	638	Wing	1 ea	49	46	159	10	5	<1	11	39	157
		Fried, flour coated:[78]										
10	639	Breast (4.2 oz with bones)	1 ea	98	57	218	31	2	<1	9	88	74
10	1212	Breast, without skin	1 ea	86	60	161	29	<1	0	4	78	68
10	640	Drumstick (2.6 oz with bones)	1 ea	49	57	120	13	1	<1	7	44	44
10	641	Thigh	1 ea	62	54	162	17	2	<1	9	60	55
10	1099	Thigh, without skin	1 ea	52	59	113	15	1	<1	5	53	49
10	642	Wing	1 ea	32	49	103	8	1	<1	7	26	25
		Roasted:										
10	643	All types of meat	1 c	140	64	266	41	0	0	10	125	120
10	644	Dark meat	1 c	140	63	286	38	0	0	14	130	130
10	645	Light meat	1 c	140	65	242	43	0	0	6	118	108
10	646	Breast, without skin	½ ea	86	65	142	27	0	0	3	73	64
10	647	Drumstick	1 ea	44	67	76	13	0	0	2	41	42
10	648	Thigh	1 ea	62	59	153	16	0	0	10	58	52
10	1100	Thigh, without skin	1 ea	52	63	109	14	0	0	6	49	46
10	649	Stewed, all types:	1 c	140	67	248	38	0	0	9	116	98
10	656	Canned, boneless chicken	5 oz	142	69	235	31	0	0	11	88	714
10	1102	Chicken gizzards, simmered	1 ea	22	67	34	6	<1	0	1	43	15
10	1101	Chicken hearts, simmered	1 ea	3.3	65	6	1	<1	0	<1	8	2
10	650	Chicken liver, simmered	1 ea	20	68	30	5	2	0	1	126	10

[78]Fried in vegetable shortening.

(For purposes of calculations, use "0" for t, <1, <.1, <.01, etc.)

Table D-1 Food Composition

Grp	Computer Code No.	Food Description	Measure	Wt (g)	H$_2$O (%)	Ener (cal)	Prot (g)	Carb (g)	Dietary Fiber (g)	Fat (g)	Chol (mg)	Sodi (mg)
MEATS: POULTRY and POULTRY PRODUCTS—Con.												
		DUCK, roasted:										
10	1293	Meat with skin, about 2.7 cups	½ duck	382	52	1287	73	0	0	108	320	227
10	651	Meat only, about 1.5 cups	½ duck	221	64	445	52	0	0	25	198	143
		GOOSE, domesticated, roasted:										
10	1294	Meat only, 4.2 cups	½ goose	591	57	1406	171	0	0	75	569	447
10	1295	Meat w/skin, about 5.5 cups	½ goose	774	52	2362	195	0	0	170	708	543
		TURKEY, roasted, meat only:										
10	652	Dark meat	3 oz	85	63	159	24	0	0	6	72	67
10	653	Light meat	3 oz	85	66	133	25	0	0	3	59	54
10	654	All types, chopped or diced	1 c	140	65	238	41	0	0	7	107	99
10	655	All types, sliced	3 oz	85	65	145	25	0	0	4	64	60
10	1103	Ground turkey, cooked	3.5 oz	100	60	229	24	0	0	14	69	83
		Turkey breast:										
10	1104	Barbecued	1 oz	28	70	40	6	0	0	1	16	156
10	1105	Hickory smoked	1 oz	28	70	35	6	1	0	1	13	208
10	1106	Gizzard, cooked	1 ea	67	65	109	20	<1	0	3	155	37
10	1107	Heart, cooked	1 ea	16	64	28	4	<1	0	1	36	9
10	1108	Liver, cooked	1 ea	75	66	127	18	3	0	4	469	48
		Poultry food products (see also items in sausages and lunchmeats section):										
10	658	Chicken roll, light meat	2 pce	57	69	90	11	1	0	4	28	331
10	659	Gravy and turkey, frozen package	5 oz	142	85	95	8	7	<1	4	26	787
10	660	Turkey loaf, breast meat	2 pce	42	72	46	10	0	0	1	17	608
10	661	Turkey patties, breaded, fried	1 ea	64	50	181	9	10	<1	12	40	512
10	662	Turkey, frozen, roasted, seasoned	3 oz	85	68	130	18	3	0	5	45	578
MEATS: SAUSAGES and LUNCHMEATS (see also Poultry food products)												
		Beerwurst/beer salami:										
11	1072	Beef	1 pce	23	54	75	3	<1	0	7	13	214
11	1074	Pork	1 pce	23	62	55	3	<1	0	4	13	285
11	1075	Berliner	1 pce	23	61	53	4	1	0	4	11	298
		Bologna:										
11	1297	Beef	1 pce	23	55	72	3	<1	0	7	13	230
11	663	Beef and pork	1 pce	28	54	89	3	1	0	8	16	289
65	1298	Pork	1 pce	23	61	57	4	<1	0	5	14	272
11	664	Turkey	1 pce	28	66	56	4	<1	0	4	28	248
11	665	Braunschweiger sausage	2 pce	57	48	205	8	2	0	18	89	652
11	1073	Brotwurst, link	1 ea	70	51	226	10	2	0	20	44	778
11	666	Brown-and-serve sausage links, cooked	1 ea	13	45	50	2	<1	0	5	9	105
11	1089	Cheesefurter/cheese smokie	1 ea	43	53	141	6	1	0	13	29	465
11	1090	Corned beef loaf, jellied	1 pce	28	67	46	7	0	0	2	12	294
		Frankfurters (see also #657):										
11	1077	Beef, large link, 8/pkg.	1 ea	57	54	184	6	1	0	17	27	584
11	1078	Beef and pork, large link, 8/pkg.	1 ea	57	54	183	6	1	0	17	29	639
11	667	Beef and pork, smaller link, 10/pkg.	1 ea	45	54	145	5	1	0	13	23	504
10	657	Chicken frankfurter, 10/pkg.	1 ea	45	58	115	6	3	0	9	45	616
11	668	Turkey, smaller link, 10/pkg.	1 ea	45	63	102	6	1	0	8	39	454
		Ham:										
11	669	Ham lunchmeat, canned, 3 x 2 x ½″	1 pce	21	52	70	3	<1	0	6	13	271
11	670	Chopped ham, packaged	2 pce	22	61	98	7	<1	0	8	21	573

(Computer code number is for West Diet Analysis program)

GRP KEY: 1 = BEV 2 = DAIRY 3 = EGGS 4 = FAT/OIL 5 = FRUIT 6 = BAKERY 7 = GRAIN 8 = FISH 9 = BEEF **10 = POULTRY**
11 = SAUSAGE 12 = MIXED/FAST 13 = NUTS/SEEDS 14 = SWEETS 15 = VEG/LEG 16 = MISC 22 = SOUP/SAUCE

Grp	Computer Code No.	Food Description	Measure	Wt (g)	H₂O (%)	Ener (cal)	Prot (g)	Carb (g)	Dietary Fiber (g)	Fat (g)	Chol (mg)	Sodi (mg)
		MEATS: SAUSAGES and LUNCHMEATS—Con.										
		Ham—Con.										
11	671	Ham lunchmeat, regular	2 pce	57	65	103	10	2	0	6	32	746
11	672	Ham lunchmeat, extra lean	2 pce	57	70	75	11	1	0	3	27	810
11	673	Turkey ham	2 pce	57	72	73	11	1	0	3	32	548
11	1091	Keilbasa sausage	1 pce	26	54	81	3	1	0	7	17	280
11	1092	Knockwurst sausage-link	1 ea	68	56	209	8	1	0	19	39	687
11	1093	Mortadella lunchmeat	1 pce	15	52	47	2	<1	0	4	8	187
11	1097	Olive loaf lunchmeat	2 pce	57	58	133	7	5	<1	9	22	842
11	1080	Pastrami, turkey	2 pce	57	72	74	11	1	0	4	30	569
11	1081	Pepperoni sausage, small slices	4 pce	22	27	109	5	1	0	10	8	449
11	1094	Pickle & pimento loaf	2 pce	57	57	149	7	3	<1	12	21	787
11	1082	Polish sausage	1 oz.	28	53	92	4	<1	0	8	20	248
		Pork sausage, cooked[83]:										
11	674	Link, small	1 ea	13	45	48	3	<1	0	4	11	168
11	1079	Patty	1 pce	27	45	100	5	<1	0	8	22	349
		Salami:										
11	675	Pork and beef	2 pce	57	60	143	8	1	0	11	37	604
11	676	Turkey	2 pce	57	66	111	9	<1	0	8	46	535
11	677	Dry, beef and pork	2 pce	20	35	85	5	1	0	7	16	372
		Sandwich spreads:										
11	1300	Ham salad	1 c	240	63	518	21	26	<1	37	88	2187
11	678	Pork and beef	1 tbsp	15	60	35	1	2	0	3	6	152
10	1296	Poultry sandwich spread	1 tbsp	13	60	25	2	1	0	2	4	49
		Smoked link sausage:										
11	1083	Beef and pork	1 ea	68	39	265	15	1	0	22	46	1020
11	1084	Pork	1 ea	68	52	229	9	1	0	21	48	642
11	1085	Summer sausage	1 pce	23	48	80	4	1	0	7	16	334
11	1076	Turkey breakfast sausage	1 pce	28	60	65	6	0	0	4	23	191
11	679	Vienna sausage, canned	1 ea	16	60	45	2	<1	0	4	8	152
		MIXED DISHES and FAST FOODS										
		MIXED DISHES:										
		Beef stew with vegetables:										
12	680	Homemade	1 c	245	82	220	16	15	3	11	71	292
12	1109	Canned	1 c	245	83	194	14	18	1	8	15	992
12	1116	Beef, macaroni & tomato sauce casserole	1 c	226	80	189	10	25	2	6	22	974
12	681	Beef pot pie, homemade[84]	1 pce	210	55	515	21	39	1	30	42	596
12	682	Chicken à la king, home recipe	1 c	245	68	470	27	12	1	34	221	760
12	683	Chicken and noodles, home recipe	1 c	240	71	365	22	26	1	18	103	600
12	684	Chicken chow mein, canned	1 c	250	89	95	7	18	5	1	8	725
12	685	Chicken chow mein, home recipe	1 c	250	78	255	23	10	4	11	75	718
12	686	Chicken pot pie, home recipe[84]	1 pce	232	57	545	23	42	2	31	56	594
12	1112	Chicken salad w/celery	.5 c	78	53	266	11	1	<1	25	48	199
12	687	Chili with beans, canned	1 c	255	76	286	15	30	8	14	43	1330
12	688	Chop suey with beef and pork	1 c	250	75	300	26	13	2	17	68	1053
12	689	Corn pudding[85]	1 c	250	76	271	11	32	9	13	230	138
12	690	Cole slaw[86]	1 c	120	82	84	2	15	2	3	10[87]	28
12	1110	Corned beef hash-canned	1 c	220	67	382	18	22	1	10	132	1354
12	1113	Egg salad	1 c	183	66	438	19	3	<1	39	629	428

[83]Cooked weight is half the weight of raw sausage.
[84]Crust made with vegetable shortening and enriched flour.
[85]Recipe: 55% yellow corn, 23% whole milk, 14% egg, 4% sugar, 3% salt, and 1% pepper.
[86]Recipe: 41% cabbage; 12% celery; 12% table cream; 12% sugar; 7% green pepper; 6% lemon juice; 4% onion; 3% pimento; 3% vinegar; 2% each for salt, dry mustard, and white pepper.
[87]From dairy cream in recipe.

(For purposes of calculations, use "0" for t, <1, <.1, <.01, etc.)

Table D–1   Food Composition

Grp	Computer Code No.	Food Description	Measure	Wt (g)	H₂O (%)	Ener (cal)	Prot (g)	Carb (g)	Dietary Fiber (g)	Fat (g)	Chol (mg)	Sodi (mg)
		MIXED DISHES and FAST FOODS—Con.										
		MIXED DISHES—Con.										
12	691	French toast, home recipe[88]	1 pce	65	53	123	5	15	1	4	73	189
12	1355	Green pepper, stuffed	1 ea	172	76	217	10	16	1	13	38	210
		Lasagna:										
12	1346	With meat	1 pce	245	64	398	26	30	2	20	56	783
12	1111	Without meat	1 pce	218	64	316	20	30	2	14	30	760
12	1117	Frozen entree	1 pce	205	73	275	17	19	1	12	90	967
		Macaroni and cheese:										
12	692	Canned[89]	1 c	240	80	230	9	26	1	10	24	730
12	693	Home recipe[90]	1 c	200	58	430	17	40	1	22	24	315
12	1115	Macaroni salad-no cheese	1 c	141	61	371	3	18	1	33	98	340
		Meat loaf:										
12	1120	Beef	1 pce	87	62	193	16	4	<1	12	97	392
12	1119	Beef and pork (1/3)	1 pce	87	59	212	15	5	<1	15	143	485
12	1303	Moussaka (lamb and eggplant)	1 c	250	79	250	21	16	6	11	170	1323
12	715	Potato salad with mayonnaise and egg[91]	1 c	250	76	358	7	28	4	21	44	1086
12	694	Quiche lorraine, ⅛ of 8″ quiche[84]	1 pce	176	47	600	13	29	1	48	285	653
		Spaghetti (enriched) in tomato sauce:										
		With cheese:										
12	695	Canned	1 c	250	80	190	6	39	3	2	3	955
12	696	Home recipe	1 c	250	77	260	9	37	3	9	8	955
		With meatballs:										
12	697	Canned	1 c	250	78	260	12	39	3	10	23	1220
12	698	Home recipe	1 c	248	70	330	19	39	3	12	89	1009
12	716	Spinach soufflé[92]	1 c	136	74	218	11	3	4	18	184	763
12	717	Tuna salad[93]	1 c	205	63	383	33	19	2	19	27	824
12	1121	Tuna noodle casserole, recipe	1 c	202	73	251	21	24	<1	7	52	869
12	1270	Waldorf salad	1 c	142	58	424	4	13	4	42	22	246
		FAST FOODS and SANDWICHES: see end of this appendix for additional Fast Foods.										
		Burrito:[94]										
12	699	Beef and bean	1 ea	175	54	390	21	40	5	18	52	516
12	700	Bean	1 ea	174	55	322	13	47	8	10	15	1030
		Cheeseburger:										
12	701	Regular	1 ea	112	46	300	15	28	1	15	44	672
12	702	4-oz patty	1 ea	194	46	524	30	40	2	31	104	1224
12	703	Chicken patty sandwich	1 ea	157	52	436	25	34	1	22	68	2732
12	704	Corn dog	1 ea	111	45	330	10	27	<1	20	37	1252
12	705	Enchilada, cheese	1 ea	163	63	320	10	29	3	19	44	784
12	706	English muffin with egg, cheese, bacon	1 ea	138	49	360	18	31	2	18	213	832
		Fish sandwich:										
12	707	Regular, with cheese	1 ea	140	43	420	16	39	1	23	56	667
12	708	Large, without cheese	1 ea	170	48	470	18	41	1	27	90	621

[84]Crust made with vegetable shortening and enriched flour.
[88]Recipe: 35% whole milk, 32% white bread, 29% egg, and cooked in 4% margarine.
[89]Made with corn oil.
[90]Made with margarine.
[91]Recipe: 62% potatoes; 12% egg; 8% mayonnaise; 7% celery; 6% sweet pickle relish; 2% onion; 1% each for green pepper, pimiento, salt, and dry mustard.
[92]Recipe: 29% whole milk, 26% spinach, 13% egg white, 13% cheddar cheese, 7% egg yolk, 7% butter, 4% flour, 1% salt and pepper.
[93]Made with drained chunk light tuna, celery, onion, pickle relish, and mayonnaise-type salad dressing.
[94]Made with a 10½″-diameter flour tortilla.

(Computer code number is for West Diet Analysis program)

GRP KEY: 1 = BEV 2 = DAIRY 3 = EGGS 4 = FAT/OIL 5 = FRUIT 6 = BAKERY 7 = GRAIN 8 = FISH 9 = BEEF 10 = POULTRY
11 = SAUSAGE **12 = MIXED/FAST** 13 = NUTS/SEEDS 14 = SWEETS 15 = VEG/LEG 16 = MISC 22 = SOUP/SAUCE

Grp	Computer Code No.	Food Description	Measure	Wt (g)	H₂O (%)	Ener (cal)	Prot (g)	Carb (g)	Dietary Fiber (g)	Fat (g)	Chol (mg)	Sodi (mg)
		MIXED DISHES and FAST FOODS—Con.										
		FAST FOODS and SANDWICHES—Con.										
		Hamburger with bun:										
12	709	Regular	1 ea	98	46	245	12	28	1	11	32	463
12	710	4-oz patty	1 ea	174	50	445	25	38	1	21	71	763
12	711	Hotdog/frankfurter and bun	1 ea	85	53	260	8	21	1	15	23	745
12	712	Cheese pizza, ⅛ of 15″ round[95]	1 pce	120	46	290	15	39	2	9	56	699
		SANDWICHES:										
		Avocado, cheese, tomato & lettuce:										
12	1276	On white bread, firm	1 ea	205	59	464	15	39	7	29	32	556
12	1278	On part whole wheat	1 ea	195	60	432	14	33	8	29	32	518
12	1277	On whole wheat	1 ea	209	58	459	16	39	13	29	32	660
		Bacon, lettuce & tomato sandwich:										
12	1137	On white bread, soft	1 ea	135	54	333	11	30	2	19	21	647
12	1139	On part whole wheat	1 ea	135	54	327	12	28	3	19	21	661
12	1138	On whole wheat	1 ea	149	53	355	13	34	8	20	21	803
		Cheese sandwich, grilled:										
12	1140	On white bread, soft	1 ea	117	37	399	17	28	1	24	55	1155
12	1142	On part whole wheat	1 ea	117	37	393	18	27	3	24	55	1169
12	1141	On whole wheat	1 ea	131	38	420	20	33	7	25	55	1311
		Chicken salad sandwich:										
12	1143	On white bread, soft	1 ea	99.7	44	300	10	28	1	16	25	401
12	1145	On part whole wheat	1 ea	99.7	44	294	11	27	3	16	25	415
12	1144	On whole wheat	1 ea	114	44	321	12	33	8	17	25	557
12	1146	Corned beef & swiss cheese on rye	1 ea	147	45	429	27	25	5	24	85	1045
		Egg salad sandwich:										
12	1147	On white bread, soft	1 ea	111	47	325	9	28	1	19	164	447
12	1149	On part whole wheat	1 ea	111	47	319	10	27	3	19	164	461
12	1148	On whole wheat	1 ea	125	47	346	12	33	7	20	164	603
		Ham sandwich:										
12	1279	On rye bread	1 ea	116	55	242	16	25	5	9	29	1261
12	1151	On white bread, soft	1 ea	122	54	262	16	28	1	9	29	1199
12	1153	On part whole wheat	1 ea	122	54	256	17	27	3	9	29	1213
12	1152	On whole wheat	1 ea	136	53	283	18	33	7	10	29	1355
		Ham & cheese sandwich:										
12	1280	On soft white bread	1 ea	151	51	369	22	29	1	18	56	1610
12	1282	On part whole wheat bread	1 ea	151	51	363	23	28	3	18	56	1624
12	1281	On whole wheat	1 ea	165	50	390	25	33	7	19	56	1766
12	1150	Ham & swiss on rye	1 ea	145	51	350	24	26	5	17	55	1336
		Ham salad sandwich:										
12	1154	On white bread, soft	1 ea	125	48	345	10	34	1	19	27	887
12	1156	On part whole wheat	1 ea	125	48	339	11	33	3	19	27	901
12	1155	On whole wheat	1 ea	139	47	366	12	38	7	20	27	1043
12	1157	Patty melt sandwich: ground beef & cheese on rye:	1 ea	177	45	567	32	25	5	38	107	923
		Peanut butter & jam sandwich:										
12	1158	On soft white bread	1 ea	100	27	347	12	45	3	15	0	403
12	1160	On part whole wheat	1 ea	100	27	341	12	44	5	15	0	417
12	1159	On whole wheat	1 ea	114	29	368	14	50	9	16	0	559
12	1161	Reuben sandwich, grilled: corned beef, swiss cheese, sauerkraut on rye:	1 ea	233	61	480	28	29	7	28	85	1642
		Roast beef sandwich:										
12	713	On a bun	1 ea	150	52	345	22	34	1	13	55	757
12	1162	On soft white bread	1 ea	122	51	286	17	28	1	11	30	757

[95] Crust made with vegetable shortening and enriched flour.

(For purposes of calculations, use "0" for t, <1, <.1, <.01, etc.)

Table D–1 Food Composition

Grp	Computer Code No.	Food Description	Measure	Wt (g)	H₂O (%)	Ener (cal)	Prot (g)	Carb (g)	Dietary Fiber (g)	Fat (g)	Chol (mg)	Sodi (mg)
		MIXED DISHES and FAST FOOD—Con.										
		SANDWICHES—Con.										
		Roast Beef—Con.										
12	1164	On part whole-wheat bread	1 ea	122	51	280	18	27	3	11	30	771
12	1163	On whole wheat bread	1 ea	136	50	307	19	32	7	12	30	912
		Tuna salad sandwich:										
12	1165	On soft white	1 ea	116	47	309	13	32	2	14	25	559
12	1167	On part whole-wheat bread	1 ea	116	47	303	14	31	3	14	25	573
12	1166	On whole-wheat bread	1 ea	130	47	331	15	37	8	15	25	715
		Turkey sandwich:										
12	1168	On soft white bread	1 ea	122	52	277	18	28	1	10	29	1151
12	1170	On part whole wheat	1 ea	122	52	271	18	26	3	11	29	1165
12	1169	On whole wheat	1 ea	136	51	298	20	32	7	11	29	1307
		Turkey ham sandwich:										
12	1272	On rye bread	1 ea	116	55	239	15	25	5	9	35	986
12	1273	On soft white bread	1 ea	122	55	259	16	29	1	9	35	924
12	1275	On part whole wheat	1 ea	122	54	253	16	28	3	9	35	938
12	1274	On whole wheat	1 ea	136	53	281	18	33	7	10	35	1080
12	714	Taco, corn tortilla, beef filling	1 ea	78	52	207	14	10	1	13	45	141
		Tostada:										
12	1114	With refried beans	1 ea	157	69	212	10	26	7	9	15	618
12	1118	With beans & beef	1 ea	192	67	332	18	20	4	21	62	483
12	1354	With beans & chicken	1 ea	157	67	249	19	19	4	11	53	474
		Vegetarian Foods:										
12	1175	Nuteena	1 ea	34	52	89	7	3	1	6	<1	203
12	1171	Proteena	1 pce	67	58	160	8	5	1	12	0	120
12	1172	Redi-burger	1 pce	71	56	140	17	5	2	6	0	460
12	1173	Vege-Burger	1 pce	68	57	130	14	5	1	6	0	370
12	1174	Breakfast links	.5 c	108	73	110	22	4	1	1	0	190
		NUTS, SEEDS and PRODUCTS										
		Almonds:										
13	1365	Dry roasted, salted	1 c	138	3	810	23	33	18	71	0	1076
13	718	Slivered, packed, unsalted	1 c	135	4	795	27	28	15[96]	70	0	15
		Whole, dried, unsalted:										
13	719	Cup	1 c	142	4	837	28	29	17[96]	74	0	15[97]
13	720	Ounce	1 oz	28	4	167	6	6	3[96]	15	0	3[97]
13	721	Almond butter	1 tbsp	16	1	101	2	3	1	9	0	2[98]
13	722	Brazil nuts, dry (about 7)	1 oz	28	3	186	4	4	3	19	0	<1
		Cashew nuts:										
		Dry roasted, salted										
13	723	Cup	1 c	137	2	787	21	45	8	63	0	877[99]
13	724	Ounce	1 oz	28	2	163	4	9	2	13	0	181[99]
		Oil roasted, salted:										
13	725	Cup	1 c	130	4	748	21	37	8	63	0	814[100]
13	726	Ounce	1 oz	28	4	163	5	8	2	14	0	177[100]

[96] Values reported for dietary fiber in almonds vary from 7.0 to 14.3g/100 g.

[97] Salted almonds contain 1108 mg sodium per cup, 221 mg per ounce.

[98] Salted almond butter contains 72 mg sodium per tablespoon.

[99] Dry-roasted cashews without salt contain 21 mg sodium per cup, or 4 mg per ounce.

[100] Oil-roasted cashews without salt contain 22 mg sodium per cup, or 5 mg per ounce.

(Computer code number is for West Diet Analysis program)

GRP KEY: 1=BEV   2=DAIRY   3=EGGS   4=FAT/OIL   5=FRUIT   6=BAKERY   7=GRAIN   8=FISH   9=BEEF   10=POULTRY
11=SAUSAGE   **12=MIXED/FAST**   **13=NUTS/SEEDS**   14=SWEETS   15=VEG/LEG   16=MISC   22=SOUP/SAUCE

Grp	Computer Code No.	Food Description	Measure	Wt (g)	H₂O (%)	Ener (cal)	Prot (g)	Carb (g)	Dietary Fiber (g)	Fat (g)	Chol (mg)	Sodi (mg)
		NUTS, SEEDS and PRODUCTS—Con.										
		Cashew nuts, unsalted:										
13	1366	Dry roasted	1 c	137	2	787	21	45	8	64	0	21
13	1367	Oil roasted	1 c	130	4	748	21	37	8	63	0	22
13	727	Cashew butter	1 tbsp	16	3	94	3	4	1	8	0	2[103]
13	728	European chestnuts, roasted, 1 c = approx 17 kernels	1 c	143	40	350	5	76	19	3	0	3
		Coconut:										
		Raw:										
13	729	Piece 2×2×½″	1 pce	45	47	159	2	7	5	15	0	9
13	730	Shredded/grated, unpacked[101]	1 c	80	47	283	3	12	9	27	0	16
		Dried, shredded/grated:										
13	731	Unsweetened	1 c	78	3	515	5	19	12	50	0	29
13	732	Sweetened	1 c	93	16	466	3	44	9	33	0	244
		Filberts (hazelnuts), chopped:										
13	733	Cup	1 c	115	5	727	15	18	7	72	0	3
13	734	Ounce	1 oz	28	5	179	4	4	2	18	0	1
		Macadamia nuts, oil roasted:										
		Salted:										
13	735	Cup	1 c	134	2	962	10	17	7	103	0	348[104]
13	736	Ounce	1 oz	28	2	204	2	4	1	22	0	74[104]
13	1368	Unsalted	1 c	134	2	962	10	17	7	103	0	9
		Mixed nuts:										
13	737	Dry roasted, salted	1 c	137	2	814	24	35	12	70	0	917[105]
13	738	Oil roasted, salted	1 c	142	2	876	24	30	13	80	0	926[105]
13	1369	Oil roasted, unsalted	1 c	142	2	876	24	30	13	80	0	16
		Peanuts:										
		Oil roasted, salted:										
13	739	Cup	1 c	144	2	837	38	27	13	71	0	624[106]
13	740	Ounce	1 oz	28	2	163	7	5	2	14	0	121[106]
13	1370	Oil roasted, unsalted	1 c	144	2	837	38	27	13	71	0	8.6
		Dried, unsalted:										
13	741	Cup	1 c	146	7	827	38	24	13	72	0	23
13	742	Ounce	1 oz	28	7	161	7	5	3	14	0	5
13	743	Peanut butter	1 tbsp	16	2	94	4	3	1	8	0	77[107]
		Pecans, halves:										
		Dried, unsalted:										
13	744	Cup	1 c	108	5	720	8	20	7[102]	73	0	1[108]
13	745	Ounce	1 oz	28	5	190	2	5	2[102]	19	0	<1
13	1372	Dry roasted, salted	¼ c	28	1	187	2	6	2	18	0	221
13	746	Pine nuts/piñons, dried	1 oz	28	6	161	3	5	2	17	0	20
		Pistachio nuts:										
13	747	Dried, shelled	1 oz	28	4	164	6	7	1	14	0	2[109]
13	1373	Dry roasted, salted, shelled	1 c	128	2	776	19	35	14	68	0	998

[101] 1 c packed = 130 g.
[102] Dietary fiber data calculated/derived from data on other nuts.
[103] Salted cashew butter contains 98 mg sodium per tablespoon.
[104] Macadamia nuts without salt contain 9 mg sodium per cup, or 2 mg per ounce.
[105] Mixed nuts without salt contain about 15 mg sodium per cup.
[106] Peanuts without salt contain 22 mg sodium per cup, or 4 mg per ounce.
[107] Peanut butter without added salt contains 3 mg sodium per tablespoon.
[108] Salted pecans contain 816 mg sodium per cup, or 214 mg per ounce.
[109] Salted pistachios contain approx 221 mg sodium per ounce.

(For purposes of calculations, use "0" for t, <1, <.1, <.01, etc.)

Table D–1 Food Composition

Grp	Computer Code No.	Food Description	Measure	Wt (g)	H$_2$O (%)	Ener (cal)	Prot (g)	Carb (g)	Dietary Fiber (g)	Fat (g)	Chol (mg)	Sodi (mg)
NUTS, SEEDS and PRODUCTS—Con.												
		Pumpkin kernals:										
13	748	Dried, unsalted	1 oz	28	7	154	7	5	2	13	0	5[110]
13	1374	Roasted, salted	1 c	227	7	1185	75	31	9	96	0	1305
13	749	Sesame seeds, hulled, dried	¼ c	38	5	221	10	4	6	21	0	15
		Sunflower seed kernels:										
13	750	Dry	¼ c	36	5	205	8	7	2	18	0	1
13	751	Oil roasted	¼ c	34	3	208	7	5	2	19	0	205[111]
13	752	Tahini (sesame butter)	1 tbsp	15	3	91	3	3	2	8	0	5
		Black walnuts, chopped:										
13	753	Cup	1 c	125	4	759	30	15	7	71	0	1
13	754	Ounce	1 oz	28	4	172	7	3	2	16	0	0
		English walnuts, chopped:										
13	755	Cup	1 c	120	4	770	17	22	7	74	0	12
13	756	Ounce	1 oz	28	4	182	4	5	2	18	0	3
SWEETENERS and SWEETS: see also Dairy (milk desserts) and Baked Goods												
14	757	Apple butter	2 tbsp	35	52	66	<1	17	<1	<1	0	1
14	1124	Butterscotch topping	3 tbsp	50	33	156	1	41	0	<1	0	111
		Cake frosting:										
14	1127	Canned, average of all types	2.5 tbsp	39	15	160	0	24	0	7	0	91
14	1123	Prepared from mix	2.5 tbsp	39	15	167	0	28	0	6	0	84
		Candy:										
14	1128	Almond Joy® candy bar	1 oz	28	7	151	2	19	1.9	8	0	—
14	758	Caramel, plain or chocolate	1 oz	28	8	115	1	22	<1	3	1	64
		Chocolate (see also, #784, 785, 971):										
		Milk chocolate:										
14	759	Plain	1 oz	28	1	145	2	16	1	9	6	23
14	760	With almonds	1 oz	28	2	150	3	15	1	10	5	23
14	761	With peanuts	1 oz	28	1	155	5	10	2	12	3	19
14	762	With rice cereal	1 oz	28	2	140	2	18	1	7	6	46
14	763	Semisweet chocolate chips	1 c	170	1	860	7	97	5	61	0	24
14	764	Sweet dark chocolate	1 oz	28	1	150	1	16	1	10	0	5
14	1133	English toffee candy bar	1 ea	32	2	220	1	11	<1	19	0	90
14	765	Fondant candy, uncoated(mints, candy corn, other)	1 oz	28	3	105	0	27	0	0	0	57
14	766	Fudge, chocolate	1 oz	28	8	115	1	21	2	3	1	54
14	767	Gum drops	1 oz	28	12	98	0	25	0	<1	0	10
14	768	Hard candy, all flavors	1 oz	28	1	109	0	28	0	0	0	7
14	769	Jelly beans	1 oz	28	6	104	t	26	0	<.1	0	7
14	1134	M&M's Plain choc. candies®	48 grm	48	1	237	3	33	<1	10	0	41
14	1135	M&M's Peanut choc. candies®	47 grm	47.3	2	240	5	28	1	12	0	29
14	1130	MARS® bar	1 ea	50	7	240	4	30	1	11	0	85
14	1129	MILKY WAY® candy bar	1 ea	60	7	260	3	43	<1	9	14	140
14	1132	REESE's® peanut butter cup	2 ea	45	4	240	6	22	2	14	3	92
14	1131	SNICKERS® candy bar, 2.2oz size	1 ea	61.2	7	290	7	37	2	14	0	170
14	1125	Caramel topping	3 tbsp	50	31	155	1	39	<1	—	0	152
14	771	Gelatin salad/dessert	½ c	120	84	70	2	17	<1	0	0	55
		Honey:										
14	772	Cup	1 c	339	17	1030	1	279	0	0	0	17
14	773	Tablespoon	1 tbsp	21	17	65	<.1	17	0	0	0	1

[110]Salted pumpkin/squash kernels contain approximately 163 mg sodium per ounce.

[111]Unsalted sunflower seeds contain 1 mg sodium per ¼ cup.

(Computer code number is for West Diet Analysis program)

GRP KEY: 1 = BEV 2 = DAIRY 3 = EGGS 4 = FAT/OIL 5 = FRUIT 6 = BAKERY 7 = GRAIN 8 = FISH 9 = BEEF 10 = POULTRY
11 = SAUSAGE 12 = MIXED/FAST **13 = NUTS/SEEDS 14 = SWEETS 15 = VEG/LEG** 16 = MISC 22 = SOUP/SAUCE

Grp	Computer Code No.	Food Description	Measure	Wt (g)	H2O (%)	Ener (cal)	Prot (g)	Carb (g)	Dietary Fiber (g)	Fat (g)	Chol (mg)	Sodi (mg)
		SWEETENERS and SWEETS—Con.										
		Jams or preserves:										
14	774	Tablespoon	1 tbsp	20	29	54	<1	14	<1	<.1	0	2
14	775	Packet	1 ea	14	29	38	<.1	10	<1	<.1	0	1
		Jellies:										
14	776	Tablespoon	1 tbsp	18	28	49	<.1	13	<1	<.1	0	4
14	777	Packet	1 ea	14	28	39	<.1	10	<1	<.1	0	3
14	1136	Marmalade	1 tbsp	20	29	52	<1	14	<1	0	0	4
14	770	Marshmallows	4 ea	28	17	90	t	23	0	0	0	25
14	1126	Marshmallow creme topping	3 tbsp	50	20	158	<1	40	0	0	0	29
14	778	Popsicles, 3 oz when fluid	1 ea	95	80	70	0	18	0	0	0	11
		Sugars:										
14	779	Brown sugar	1 c	220	2	820	0	212	0	0	0	97
		White sugar, granulated:										
14	780	Cup	1 c	200	1	770	0	199	0	0	0	5
14	781	Tablespoon	1 tbsp	12	1	45	0	12	0	0	0	t
14	782	Packet	1 ea	6	1	25	0	6	0	0	0	t
14	783	White sugar, powdered, sifted	1 c	100	<1	385	0	99	0	0	0	2
		Syrups:										
		Chocolate:										
14	784	Thin type	2 tbsp	38	37	85	1	22	1	<1	0	36
14	785	Fudge type	2 tbsp	38	25	125	2	21	1	5	0	42
14	786	Molasses, blackstrap	2 tbsp	40	24	85	0	22	0	0	0	38
14	787	Pancake table syrup (corn and maple)	¼ c	84	25	244	0	64	0	0	0	38
		VEGETABLES AND LEGUMES										
15	788	Alfalfa seeds, sprouted	1 c	33	91	10	1	1	1	<1	0	2
15	789	Artichokes, cooked globe (300 g with refuse)	1 ea	120	84	60	4	13	10	<1	0	114
		Artichoke hearts:										
15	1177	Cooked from frozen	9 oz	240	87	108	7	22	18	1	0	127
15	1176	Marinated	6 oz	170	59	168	4	13	11	14	0	900
		Asparagus, green, cooked:										
		From raw:										
15	790	Cuts and tips	½ c	90	92	23	2	4	2	<1	0	4
15	791	Spears, ½″ diam at base	4 spears	60	92	15	2	3	1	<1	0	2
		From frozen:										
15	792	Cuts and tips	1 c	180	91	50	5	9	3	1	0	7
15	793	Spears, ½″ diam at base	4 spears	60	91	17	2	3	1	<1	0	2
15	794	Canned, spears, ½″ diam at base	4 spears	80	95	11	2	2	1	1	0	278[113]
15	795	Bamboo shoots, canned, drained slices	1 c	131	94	25	2	4	3	1	0	9
		Beans (see also Great northern, #855; Kidney beans, #860; Navy beans, #876; Pinto beans, #898; Refried beans, #921; Soybeans, #925):										
15	796	Black beans, cooked	1 c	172	66	227	15	41	15	1	0	1
		Canned beans (white/navy):										
15	803	Beans w/pork and tomato sauce	1 c	253	73	247	13	49	14	3	17	45
15	804	Beans w/pork and sweet sauce	1 c	253	71	282	13	53	14	4	17	1113
15	805	Beans with frankfurters	1 c	257	70	366	17	40	18	17	15	849
		Lima beans:										
15	797	Thick seeded (Fordhooks), cooked from frozen	½ c	85	74	85	5	16	5	<1	0	1105

[113]Special dietary pack contains 3 mg sodium.

(For purposes of calculations, use "0" for t, <1, <.1, <.01, etc.)

Table D–1 Food Composition

Grp	Computer Code No.	Food Description	Measure	Wt (g)	H$_2$O (%)	Ener (cal)	Prot (g)	Carb (g)	Dietary Fiber (g)	Fat (g)	Chol (mg)	Sodi (mg)
		VEGETABLES and LEGUMES—Con.										
		Lima Beans—Con.										
15	798	Thin seeded (baby), cooked from frozen	½ c	90	72	94	6	18	8	<1	0	26
15	799	Cooked from dry, drained	1 c	188	70	217	15	39	18	1	0	4
		Snap beans/green beans, cuts and french style:										
15	800	Cooked from raw	1 c	125	89	44	2	10	3	<1	0	4
15	801	Cooked from frozen	1 c	135	92	36	2	8	4	<1	0	17
15	802	Canned, drained	1 c	136	93	26	2	6	2	<1	0	339[116]
		Bean sprouts (mung):										
15	806	Raw	1 c	104	90	31	3	6	3	<1	0	6
15	807	Cooked, stir fried	1 c	124	84	62	5	13	3	<1	0	14
15	808	Cooked, boiled, drained	1 c	124	93	26	3	5	3	<1	0	12
		Beets:										
		Cooked from fresh:										
15	809	Sliced or diced	½ c	85	91	26	1	6	2	<.1	0	42
15	810	Whole beets, 2″ diam	2 beets	100	91	31	1	7	2	<.1	0	49
		Canned:										
15	811	Sliced or diced	½ c	85	91	27	1	6	2	<1	0	233[118]
15	812	Pickled slices	½ c	114	82	74	1	19	2	<1	0	301
15	813	Beet greens, cooked, drained	1 c	144	89	40	4	8	3	<1	0	346
		Black-eyed peas: see Peas										
		Broccoli:										
15	817	Raw, chopped	1 c	88	91	24	3	5	3	<1	0	24
15	818	Raw, spears	1 spear	151	91	42	5	8	6	1	0	41
		Cooked from raw:										
15	819	Spears	1 spear	180	91	50	5	9	7	<1	0	47
15	820	Chopped	1 c	156	91	44	5	8	6	<1	0	40
		Cooked from frozen:										
15	821	Spear, small piece	1 spear	30	91	8	1	2	1	<.1	0	7
15	822	Chopped	1 c	184	91	51	6	10	6	<1	0	44
		Brussels sprouts:										
15	823	Cooked from raw	1 c	156	87	60	6	14	6	1	0	17
15	824	Cooked from frozen	1 c	155	87	65	6	13	5	1	0	36
		Cabbage, common varieties:										
15	825	Raw, shredded or chopped	1 c	70	92	16	1	4	2	<1	0	12
15	826	Cooked, drained	1 c	150	94	32	1	7	4	<1	0	29
		Chinese cabbage:										
15	1178	Bok-choy, raw, shredded	1 c	70	95	9	1	2	1	<1	0	<1
15	827	Bok choy, cooked, drained	1 c	170	96	20	3	3	3	<1	0	57
15	828	Pe-Tsai, raw, chopped	1 c	76	94	11	1	2	2	<1	0	7
		Cabbage, red, coarsely chopped:										
15	829	Raw	1 c	70	92	19	1	4	2	<1	0	8
15	830	Cooked	½ c	75	94	16	1	3	4	<1	0	6
15	831	Savoy cabbage, coarsely chopped, raw	1 c	70	91	20	1	4	2	<.1	0	20

[116]Dietary pack contains 3 mg Sodium per cup.
[118]Dietary pack contains 39 mg Sodium.

(Computer code number is for West Diet Analysis program)

GRP KEY: 1 = BEV 2 = DAIRY 3 = EGGS 4 = FAT/OIL 5 = FRUIT 6 = BAKERY 7 = GRAIN 8 = FISH 9 = BEEF 10 = POULTRY
11 = SAUSAGE 12 = MIXED/FAST 13 = NUTS/SEEDS 14 = SWEETS **15 = VEG/LEG** 16 = MISC 22 = SOUP/SAUCE

Grp	Computer Code No.	Food Description	Measure	Wt (g)	H$_2$O (%)	Ener (cal)	Prot (g)	Carb (g)	Dietary Fiber (g)	Fat (g)	Chol (mg)	Sodi (mg)
		VEGETABLES and LEGUMES—Con.										
		Carrots:										
		Raw:										
15	832	Whole, 7½ × 1⅛″	1 carrot	72	88	31	1	7	2	<1	0	25
15	833	Grated	½ c	55	88	24	1	6	2	<1	0	19
		Cooked, sliced, drained:										
15	834	Cooked from raw	½ c	78	87	35	1	8	3	<1	0	52
15	835	Cooked from frozen	½ c	73	90	26	1	6	3	<.1	0	43
15	836	Canned, sliced, drained	½ c	73	93	17	<1	4	1	<1	0	176[120]
15	837	Carrot juice	½ c	123	89	49	1	11	2	<1	0	36
		Cauliflower:										
15	838	Raw, flowerets	½ c	50	92	12	1	2	1	<.1	0	7
		Cooked, drained, flowerets:										
15	839	From raw	½ c	62	92	15	1	3	1	<1	0	4
15	840	From frozen	1 c	180	94	34	3	7	3	<1	0	33
		Celery, pascal type, raw:										
15	841	Large outer stalk, 8 × 1½″ (at root end)	1 stalk	40	95	6	<1	1	1	<.1	0	35
15	842	Diced	½ c	60	95	11	<1	2	1	<.1	0	55
		Chard, swiss:										
15	1179	Raw, chopped	1 c	36	93	7	1	1	1	<1	0	77
15	1180	Cooked	1 c	175	93	35	3	7	4	<1	0	313
		Chick-peas (see Garbanzo, #854)										
		Collards, cooked, drained:										
15	843	From raw	1 c	128	92	35	2	8	4	<1	0	21
15	844	From frozen	1 c	170	88	63	3	14	6	1	0	37
		Corn:										
		Cooked, drained:										
15	845	From raw, on cob, 5″ long	1 ear	77	70	83	3	19	3	1	0	13
15	846	From frozen, on cob, 3½″ long	1 ear	63	73	59	2	14	3	<1	0	3
15	847	Kernels, cooked from frozen	½ c	82	76	67	2	17	3	<.1	0	4
		Canned:										
15	848	Cream style	½ c	128	79	93	2	23	2	<1	0	365[122]
15	849	Whole kernel, vacuum pack	1 c	210	77	166	5	41	3	1	0	572[123]
		Cowpeas; (see Black-eyed peas, #814−816)										
15	850	Cucumbers with peel, ⅛″ thick, 2⅛″ diam	6 slices	28	96	4	<1	1	<1	<.1	0	1
		Dandelion greens:										
15	851	Raw	1 c	55	86	25	1	5	1	<1	0	42
15	852	Chopped, cooked, drained	1 c	105	90	35	2	7	1	1	0	46
15	853	Eggplant, cooked	1 c	160	92	45	1	11	6	<1	0	5
15	854	Garbanzo beans (chick-peas), cooked	1 c	164	60	269	15	45	11	4	0	11
15	855	Great northern beans, cooked	1 c	177	69	210	15	37	11	1	0	4
15	856	Escarole/curly endive, chopped	1 c	50	94	9	1	2	1	<1	0	11
15	857	Jerusalem artichokes, raw slices	1 c	150	78	114	3	26	2	<.1	0	6
		Kale, cooked, drained:										
15	858	From raw	1 c	130	91	42	3	7	4	1	0	30
15	859	From frozen	1 c	130	90	39	4	7	3	1	0	20
15	860	Kidney beans, canned	1 c	256	77	216	13	39	19	<1	0	889
		Kohlrabi:										
15	1181	Raw slices	1 c	140	91	38	2	9	2	<1	0	28
15	861	Cooked	1 c	165	90	48	3	11	2	<1	0	34

[120]Dietary pack contains 31 mg sodium.
[122]Dietary pack contains 4 mg sodium per ½ cup.
[123]Dietary pack contains 6 mg sodium per cup.

(For purposes of calculations, use "0" for t, <1, <.1, <.01, etc.)

Table D–1 Food Composition

Grp	Computer Code No.	Food Description	Measure	Wt (g)	H$_2$O (%)	Ener (cal)	Prot (g)	Carb (g)	Dietary Fiber (g)	Fat (g)	Chol (mg)	Sodi (mg)
		VEGETABLES and LEGUMES—Con.										
		Leeks:										
15	1183	Raw, chopped	1 c	104	83	63	2	15	2	<1	0	21
15	1182	Cooked, chopped	.5 c	52	91	16	<1	4	2	<1	0	5
15	862	Lentils, cooked from dry	1 c	198	70	230	18	40	10	1	0	4
		Lentils, sprouted:										
15	1288	Stir fried	3.5 oz	100	69	101	9	21	4	<1	0	9
15	1289	Raw	1 c	77	67	81	7	17	3	<1	0	8
		Lettuce:										
		Butterhead/Boston types:										
15	863	Head, 5″ diam	1 head	163	96	21	2	4	3	<1	0	8
15	864	Leaves, 2 inner or outer	2 leaves	15	96	2	<1	<1	<1	<.1	0	1
		Iceberg/crisphead:										
15	865	Head, 6″ diam	1 head	539	96	70	5	11	9	1	0	48
15	866	Wedge, ¼ of head	1 wedge	135	96	18	1	3	2	<1	0	12
15	867	Chopped or shredded	1 c	56	96	7	1	1	1	<1	0	5
15	868	Loose leaf, chopped	1 c	56	94	10	1	2	1	<1	0	5
		Romaine:										
15	869	Chopped	1 c	56	95	9	1	1	1	<1	0	4
15	870	Inner leaf	1 leaf	10	95	2	<1	<1	<1	<.1	0	1
		Mushrooms:										
15	871	Raw, sliced	½ c	35	92	9	1	2	1	<1	0	1
15	872	Cooked from raw, pieces	½ c	78	91	21	2	4	2	<1	0	2
15	873	Canned, drained	½ c	78	91	19	1	4	2	<1	0	332
		Mustard greens:										
15	874	Cooked from raw	1 c	140	94	21	3	3	3	<1	0	22
15	875	Cooked from frozen	1 c	150	94	29	3	5	3	<1	0	38
15	876	Navy beans, cooked from dry	1 c	182	63	259	16	43	16	1	0	2
		Okra, cooked:										
15	877	From fresh pods	8 pods	85	90	27	2	6	2	<1	0	4
15	878	From frozen slices	½ c	92	91	34	2	8	2	<1	0	3
		Onions:										
15	879	Raw, chopped	1 c	160	90	61	2	14	3	<1	0	5
15	880	Raw, sliced	1 c	115	90	44	1	10	2	<1	0	3
15	881	Cooked, drained, chopped	½ c	105	88	46	1	11	2	<1	0	3
15	882	Dehydrated flakes	¼ c	14	4	45	1	12	1	<.1	0	3
		Spring onions:										
15	883	Chopped, bulb and top	½ c	50	90	16	1	4	1	.1	0	8
15	1185	Green tops only, chopped,	1 c	100	92	34	2	6	3	<1	0	7
15	1184	White part only, chopped	1 c	100	92	50	1	10	3	<1	0	7
15	884	Onion rings, breaded, prepared f/frozen	2 rings	20	29	81	1	8	<1	5	0	75
		Parsley:										
15	885	Raw, chopped	½ c	30	88	10	1	2	2	<.1	0	12
15	886	Raw, sprigs	10 sprigs	10	88	3	<1	1	1	<.1	0	4
15	887	Freeze dried	¼ c	1	2	4	<1	1	1	<.1	0	5
15	888	Parsnips, sliced, cooked	1 c	156	78	125	2	30	5	1	0	16
		Peas:										
		Black-eyed peas, cooked:										
15	814	From dry, drained	1 c	171	70	198	13	36	21	1	0	6
15	815	From fresh, drained	1 c	165	76	160	5	33	12	1	0	7
15	816	From frozen, drained	1 c	170	66	224	14	40	14	1	0	9
15	889	Edible-pod, peas, cooked	1 c	160	89	67	5	11	4	<1	0	6

(Computer code number is for West Diet Analysis program)

GRP KEY: 1 = BEV   2 = DAIRY   3 = EGGS   4 = FAT/OIL   5 = FRUIT   6 = BAKERY   7 = GRAIN   8 = FISH   9 = BEEF   10 = POULTRY   11 = SAUSAGE   12 = MIXED/FAST   13 = NUTS/SEEDS   14 = SWEETS   **15 = VEG/LEG**   16 = MISC   22 = SOUP/SAUCE

Grp	Computer Code No.	Food Description	Measure	Wt (g)	H₂O (%)	Ener (cal)	Prot (g)	Carb (g)	Dietary Fiber (g)	Fat (g)	Chol (mg)	Sodi (mg)
		VEGETABLES and LEGUMES—Con.										
		Peas—Con.										
		Green peas:										
15	890	Canned, drained	½ c	85	82	59	4	11	4	<1	0	186[128]
15	891	Cooked from frozen	½ c	80	80	63	4	11	4	<1	0	70
15	892	Split, green, cooked from dry	1 c	196	69	231	16	41	10	1	0	4
		Peas and carrots:										
15	1187	Cooked from frozen	½ c	80	86	38	2	8	3	<1	0	55
15	1186	Canned, with liquid	½ c	128	88	48	3	11	4	<1	0	332
		Peppers, hot:										
15	893	Hot green chili, canned	½ c	68	92	17	1	4	1	<.1	0	10
15	894	Hot green chili, raw	1 pepper	45	88	18	1	4	1	<.1	0	3
15	895	Jalapenos, chopped, canned	½ c	68	90	17	1	3	2	<1	0	995
		Peppers, sweet, green:										
15	896	Whole pod (90 g with refuse), raw	1 pod	74	92	20	1	5	1	<1	0	1
15	897	Cooked, chopped (1 pod cooked = 73 g)	½ c	68	92	19	1	5	1	<1	0	1
		Peppers, sweet, red:										
15	1286	Raw, chopped	½ c	50	92	14	<1	3	1	<1	0	1
15	1287	Cooked, chopped	½ c	68	92	19	1	5	1	<1	0	1
15	898	Pinto beans, cooked from dry	1 c	171	64	235	14	44	20	1	0	3
15	1191	Poi - two finger	1 c	240	72	269	1	65	6	<1	0	28
		Potatoes:[125]										
		Baked in oven, 4¾ × 2⅓″ diam:										
15	899	With skin	1 potato	202	71	220	5	51	5	<1	0	16
15	900	Flesh only	1 potato	156	75	145	3	34	2	<1	0	8
15	901	Skin only	1 ea	58	47	115	2	27	2	<.1	0	12
		Baked in microwave, 4¾ × 2⅓″ diam:										
15	902	With skin	1 potato	202	72	212	5	49	5	<1	0	16
15	903	Flesh only	1 potato	156	74	156	3	36	2	<1	0	11
15	904	Skin only	1 ea	58	64	77	3	17	2	<.1	0	9
		Boiled, about 2½″ diam:										
15	905	Peeled after boiling	1 potato	136	77	119	3	27	2	<1	0	6
15	906	Peeled before boiling	1 potato	135	78	116	2	27	2	<1	0	7
		French fried, strips 2-3½″ long, frozen:										
15	907	Oven heated	10 strips	50	53	111	2	17	1	4	0	15
15	908	Fried in veg oil	10 strips	50	38	158	2	20	1	8	0	108
15	1188	Fried in veg. and animal oil	10 strips	50	38	158	2	20	1	8	0	108
15	909	Hashed brown, from frozen	1 c	156	56	340	5	44	3	18	0	53
		Mashed:										
15	910	Home recipe with milk[126]	1 c	210	78	162	4	37	3	1	4	636
15	911	Home recipe with milk and margarine	1 c	210	76	222	4	35	3	9	4[130]	619
15	912	Prepared from flakes; water, milk, margarine, salt added	1 c	215	76	239	4	28	2	13	4[130]	733
		Potato products, prepared:										
		Au gratin:										
15	913	From dry mix	1 c	245	79	228	6	32	4	10	12	1076
15	914	From home recipe[127]	1 c	245	74	322	12	28	4	19	56[131]	1064

[125] Vitamin C varies with length of storage. After 3 months of storage approximately two-thirds of the ascorbic acid remains; after 6 to 7 months, about one-third remains.
[126] Recipe: 84% potatoes, 15% whole milk, 1% salt.
[127] Recipe: 55% potatoes, 30% whole milk, 9% cheddar cheese, 3% butter, 2% flour, 1% salt.
[128] Dietary pack contains 1.7 mg sodium.
[130] Data is for margarine; if butter is used, cholesterol = 25 mg for 29 total mg.
[131] Data is for butter; if margarine is used, cholesterol = 37 mg.

(For purposes of calculations, use "0" for t, <1, <.1, <.01, etc.)

Table D–1   Food Composition

Grp	Computer Code No.	Food Description	Measure	Wt (g)	H₂O (%)	Ener (cal)	Prot (g)	Carb (g)	Dietary Fiber (g)	Fat (g)	Chol (mg)	Sodi (mg)
		VEGETABLES and LEGUMES—Con.										
		Potato Products—Con.										
		Potato salad (see Mixed Dishes #715)										
		Scalloped:										
15	915	From dry mix	1 c	245	79	228	5	31	3	11	27	835
15	916	Home recipe[132]	1 c	245	81	210	7	26	3	9	29[133]	821
15	1192	Potato puffs, cooked from frozen	.5 c	62	53	138	2	19	1	7	0	462
15	917	Potato chips (14 chips = about 1 oz)	14 chips	28	2	148	2	15	1	10	0	133[134]
		Pumpkin:										
15	918	Cooked from raw, mashed	1 c	245	94	50	2	12	4	<1	0	3
15	919	Canned	1 c	245	90	83	3	20	5	1	0	12
15	920	Red radishes	10 radishes	45	95	7	<1	2	1	<1	0	11
15	921	Refried beans, canned	1 c	253	72	270	16	47	22	3	0	1071
15	1375	Rutabaga, cooked cubes	.5 c	85	90	29	1	7	1	<1	0	15
15	922	Sauerkraut, canned with liquid	1 c	236	92	44	2	10	4	<1	0	1561
		Seaweed:										
15	923	Kelp, raw	1 oz	28	82	12	1	3	1	<1	0	66
15	924	Spirulina, dried	1 oz	28	5	82	16	7	1	2	0	297
15	925	Soybeans, cooked from dry	1 c	172	63	298	29	17	5	15	0	1
		Soybean products:										
15	926	Miso	½ c	138	46	283	16	39	7	8	0	5032
15	927	Tofu	½ c	124	85	94	10	2	2	6	0	9
		Spinach:										
15	928	Raw, chopped	1 c	56	92	12	2	2	2	<1	0	44
		Cooked, drained:										
15	929	From raw	1 c	180	91	41	5	7	4	<1	0	126
15	930	From frozen (leaf)	1 c	190	90	53	6	10	5	<1	0	163
15	931	Canned, drained solids	1 c	214	92	50	6	7	6	1	0	683[135]
		Spinach soufflé (Mixed Dishes)										
		Squash, summer varieties, cooked slices:										
15	932	Varieties averaged	1 c	180	94	36	2	8	3	1	0	2
15	933	Crookneck	1 c	180	94	36	2	8	3	1	0	2
15	934	Zucchini	1 c	180	95	29	1	7	4	<.1	0	5
		Squash, winter varieties, cooked:										
		Average of all varieties, baked:										
15	935	Mashed	1 c	245	89	96	2	21	7	2	0	2
15	936	Baked cubes	1 c	205	89	79	2	18	6	1	0	3
		Acorn squash:										
15	937	Baked, mashed	1 c	245	83	137	3	36	7	<1	0	11
15	1218	Boiled, mashed	1 c	245	90	83	2	22	6	<1	0	6
15	938	Butternut, baked cubes	1 c	205	88	83	2	22	6	<1	0	7
		Butternut squash:										
15	1219	Baked, mashed	1 c	245	88	99	2	26	7	<1	0	8
15	1193	Cooked from frozen	1 c	240	88	94	3	24	7	<1	0	4
		Hubbard squash:										
15	1194	Baked, mashed	1 c	240	85	120	6	26	6	1	0	19
15	1195	Boiled, mashed	1 c	236	91	70	4	15	7	1	0	12
15	1196	Spaghetti squash, baked or boiled	1 c	155	92	45	1	10	4	<1	0	28
15	1189	Succotash, cooked from frozen	1 c	170	74	158	7	34	9	2	0	77

[132]Recipe: 59% potatoes, 36% whole milk, 2% butter, 2% flour, 1% salt.
[133]Data is for butter; if margarine is used cholesterol = 15 mg.
[134]If no salt added, sodium = 2 mg.
[135]Dietary pack contains 58 mg sodium.

(Computer code number is for West Diet Analysis program)

GRP KEY: 1 = BEV   2 = DAIRY   3 = EGGS   4 = FAT/OIL   5 = FRUIT   6 = BAKERY   7 = GRAIN   8 = FISH   9 = BEEF   10 = POULTRY
11 = SAUSAGE   12 = MIXED/FAST   13 = NUTS/SEEDS   14 = SWEETS   **15 = VEG/LEG**   **16 = MISC**   22 = SOUP/SAUCE

Grp	Computer Code No.	Food Description	Measure	Wt (g)	H₂O (%)	Ener (cal)	Prot (g)	Carb (g)	Dietary Fiber (g)	Fat (g)	Chol (mg)	Sodi (mg)
		VEGETABLES and LEGUMES—Con.										
		Sweet potatoes:										
		Cooked, 5 × 2″ diam:										
15	939	Baked in skin, peeled	1 potato	114	73	118	2	28	3	<1	0	12
15	940	Boiled without skin	1 potato	151	73	160	2	37	5	<1	0	20
15	941	Candied, 2½ × 2″	1 pce	105	67	144	1	29	2	3	0[137]	73
		Canned:										
15	942	Solid pack, mashed	1 c	265	74	258	5	59	6	<1	0	191
15	943	Vacuum pack, mashed	1 c	255	76	233	4	54	5	1	0	136
15	944	Vacuum pack, 2¾ × 1″	1 pce	40	76	36	1	8	1	<1	0	21
		Tomatoes:										
15	945	Raw, whole, 2⅗″ diam	1 tomato	123	94	26	1	6	2	<1	0	11
15	946	Raw, chopped	1 c	180	94	38	2	8	3	<1	0	16
15	947	Cooked from raw	1 c	240	92	65	3	14	4	1	0	26
15	948	Canned, solids and liquid	1 c	240	94	47	2	10	3	1	0	390[140]
15	949	Tomato juice, canned	1 c	244	94	42	2	10	2	<1	0	881[141]
		Tomato products, canned:										
15	950	Paste	1 c	262	74	220	10	49	11	2	0	170[142]
15	951	Puree	1 c	250	87	102	4	25	6	<1	0	49[143]
15	952	Sauce	1 c	245	89	74	3	18	4	<1	0	1481[144]
15	953	Turnips, cubes, cooked from raw	½ c	78	94	14	1	4	2	<1	0	39
		Turnip greens, cooked:										
15	954	From raw (leaves and stems)	1 c	144	94	29	2	6	4	<1	0	41
15	955	From frozen (chopped)	½ c	82	90	24	3	4	4	<1	0	12
15	956	Vegetable juice cocktail, canned	1 c	242	94	46	2	11	2	<1	0	883
		Vegetables, mixed:										
15	957	Canned, drained	1 c	163	87	77	4	15	6	<1	0	243
15	958	Frozen, cooked, drained	1 c	182	83	107	5	24	7	<1	0	64
		Water chestnuts, canned:										
15	959	Slices	½ c	70	86	35	1	9	2	<.1	0	6
15	960	Whole	4 ea	28	86	14	<1	4	1	<1	0	2
15	1190	Watercress, fresh, chopped	.5 c	17	95	2	<1	<1	<1	<1	0	7
		MISCELLANEOUS										
		Baking powders for home use:										
		Sodium aluminum sulfate:										
16	962	With monocalcium phosphate monohydrate	1 tsp	3	2	5	t	1	0	0	0	329
16	963	With monocalcium phosphate monohydrate, calcium sulfate	1 tsp	3	1	5	t	1	0	0	0	290
16	964	Straight phosphate	1 tsp	4	2	5	t	1	0	0	0	312
16	965	Low sodium	1 tsp	4	1	5	t	1	0	0	0	t
16	1204	Baking soda	1 tsp	3	1	0	0	0	0	0	0	821
16	966	Basil, ground	1 tbsp	5	6	11	1	3	1	<1	0	2
16	961	Carob flour	1 c	103	3	185	5	92	34	1	0	36

[137] For recipe using margarine; if butter is used, cholesterol = 8 mg.
[140] Dietary pack contains 31 mg sodium.
[141] If no salt is added, sodium content is 24 mg.
[142] If salt is added, sodium content is 2070 mg.
[143] If salt is added, sodium content is 998 mg.
[144] With salt added.

(For purposes of calculations, use "0" for t, <1, <.1, <.01, etc.)

Table D-1 Food Composition

Grp	Computer Code No.	Food Description	Measure	Wt (g)	H₂O (%)	Ener (cal)	Prot (g)	Carb (g)	Dietary Fiber (g)	Fat (g)	Chol (mg)	Sodi (mg)
		MISCELLANEOUS—Con.										
		Catsup:										
16	967	Cup	1 c	245	67	255	4	67	4	1	0	2906
16	968	Tablespoon	1 tbsp	15	67	16	<1	4	<1	<.1	0	178
16	1200	Cayenne (red pepper)	1 tbsp	5.3	8	17	1	3	2	1	0	7
16	969	Celery seed	1 tsp	2	6	9	<1	1	<1	1	0	4
16	970	Chili powder	1 tsp	3	8	8	<1	1	1	<1	0	26
		Chocolate:										
16	971	Baking, unsweetened	1 oz	28	2	145	4	7	4	15	0	1
		For other chocolate items, see Sweeteners and Sweets										
16	972	Coriander, fresh	¼ c	4	93	<1	<1	<1	<1	<.1	0	1
16	1197	Cornstarch	1 tbsp	8	8	20	<.1	5	<.1	<.1	0	.5
16	973	Cinnamon	1 tsp	2	10	6	<1	2	1	<.1	0	1
16	974	Curry powder	1 tsp	2	10	6	<1	1	<1	<1	0	1
16	1202	Dill weed, dried	1 tbsp	3.1	7	8	1	2	<1	<1	0	6
		Garlic:										
16	975	Cloves	4 cloves	12	59	18	1	4	<1	<.1	0	2
16	976	Powder	1 tsp	3	6	9	<1	2	<1	<.1	0	1
16	977	Gelatin, dry, plain	1 envelope	7	13	25	6	0	1	0	0	6
16	978	Ginger root, raw, sliced	5 slices	11	87	8	<1	2	<1	<1	0	1
16	1198	Horseradish, prepared	1 tbsp	15	87	6	<1	1	<1	<1	0	14
16	1199	Hummous/Humous	1 c	246	65	420	33	50	4	21	0	599
16	979	Mustard, prepared, (1 packet = 1 tsp)	1 tsp	5	80	4	<1	<1	<1	<1	0	63
		Miso (see #926 under Vegetables and Legumes, Soybean products):										
		Olives:										
16	980	Green	10 olives	39	78	45	<1	<1	1	6	0	936
16	981	Ripe, pitted	10 olives	45	80	52	<1	3	1.5	5	0	392
16	982	Onion powder	1 tsp	2.1	5	5	<1	2	<1	<.1	0	1
16	983	Oregano, ground	1 tsp	2	7	5	<1	1	<1	<1	0	<1
16	984	Paprika	1 tsp	2	10	6	<1	1	<1	<1	0	1
16	985	Pepper, black	1 tsp	2	11	5	<1	1	<1	<.1	0	1
		Pickles:										
16	986	Dill, medium, 3¾ × 1¼″ diam	1 pickle	65	92	12	<1	3	1	<1	0	833
16	987	Fresh pack, slices, 1½″ diam × ¼″	4 slices	30	79	20	<1	5	<1	<.1	0	201
16	988	Sweet, medium	1 pickle	35	65	41	<1	11	<1	.1	0	329
16	989	Pickle relish, sweet	1 tbsp	15	63	20	<.1	5	<1	<.1	0	107
16	1201	Sage-ground	1 tbsp	2	8	6	<1	1	<1	<1	0	0
		Popcorn (see Grain Products, #539-541)										
22	1347	Salsa, from recipe	.85 c	184	91	79	2	9	3	5	0	191
16	990	Salt	1 tsp	6	0	0	0	0	0	0	0	2132
		Salt substitute:										
16	1205	Morton Salt Substitute	1 tbsp	6	0	0	0	<1	0	0	0	t
16	1206	No Salt, packet, Norcliff Thayer	1 packet	.75	0	0	0	0	0	0	0	0
16	1207	Light Salt, Morton	1 tsp	6	0	0	0	0	0	0	0	1100
16	991	Vinegar, cider	1 tbsp	15	94	2	0	1	0	0	0	t
		Yeast:										
16	992	Baker's, dry, active, package	1 package	7	5	20	3	3	2	<1	0	4
16	993	Brewer's, dry	1 tbsp	8	5	25	3	3	3	<.1	0	10

(Computer code number is for West Diet Analysis program)

GRP KEY: 1 = BEV   2 = DAIRY   3 = EGGS   4 = FAT/OIL   5 = FRUIT   6 = BAKERY   7 = GRAIN   8 = FISH   9 = BEEF   10 = POULTRY
11 = SAUSAGE   12 = MIXED/FAST   13 = NUTS/SEEDS   14 = SWEETS   15 = VEG/LEG   **16 = MISC   22 = SOUP/SAUCE**

Grp	Computer Code No.	Food Description	Measure	Wt (g)	H$_2$O (%)	Ener (cal)	Prot (g)	Carb (g)	Dietary Fiber (g)	Fat (g)	Chol (mg)	Sodi (mg)
		SOUPS, SAUCES, AND GRAVIES										
		SOUPS, canned, condensed:										
		Unprepared, condensed:										
22	1210	Cream of celery	1 c	251	85	180	3	18	1	11	28	1899
22	1215	Cream of chicken	1 c	251	82	233	7	19	<1	15	20	1973
22	1216	Cream of mushroom	1 c	251	81	257	4	19	<1	19	3	2032
22	1220	Onion	1 c	246	86	114	8	16	1	3	0	2116
		Prepared with equal volume of whole milk:										
22	994	Clam chowder, New England	1 c	248	85	163	9	17	1	7	22	992
22	1209	Cream of celery	1 c	248	87	165	6	15	<1	10	32	1010
22	995	Cream of chicken	1 c	248	85	191	7	15	<1	12	27	1046
22	996	Cream of mushroom	1 c	248	85	205	6	15	<1	14	20	1076
22	1214	Cream of potato	1 c	248	87	148	6	17	<1	6	22	1060
22	1213	Oyster stew	1 c	245	89	134	6	10	0	8	32	1040
22	997	Tomato	1 c	248	85	160	6	22	<1	6	17	932
		Prepared with equal volume of water:										
22	998	Bean with bacon	1 c	253	84	173	8	23	3	6	3	952
22	999	Beef broth, bouillon, consommé	1 c	240	98	16	3	<1	0	1	1	782
22	1000	Beef noodle	1 c	244	92	84	5	9	<1	3	5	952
22	1001	Chicken noodle	1 c	241	92	75	4	9	1	2	7	900
22	1002	Chicken rice	1 c	241	94	60	4	7	1	2	7	815
22	1208	Chili beef soup	1 c	250	85	169	7	22	1	7	12	1035
22	1003	Clam chowder, Manhatten	1 c	244	92	78	2	12	1	2	2	578
22	1004	Cream of chicken	1 c	244	91	115	3	9	<1	7	10	986
22	1005	Cream of mushroom	1 c	244	90	130	2	9	1	9	2	1032
22	1006	Minestrone	1 c	241	91	80	4	11	1	3	2	911
22	1211	Onion soup-canned	1 c	241	93	57	4	8	<1	2	0	1053
22	1007	Split pea with ham	1 c	253	82	189	10	28	1	4	8	1008
22	1008	Tomato	1 c	244	90	86	2	17	<1	2	0	872
22	1009	Vegetable beef	1 c	244	92	79	6	10	1	2	5	956
22	1010	Vegetarian vegetable	1 c	241	92	70	2	12	2	2	0	823
		SOUPS, dehydrated:										
		Unprepared, dry products:										
22	1011	Bouillon	1 packet	6	3	14	1	1	<1	1	1	1019
22	1012	Onion	1 packet	7	4	20	1	4	<1	<1	<1	627
		Prepared with water:										
22	1299	Beef broth/bouillon	1 c	244	97	20	1	2	<1	1	0	1362
22	1376	Chicken broth/bouillon	1 c	244	97	21	1	1	<1	1	1	1484
22	1013	Chicken noodle	¾ c	188	94	40	2	6	<1	1	2	957
22	1122	Cream of chicken	1 c	261	91	107	2	13	1	5	3	1184
22	1014	Onion	¾ c	184	96	20	1	4	<1	<1	0	635
22	1217	Split pea	1 c	255	87	133	8	23	1	2	3	1220
22	1015	Tomato vegetable	¾ c	189	94	41	1	8	<1	1	0	856
		SAUCES										
		From dry mixes, prepared with milk:										
22	1016	Cheese sauce	1 c	279	77	305	16	23	<1	17	53	1565
22	1017	Hollandaise	1 c	259	84	240	5	14	—	20	52	1564
22	1019	White sauce	1 c	264	81	240	10	21	<1	13	34	797
		From home recipe:										
22	1019	White sauce, medium[146]	1 c	250	73	395	10	24	<1	30	32	888
		Ready to serve:										
22	1020	Barbeque sauce	1 tbsp	16	81	10	<1	2	<1	<1	0	128
22	1021	Soy sauce	1 tbsp	18	71	9	1	2	0	t	0	1029

[146] Made with enriched flour, margarine, and whole milk.

(For purposes of calculations, use "0" for t, <1, <.1, <.01, etc.)

Table D-1 Food Composition

Grp	Computer Code No.	Food Description	Measure	Wt (g)	H$_2$O (%)	Ener (cal)	Prot (g)	Carb (g)	Dietary Fiber (g)	Fat (g)	Chol (mg)	Sodi (mg)
		SOUPS, SAUCES and GRAVIES—Con.										
		SOUPS—Con.										
		Spaghetti sauce: canned:										
22	1377	Plain	1 c	249	75	272	5	40	3	12	0	1236
22	1378	With meat	.8 c	206	75	220	8	27	1	10	17	1045
22	1379	With mushrooms	.75 c	185	75	162	2	9	2	5	0	744
22	1380	Teriyaki sauce	1 tbsp	18	84	15	1	3	0	<1	0	690
		GRAVIES:										
		Canned:										
22	1022	Beef	1 c	233	87	123	9	11	<1	5	7	1305
22	1023	Chicken	1 c	238	85	189	5	13	<1	14	5	1375
22	1024	Mushroom	1 c	238	89	120	3	13	<1	6	0	1357
		From dry mix:										
22	1025	Brown	1 c	258	92	75	2	13	<1	2	3	1076
22	1026	Chicken	1 c	260	91	85	3	14	<1	2	3	1134

(Computer code number is for West Diet Analysis program)

GRP KEY: 1 = BEV   2 = DAIRY   3 = EGGS   4 = FAT/OIL   5 = FRUIT   6 = BAKERY   7 = GRAIN   8 = FISH   9 = BEEF   10 = POULTRY
11 = SAUSAGE   **12 = MIXED/FAST**   13 = NUTS/SEEDS   14 = SWEETS   15 = VEG/LEG   16 = MISC   **22 = SOUP/SAUCE**

Grp	Computer Code No.	Food Description	Measure	Wt (g)	H$_2$O (%)	Ener (cal)	Prot (g)	Carb (g)	Dietary Fiber (g)	Fat (g)	Chol (mg)	Sodi (mg)
ARBY'S												
12	1402	Bac'n Cheddar, deluxe	1 ea	226	56	526	27	33	<1	37	83	1672
		Roast beef sandwiches:										
12	1403	Regular	1 ea	147	51	353	22	32	<1	15	39	588
12	1404	Junior	1 ea	86	48	218	12	22	<1	9	20	345
12	1405	Super	1 ea	234	58	501	25	50	<1	22	40	798
12	1406	Deluxe	1 ea	247	62	486	26	43	<1	23	59	1288
12	1407	Beef 'n Cheddar	1 ea	197	57	455	26	28	<1	27	63	955
		Chicken sandwiches:										
12	1408	Chicken breast sandwich	1 ea	195	52	509	26	36	<1	29	83	1082
12	1409	Chicken salad sandwich	1 ea	156	53	386	18	33	<1	20	30	630
12	1410	Chicken salad & croissant	1 ea	150	50	472	22	16	<1	36	12	725
12	1411	Chicken club sandwich	1 ea	210	44	621	26	57	<1	32	108	1300
12	1412	Hot ham and cheese sandwich	1 ea	156	62	292	23	19	<1	14	45	1350
12	1413	Turkey deluxe sandwich	1 ea	197	61	375	24	33	<1	17	39	1047
		Baked potatoes:										
12	1414	Plain	1 ea	312	75	290	8	66	6	<1	0	12
12	1415	Deluxe, w/butter & sour cream	1 ea	340	74	648	18	59	6	38	72	475
12	1416	W/broccoli & cheese	1 ea	340	70	541	13	72	6	22	24	475
12	1417	W/mushrooms & cheese	1 ea	321	70	506	16	61	6	22	21	635
12	1418	Taco	1 ea	425	70	619	23	73	6	27	145	1065
		Milkshakes:										
12	1419	Chocolate	1 ea	340	74	451	10	77	<1	12	36	341
12	1420	Jamocha	1 ea	326	75	368	9	59	0	11	35	262
12	1421	Vanilla	1 ea	312	75	330	11	46	0	12	32	281

Source: Arby's Inc., Atlanta Georgia for the basic nutrients. Values for dietary fiber and percent water are estimates calculated from known values for major ingredients.

Grp	Computer Code No.	Food Description	Measure	Wt (g)	H$_2$O (%)	Ener (cal)	Prot (g)	Carb (g)	Dietary Fiber (g)	Fat (g)	Chol (mg)	Sodi (mg)
BURGER KING												
		Croissant sandwiches:										
12	1422	With egg, bacon & cheese	1 ea	119	49	335	15	20	<1	24	249	762
12	1423	With egg, sausage & cheese	1 ea	163	49	538	19	20	<1	41	293	1042
12	1424	With egg, ham & cheese	1 ea	145	58	335	18	20	<1	20	262	987
		Whopper sandwiches:										
12	1425	Whopper	1 ea	265	57	640	27	42	<1	41	94	842
12	1426	Whopper w/ cheese	1 ea	289	57	723	31	43	<1	48	117	1126
12	1427	Double beef	1 ea	351	56	850	46	52	<1	52	188	1080
12	1428	Double w/cheese	1 ea	374	55	950	51	54	<1	60	211	1535
12	1429	Whopper, Junior	1 ea	136	52	370	15	31	<1	17	41	486
12	1430	Whopper, Junior w/cheese	1 ea	158	55	420	17	32	<1	20	52	628
12	1431	Hamburger	1 ea	109	46	275	15	29	<1	12	37	509
12	1432	Cheeseburger	1 ea	120	45	317	17	30	<1	15	48	651
12	1433	Bacon double cheeseburger	1 ea	159	41	510	33	27	<1	31	104	728
12	1434	Chicken sandwich	1 ea	230	46	688	26	56	<1	40	82	1423
12	1435	Chicken tenders	1 ea	95	50	204	20	10	0	10	47	636
12	1436	Ham & cheese sandwich	1 ea	230	59	471	24	44	<1	23	70	1534
12	1437	Whaler fish sandwich	1 ea	189	45	488	19	45	<1	27	84	592
12	1438	Whaler sandwich w/cheese	1 ea	201	45	530	21	46	<1	30	95	734
12	1439	French fries, regular	1 svg	74	37	227	3	24	<1	13	14	160
12	1440	Onion rings, regular	1 svg	79	37	274	4	28	<1	16	0	665
		Milkshakes:										
12	1441	Chocolate, medium	1 ea	273	76	320	8	46	<1	12	—	202
12	1442	Vanilla, medium	1 ea	273	74	321	9	49	<1	10	—	205

(For purposes of calculations, use "0" for t, <1, <.1, <.01, etc.)

Table D–1 Food Composition

Grp	Computer Code No.	Food Description	Measure	Wt (g)	H₂O (%)	Ener (cal)	Prot (g)	Carb (g)	Dietary Fiber (g)	Fat (g)	Chol (mg)	Sodi (mg)
		BURGER KING—Con.										
		Pies:										
12	1443	Apple pie	1 ea	125	51	305	3	44	<1	12	4	412
12	1444	Cherry pie	1 ea	128	42	357	4	55	<1	13	6	204
12	1445	Pecan pie	1 ea	113	20	459	5	64	1	20	4	374

Source: Burger King Corporation for basic nutrients. Values for dietary fiber and percent water, calculated from known values for major ingredients.

Grp	Computer Code No.	Food Description	Measure	Wt (g)	H₂O (%)	Ener (cal)	Prot (g)	Carb (g)	Dietary Fiber (g)	Fat (g)	Chol (mg)	Sodi (mg)
		DAIRY QUEEN										
		Ice cream cones:										
12	1446	Small	1 ea	85	65	140	3	22	0	4	10	45
12	1447	Regular	1 ea	142	65	240	6	38	0	7	15	80
12	1448	Large	1 ea	213	65	340	9	57	0	10	25	115
		Dipped ice cream cones:										
12	1449	Small	1 ea	92	58	190	3	25	<1	9	10	55
12	1450	Regular	1 ea	156	58	340	6	42	<1	16	20	100
12	1451	Large	1 ea	234	58	510	9	64	<1	24	30	145
		Sundaes:										
12	1452	Small	1 ea	106	60	190	3	33	<1	4	10	75
12	1453	Regular	1 ea	177	60	310	5	56	<1	8	20	120
12	1454	Large	1 ea	248	60	440	8	78	<1	10	30	165
12	1455	Banana split	1 ea	383	67	540	9	103	<1	11	30	150
12	1456	Peanut buster parfait	1 ea	305	52	740	16	94	<1	34	30	250
12	1457	Hot fudge brownie delight	1 ea	266	55	600	9	85	<1	25	20	225
12	1458	Strawberry shortcake	1 ea	312	61	540	10	100	<1	11	25	215
12	1459	Buster bar	1 ea	149	45	460	10	41	<1	29	10	175
12	1460	Dilly bar	1 ea	85	55	210	3	21	<1	13	10	50
12	1461	DQ ice cream sandwich	1 ea	60	47	140	3	24	<1	4	5	40
		Milkshakes:										
12	1462	Small	1 ea	291	63	490	10	82	<1	13	35	180
12	1463	Regular	1 ea	418	63	710	14	120	<1	19	50	260
12	1464	Large	1 ea	489	63	831	16	140	<1	22	60	304
		Malted milkshakes:										
12	1465	Small	1 ea	291	60	520	10	91	<1	13	35	180
12	1466	Regular	1 ea	418	60	760	14	134	<1	18	50	260
12	1467	Large	1 ea	489	60	889	16	157	<1	21	60	304
12	1468	Float	1 ea	397	76	410	5	82	0	7	20	85
12	1469	Freeze	1 ea	397	72	500	9	89	0	12	30	180
		Mr. Misty:										
12	1470	Regular	1 ea	330	81	250	0	63	0	0	0	10
12	1471	Kiss	1 ea	89	81	70	0	17	0	0	0	10
12	1472	Freeze	1 ea	411	72	500	9	91	0	12	30	140
12	1473	Float	1 ea	411	78	390	5	74	0	7	20	95
12	1474	Chicken sandwich	1 ea	202	46	608	27	46	<1	34	78	725
12	1475	Fish filet sandwich	1 ea	177	52	430	20	45	<1	18	40	674
12	1476	Fish filet sandwich w/cheese	1 ea	191	51	483	23	46	<1	22	49	870
		Hamburgers:										
12	1477	Single	1 ea	148	51	360	21	33	<1	16	45	630
12	1478	Double	1 ea	210	52	530	36	33	<1	28	85	660
12	1479	Triple	1 ea	272	52	710	51	33	<1	45	135	690
		Cheeseburgers:										
12	1480	Single	1 ea	162	51	410	24	33	<1	20	50	790
12	1481	Double	1 ea	239	51	650	43	34	<1	37	95	980
12	1482	Triple	1 ea	301	52	820	58	34	<1	50	145	1010

(Computer code number is for West Diet Analysis program)

GRP KEY: 1 = BEV 2 = DAIRY 3 = EGGS 4 = FAT/OIL 5 = FRUIT 6 = BAKERY 7 = GRAIN 8 = FISH 9 = BEEF 10 = POULTRY
11 = SAUSAGE **12 = MIXED/FAST** 13 = NUTS/SEEDS 14 = SWEETS 15 = VEG/LEG 16 = MISC 22 = SOUP/SAUCE

Grp	Computer Code No.	Food Description	Measure	Wt (g)	H₂O (%)	Ener (cal)	Prot (g)	Carb (g)	Dietary Fiber (g)	Fat (g)	Chol (mg)	Sodi (mg)
		DAIRY QUEEN—Con.										
		Hotdogs:										
12	1483	Regular	1 ea	100	50	280	11	21	<1	16	45	830
12	1484	With cheese	1 ea	114	49	330	15	21	<1	21	55	990
12	1485	With chili	1 ea	128	55	320	13	23	2	20	55	985
		Super hotdogs:										
12	1486	Regular	1 ea	175	48	520	17	44	<1	27	80	1365
12	1487	With cheese	1 ea	196	48	580	22	45	<1	34	100	1605
12	1488	With chili	1 ea	218	53	570	21	47	2	32	100	1595
12	1489	French fries, small	1 svg	71	47	200	2	25	<1	10	10	115
12	1490	French fries, large	1 svg	113	47	320	3	40	<1	16	15	185
12	1491	Onion Rings	1 svg	85	28	280	4	31	<1	16	15	140

Source: International Dairy Queen Inc., Minneapolis, MN for basic nutrients. Values for dietary fiber and percent water, calculated from known values for the major ingredients.

Grp	Computer Code No.	Food Description	Measure	Wt (g)	H₂O (%)	Ener (cal)	Prot (g)	Carb (g)	Dietary Fiber (g)	Fat (g)	Chol (mg)	Sodi (mg)
		JACK IN THE BOX										
12	1492	Breakfast Jack sandwich	1 ea	126	49	307	18	30	<1	13	203	871
12	1493	Canadian crescent	1 ea	134	42	472	19	25	<1	31	226	851
12	1494	Sausage crescent	1 ea	156	38	584	22	28	<1	43	187	1012
12	1495	Supreme crescent	1 ea	146	38	547	20	27	<1	40	178	1053
12	1496	Pancakes breakfast platter	1 ea	231	45	612	15	87	<1	22	99	888
12	1497	Scrambled egg breakfast platter	1 ea	249	51	662	24	52	<1	40	354	1188
12	1498	Hamburger	1 ea	98	44	276	13	30	<1	12	29	521
12	1499	Cheeseburger	1 ea	113	44	323	16	32	<1	15	42	749
12	1500	Jumbo Jack	1 ea	205	57	485	26	38	<1	26	64	905
12	1501	Jumbo Jack w/cheese	1 ea	246	56	630	32	45	<1	35	110	1665
12	1502	Bacon cheeseburger supreme	1 ea	231	45	724	34	44	<1	46	70	1307
12	1503	Swiss & baconburger	1 ea	231	52	643	33	31	<1	43	99	1354
12	1504	Ham & swiss burger	1 ea	203	44	638	36	37	<1	39	117	1330
12	1505	Chicken supreme	1 ea	228	52	601	31	39	<1	36	60	1582
12	1506	Moby Jack sandwich	1 ea	137	40	444	16	39	<1	25	47	820
12	1583	Double cheeseburger	1 ea	149	64	467	21	33	—	27	72	842
		Tacos:										
12	1508	Regular	1 ea	81	57	191	8	16	<1	11	21	460
12	1509	Super	1 ea	135	63	288	12	21	<1	17	37	765
12	1513	Taco salad	1 ea	358	81	377	31	10	1	24	102	1436
12	1516	French fries	1 svg	68	40	221	2	27	<1	12	8	164
12	1517	Hash brown potatoes	1 svg	62	60	116	2	11	<1	7	3	211
12	1518	Onion rings	1 svg	108	28	382	5	39	<1	23	27	407
		Milkshakes:										
12	1519	Chocolate	1 ea	322	77	330	11	55	0	7	25	270
12	1520	Strawberry	1 ea	328	77	320	10	55	0	7	25	240
12	1521	Vanilla	1 ea	317	76	320	10	57	0	6	25	230
12	1522	Apple turnover	1 ea	119	38	410	4	45	<1	24	15	350

Source: Jack in the Box Restaurants, Foodmaker, Inc., San Diego, CA for basic nutrients. Some values for dietary fiber are calculated from known values for major ingredients.

(For purposes of calculations, use "0" for t, <1, <.1, <.01, etc.)

Table D–1 Food Composition

Grp	Computer Code No.	Food Description	Measure	Wt (g)	H₂O (%)	Ener (cal)	Prot (g)	Carb (g)	Dietary Fiber (g)	Fat (g)	Chol (mg)	Sodi (mg)
		KENTUCKY FRIED CHICKEN										
		Original Recipe:										
12	1253	Center breast	1 ea	95	52	236	24	7	<1	14	87	631
12	1251	Side breast	1 ea	69	39	199	16	7	<1	12	70	558
12	1250	Drumstick	1 ea	47	53	117	12	3	<1	7	63	207
12	1252	Thigh	1 ea	88	49	257	18	7	<1	18	109	566
12	1249	Wing	1 ea	42	44	136	10	4	<1	9	55	302
		Dinners:										
12	1254	2 pce dinner, white	1 ea	322	64	604	30	48	1	32	133	1528
12	1255	2 pce dinner, dark	1 ea	346	65	643	35	46	1	35	180	1441
12	1256	2 pce dinner, combination	1 ea	341	63	661	33	48	1	38	172	1536
		Extra crispy recipe:										
12	1261	Center breast	1 ea	104	39	297	24	14	<1	16	79	584
12	1259	Side breast	1 ea	84	39	286	17	14	<1	18	65	564
12	1258	Drumstick	1 ea	58	51	155	13	5	<1	9	66	263
12	1260	Thigh	1 ea	107	45	343	20	13	<1	23	109	549
12	1257	Wing	1 ea	53	36	201	11	9	<1	14	59	312
		Dinners:										
12	1262	2 pce dinner, white	1 ea	348	60	755	33	60	1	43	132	1544
12	1263	2 pce dinner, dark	1 ea	375	62	765	38	55	1	54	183	1480
12	1264	2 pce dinner, combination	1 ea	371	60	902	36	58	1	48	176	1529
12	1265	Mashed potatoes	⅓ c	80	81	60	2	12	<1	1	<1	228
12	1266	Chicken gravy	⅓ c	78	76	59	2	4	<1	4	2	398
12	1267	Dinner roll	1 ea	21	31	61	2	11	<1	1	1	118
12	1268	Corn on the cob	1 ea	143	70	176	5	32	2	3	<1	12
12	1269	Coleslaw	⅓ c	79	76	103	1	12	<1	6	4	171
12	1381	Kentucky nuggets	1 ea	16	44	46	3	2	<1	3	12	140
		Kentucky nugget sauces:										
12	1382	Barbeque	2 tbsp	30	51	35	<1	7	—	1	1	450
12	1383	Sweet & sour	2 tbsp	30	50	58	<1	13	—	1	1	148
12	1384	Honey	1 tbsp	15	50	49	0	12	—	<1	t	10
12	1385	Mustard	2 tbsp	30	52	36	1	6	—	1	1	346
12	1386	Kentucky fries	1 svg	119	45	268	5	33	<1	13	1	81
12	1387	Mashed potatoes & gravy	⅓ c	86	80	62	2	10	<1	1	1	297
12	1388	Buttermilk biscuit	1 ea	75	27	269	5	32	<1	14	1	521
12	1389	Potato salad	⅓ c	90	76	141	2	13	1	9	11	396
12	1390	Baked beans	⅓ c	89	71	105	5	18	6	1	1	387
12	1391	Chicken Little sandwich	1 ea	57	52	177	6	17	1	9	20	398

Source: Kentucky Fried Chicken Corporation

Grp	Computer Code No.	Food Description	Measure	Wt (g)	H₂O (%)	Ener (cal)	Prot (g)	Carb (g)	Dietary Fiber (g)	Fat (g)	Chol (mg)	Sodi (mg)
		LONG JOHN SILVER'S										
		Fish, batter fried:										
12	1523	Fish & fryes, 3 pce	1 ea	350	55	853	43	64	<1	48	106	2025
12	1524	Fish & fryes, 2 pce	1 ea	260	53	651	30	53	<1	36	75	1352
12	1525	Fish dinner, 3 pce	1 ea	540	60	1180	47	93	<1	70	119	2797
		Fish, breaded & fried:										
12	1526	Fish dinner, 3 pce	1 ea	450	60	940	35	84	<1	52	101	1900
12	1527	Fish dinner, 2 pce	1 ea	400	60	818	26	76	<1	46	76	1526
		Chicken:										
12	1528	Chicken plank dinner, 3 pce	1 ea	370	60	885	32	72	<1	51	25	1918
12	1529	Chicken plank dinner, 4 pce	1 ea	440	60	1037	41	82	<1	59	25	2433
12	1530	Chicken nugget dinner, 6 pce	1 ea	300	60	699	23	54	<1	45	25	853
12	1531	Clam chowder	1 svg	185	85	128	7	15	<1	5	17	611
12	1532	Clam dinner	1 ea	460	60	955	22	100	<1	58	27	1543
12	1533	Fish & chicken dinner	1 ea	460	60	935	36	73	<1	55	56	2076

(Computer code number is for West Diet Analysis program)

GRP KEY: 1 = BEV 2 = DAIRY 3 = EGGS 4 = FAT/OIL 5 = FRUIT 6 = BAKERY 7 = GRAIN 8 = FISH 9 = BEEF 10 = POULTRY
11 = SAUSAGE **12 = MIXED/FAST** 13 = NUTS/SEEDS 14 = SWEETS 15 = VEG/LEG 16 = MISC 22 = SOUP/SAUCE

	Computer Code			Wt	H₂O	Ener	Prot	Carb	Dietary Fiber	Fat	Chol	Sodi
Grp	No.	Food Description	Measure	(g)	(%)	(cal)	(g)	(g)	(g)	(g)	(mg)	(mg)
LONG JOHN SILVER'S—Con.												
12	1534	Oyster dinner	1 ea	360	60	789	17	78	<1	45	55	763
12	1535	Scallop dinner	1 ea	320	60	747	17	66	<1	45	37	1579
12	1536	Seafood platter	1 ea	410	60	976	29	85	<1	58	95	2161
12	1537	Batter fried shrimp dinner	1 ea	300	60	711	17	60	<1	45	127	1297
12	1538	Fish sandwich platter	1 ea	400	60	835	30	84	<1	42	75	1402
		Salads:										
12	1539	Ocean chef	1 ea	320	85	229	27	13	2	8	64	986
12	1540	Seafood	1 ea	480	85	426	19	22	2	30	113	1086
12	1541	Cole slaw	1 svg	98	70	182	1	11	<1	15	12	367
12	1542	Fries	1 svg	85	42	247	4	31	.1	12	13	.6
12	1543	Hush puppies	1 ea	47	37	145	3	18	<1	7	—	405

Source: Long John Silver's Inc., Lexington, KY.

		McDONALD'S										
		Sandwiches:										
12	1221	Big Mac	1 ea	215	48	562	25	42	1	32	103	950
12	1591	McDLT Sandwich	1 ea	288	59	674	28	46	1.4	42	112	1170
12	1222	Quarter Pounder	1 ea	166	49	414	23	34	1	21	86	660
12	1223	Quarter Pounder w/cheese	1 ea	194	48	517	28	35	1	29	118	1150
12	1224	Filet-O-Fish sandwich	1 ea	142	44	442	14	38	<1	26	50	1030
12	1225	Hamburger	1 ea	102	46	257	12	31	<1	10	37	460
12	1226	Cheeseburger	1 ea	114	45	308	15	31	<1	14	53	750
12	1227	French fries	1 svg	68	37	220	3	26	<1	12	9	110
12	1228	Chicken McNuggets	6 ea	113	49	288	19	17	<1	16	65	520
		Sauces:										
12	1229	Barbeque	1 ea	32	51	53	<1	12	<1	<1	0	340
12	1230	Mustard	1 ea	30	53	66	1	11	<1	4	5	250
12	1231	Sweet & sour	1 ea	32	50	57	<1	14	<1	<1	0	190
		Milkshakes:										
12	1232	Chocolate	10 fl oz	303	70	388	11	63	<1	11	41	240
12	1233	Strawberry	10 fl oz	303	72	384	10	63	<1	10	41	170
12	1234	Vanilla	10 fl oz	303	73	354	10	56	<1	10	41	170
		Sundaes:										
12	1235	Hot fudge	1 ea	169	60	313	7	50	<1	9	28	160
12	1236	Strawberry	1 ea	171	62	283	6	48	<1	7	27	85
12	1237	Caramel	1 ea	174	57	343	7	58	<1	9	35	160
12	1238	Soft ice cream cone	1 ea	86	65	144	4	22	<1	5	16	70
		Pies:										
12	1239	Fried Apple	1 ea	85	45	262	2	30	<1	15	6	240
12	1240	Fried Cherry	1 ea	88	44	260	2	32	<1	14	8	427
		Cookies, package:										
12	1241	McDonaldland cookies	1 pkg	65	3	288	4	47	<1	9	0	300
12	1242	Chocolate chip cookies	1 pkg	65	3	325	4	42	2	16	4	280
		Breakfast items:										
12	1243	English muffin, w/butter	1 ea	59	42	169	5	27	<1	5	9	270
12	1244	Egg McMuffin	1 ea	138	51	293	18	28	<1	12	299	740
12	1245	Hot cakes w/butter & syrup	1 ea	176	46	413	8	74	<1	9	21	640
12	1246	Scrambled eggs	1 ea	100	70	157	12	1	<1	11	545	290
12	1247	Sausage	1 svg.	48	43	180	8	0	<1	16	48	350
12	1248	Hash brown potato patty	1 ea	53	56	131	1	15	1	7	9	330
12	1392	Sausage McMuffin	1 ea	117	38	372	17	27	<1	22	64	830
12	1393	Sausage McMuffin w/egg	1 ea	167	47	451	23	28	<1	27	336	980
12	1394	Biscuit with spread	1 ea	75	27	260	5	32	<1	13	1	730

(For purposes of calculations, use "0" for t, <1, <.1, <.01, etc.)

Table D–1 Food Composition

Grp	Computer Code No.	Food Description	Measure	Wt (g)	H₂O (%)	Ener (cal)	Prot (g)	Carb (g)	Dietary Fiber (g)	Fat (g)	Chol (mg)	Sodi (mg)
		McDONALD'S—Con.										
		Breakfast Items Con.										
12	1395	Biscuit w/sausage	1 ea	123	32	440	13	32	<1	29	49	1080
12	1396	Biscuit w/sausage & egg	1 ea	180	43	529	20	33	<1	35	358	1250
12	1397	Biscuit w/bacon, egg & cheese	1 ea	156	41	449	17	33	<1	27	336	1230
		Salads:										
12	1398	Chef salad	1 ea	283	84	231	21	8	2	13	152	850
12	1399	Shrimp salad	1 ea	262	88	104	14	6	2	3	193	480
12	1400	Garden salad	1 ea	213	91	112	7	8	2	7	107	160
12	1401	Chicken salad oriental	1 ea	244	88	141	23	5	2	3	78	230

Source: McDonald's Corporation, Oak Brook, Illinois. Some values for Salads estimated from known values for major ingredients.

Grp	No.	Food Description	Measure	Wt (g)	H₂O (%)	Ener (cal)	Prot (g)	Carb (g)	Fiber (g)	Fat (g)	Chol (mg)	Sodi (mg)
		TACO BELL										
		Burritos:										
12	1544	Bean	1 ea	191	58	357	13	54	8	10	9	888
12	1545	Beef	1 ea	191	58	403	22	39	2	17	57	1051
12	1546	Bean & beef	1 ea	191	58	381	17	46	5	14	36	958
12	1547	Burrito supreme	1 ea	241	66	413	18	46	5	18	33	921
12	1548	Double beef supreme	1 ea	255	66	457	24	42	2	22	57	1053
12	1549	Enchirito	1 ea	213	61	382	20	31	5	20	54	1243
12	1550	Fajita (steak taco)	1 ea	135	65	234	15	20	2	11	14	485
		Tacos:										
12	1551	Regular	1 ea	78	55	183	10	11	1	11	32	276
12	1552	Taco bellgrande	1 ea	163	63	355	18	18	2	23	56	472
12	1553	Taco light	1 ea	170	59	410	19	18	2	29	56	594
12	1554	Soft taco	1 ea	92	52	228	12	18	2	12	32	516
		Tostadas:										
12	1555	Regular	1 ea	156	67	243	10	27	7	11	16	596
12	1556	Beefy tostada	1 ea	198	69	322	15	22	4	20	40	764
12	1557	Bellbeefer	1 ea	177	63	312	17	32	<1	13	39	855
12	1558	Mexican pizza	1 ea	223	55	575	21	40	5	48	81	1364
12	1559	Taco salad with salsa	1 ea	595	73	941	36	63	5	61	80	1662
		Nachos:										
12	1560	Regular	1 ea	106	40	356	7	38	<1	19	9	423
12	1561	Bellgrande	1 ea	287	58	649	22	61	6	35	36	997
12	1562	Pintos & cheese	1 ea	128	69	190	9	19	7	9	16	642
12	1563	Taco sauce	1 ea	3.7	96	2	<1	<1	<1	<1	0	126
12	1564	Salsa	1 ea	9.7	95	18	1	4	1	<1	0	376
12	1565	Cinnamon Crispas	1 ea	47.3	1	259	3	27	<1	15	1	127

Source: Taco Bell Corporation, California for most nutrient values. Values for dietary fiber and percentage water are estimates calculated from known values of major ingredients.

Grp	No.	Food Description	Measure	Wt (g)	H₂O (%)	Ener (cal)	Prot (g)	Carb (g)	Fiber (g)	Fat (g)	Chol (mg)	Sodi (mg)
		WENDY's										
		Hamburgers:										
12	1566	Single, on white bun, no toppings	1 ea	119	41	350	21	29	<1	16	65	420
12	1568	Double, on white bun, no toppings	1 ea	197	44	560	41	32	<1	34	125	575
12	1569	Big classic	1 ea	241	63	470	26	36	2	25	80	900
		Cheeseburgers:										
12	1570	Bacon cheeseburger	1 ea	147	46	460	29	23	<1	28	65	860
12	1571	Single, w/all toppings	1 ea	215	50	548	30	32	2	33	84	864
12	1572	Double, w/all toppings	1 ea	291	50	735	48	27	2	48	165	883

(Computer code number is for West Diet Analysis program)

GRP KEY: 1＝BEV 2＝DAIRY 3＝EGGS 4＝FAT/OIL 5＝FRUIT 6＝BAKERY 7＝GRAIN 8＝FISH 9＝BEEF 10＝POULTRY
11＝SAUSAGE **12＝MIXED/FAST** 13＝NUTS/SEEDS 14＝SWEETS 15＝VEG/LEG 16＝MISC 22＝SOUP/SAUCE

Grp	Computer Code No.	Food Description	Measure	Wt (g)	H$_2$O (%)	Ener (cal)	Prot (g)	Carb (g)	Dietary Fiber (g)	Fat (g)	Chol (mg)	Sodi (mg)
		WENDY'S—Con.										
		Baked potatoes:										
12	1573	Plain	1 ea	250	75	250	6	52	5	<1	0	60
12	1574	W/bacon & cheese	1 ea	350	71	570	19	57	5	30	22	180
12	1575	W/broccoli & cheese	1 ea	365	74	500	13	54	5	25	22	2.19
12	1576	W/cheese	1 ea	350	71	590	17	55	5	34	22	2.22
12	1577	W/chili & cheese	1 ea	400	72	510	22	63	8	20	22	810
12	1578	W/sour cream & chives	1 ea	310	71	460	7	53	5	24	15	230
12	1579	Chili	1 c	256	77	230	21	16	5	9	30	960
12	1580	French fries	1 svg	106	43	306	4	38	<1	15	15	105
12	1581	Frosty dairy dessert	1 c	216	35	354	7	53	0	13	45	194
12	1582	Chocolate chip cookie	1 ea	64	5	320	3	40	1	17	5	235

Source: Wendy's International, for most nutrient values. Some of the values for dietary fiber and percentage water
for estimates calculated from known values of major ingredients.

(For purposes of calculations, use "0" for t, <1, <.1, <.01, etc.)

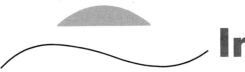

Index

This index lists primarily topics that received significant mention in the text. Pages inclusive (for example 53-56) indicate major discussions; pages in **bold** refer to defined terms; pages followed by *f* or *t* indicate that the listing on that page is included in a figure or table, respectively.

About the Authors

Linda Kelly DeBruyne, M.S., R.D., received her B.S. in 1980 and her M.S. in 1982 in Nutrition and Food Science with an emphasis on exercise physiology at the Florida State University. She serves on the board of directors of Nutrition and Health Associates, an information resource center in Tallahassee, Florida, where her specialty areas are fitness, sports medicine, and life-cycle nutrition. Her other textbooks are *Life Cycle Nutrition: Conception through Adolescence* and *Life Span Nutrition: Conception through Life*. She is a member of the American Alliance for Health, Physical Education, Recreation, and Dance, and the American Dietetic Association.

Frances Sienkiewicz Sizer, M.S., R.D., attended Florida State University where, in 1980, she received her B.S., and in 1982, her M.S. in nutrition. She has counseled clients in the University's stress-reduction clinic and served as a consultant to schools and alcoholism programs in Florida. She now devotes full time to research and writing in nutrition, fitness, and health. Her publications include the textbooks *Nutrition: Concepts and Controversies* (now entering its fifth edition), *Life Choices:*

Health Concepts and Strategies, and *Essential Life Choices: Health Concepts and Strategies;* a series of monographs for health professionals; and articles for popular and professional press. She is a member of the American Public Health Association, the American Alliance for Health, Physical Education, Recreation, and Dance, and the Association for the Advancement of Health Education.

Eleanor Noss Whitney, Ph.D., R.D., received her B.A. in Biology from Radcliffe College in 1960 and her Ph.D. in Biology from Washington University, St. Louis, in 1970. Formerly on the faculty at the Florida State University, she now devotes full time to research, writing, and consulting in nutrition, health, and environmental issues. She is president of Nutrition and Health Associates, an information resource center in Tallahassee, Florida. Her publications include articles in *Science,* the *Journal of Nutrition, Genetics,* and other journals, and the textbooks *Nutrition: Concepts and Controversies, Understanding Nutrition,* and *Life Choices: Health Concepts and Strategies,* among others.

Acceptable Weight for Height Based on Body Mass Index (BMI)

To determine your acceptable weight range, find your height in the top line. Look down the column below it and find the range represented by the white band. Look to the left column to see what weights are acceptable for you.

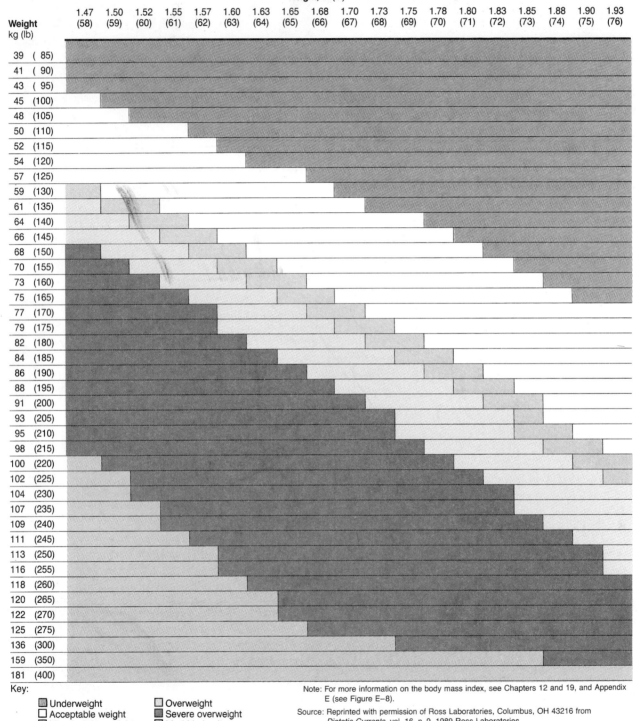

Men

Height, m (in)

Weight kg (lb)	1.47 (58)	1.50 (59)	1.52 (60)	1.55 (61)	1.57 (62)	1.60 (63)	1.63 (64)	1.65 (65)	1.68 (66)	1.70 (67)	1.73 (68)	1.75 (69)	1.78 (70)	1.80 (71)	1.83 (72)	1.85 (73)	1.88 (74)	1.90 (75)	1.93 (76)
39 (85)																			
41 (90)																			
43 (95)																			
45 (100)																			
48 (105)																			
50 (110)																			
52 (115)																			
54 (120)																			
57 (125)																			
59 (130)																			
61 (135)																			
64 (140)																			
66 (145)																			
68 (150)																			
70 (155)																			
73 (160)																			
75 (165)																			
77 (170)																			
79 (175)																			
82 (180)																			
84 (185)																			
86 (190)																			
88 (195)																			
91 (200)																			
93 (205)																			
95 (210)																			
98 (215)																			
100 (220)																			
102 (225)																			
104 (230)																			
107 (235)																			
109 (240)																			
111 (245)																			
113 (250)																			
116 (255)																			
118 (260)																			
120 (265)																			
122 (270)																			
125 (275)																			
136 (300)																			
159 (350)																			
181 (400)																			

Key:

- Underweight
- Acceptable weight
- Marginal overweight
- Overweight
- Severe overweight
- Morbid obesity

Note: For more information on the body mass index, see Chapters 12 and 19, and Appendix E (see Figure E-8).

Source: Reprinted with permission of Ross Laboratories, Columbus, OH 43216 from *Dietetic Currents*, vol. 16, p. 9, 1989 Ross Laboratories.